Edited by
Frank Emmert-Streib and
Matthias Dehmer

**Medical Biostatistics
for Complex Diseases**

Related Titles

Emmert-Streib, F., Dehmer, M. (eds.)

Analysis of Microarray Data
A Network-Based Approach

2008
ISBN: 978-3-527-31822-3

Dehmer, M., Emmert-Streib, F. (eds.)

Analysis of Complex Networks
From Biology to Linguistics

2009
ISBN: 978-3-527-32345-6

Biswas, A., Datta, S., Fine, J. P., Segal, M. R. (eds.)

Statistical Advances in the Biomedical Sciences
Clinical Trials, Epidemiology, Survival Analysis, and Bioinformatics

2008
ISBN: 978-0-471-94753-0

Knudsen, S.

Cancer Diagnostics with DNA Microarrays

2006
ISBN: 978-0-471-78407-4

Nagl, S. (ed.)

Cancer Bioinformatics: From Therapy Design to Treatment

2006
ISBN: 978-0-470-86304-6

Edited by
Frank Emmert-Streib and Matthias Dehmer

Medical Biostatistics for Complex Diseases

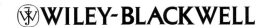

The Editors

Prof. Dr. Frank Emmert-Streib
Queen's University
Cancer Research
School of Medicine & Biomedical Sciences
97, Lisburn Road
Belfast BT9 7BL
United Kingdom

Prof. Dr. Matthias Dehmer
Universität für Gesundheitswissenschaften UMIT
Institut für Bioinformatik
Eduard Wallnöfer Zentrum 1
6060 Thaur
Austria

Cover
A heatmap of residuals diagnosing model fit in gene-set expression analysis, as described in chapter 5 by A.P. Oron. It was produced using the R open-source statistical language, via the 'heatmap' function. The reader can produce a similar heatmap by running the tutorial script for the 'GSEAlm' package, available at the Bioconductor repository: http://www.bioconductor.org/packages/2.6/bioc/vignettes/GSEAlm/inst/doc/GSEAlm.R
(Copyright 2008 by Oxford University Press).

Limit of Liability/Disclaimer of Warranty: While the publisher and authors have used their best efforts in preparing this book, they make no representations or warranties with respect to the accuracy or completeness of the contents of this book and specifically disclaim any implied warranties of merchantability or fitness for a particular purpose. No warranty can be created or extended by sales representatives or written sales materials. The Advice and strategies contained herein may not be suitable for your situation. You should consult with a professional where appropriate. Neither the publisher nor authors shall be liable for any loss of profit or any other commercial damages, including but not limited to special, incidental, consequential, or other damages.

Library of Congress Card No.: applied for

British Library Cataloguing-in-Publication Data
A catalogue record for this book is available from the British Library.

Bibliographic information published by the Deutsche Nationalbibliothek
The Deutsche Nationalbibliothek lists this publication in the Deutsche Nationalbibliografie; detailed bibliographic data are available on the Internet at http://dnb.d-nb.de.

© 2010 WILEY-VCH Verlag GmbH & Co. KGaA, Weinheim, Germany

Wiley-Blackwell is an imprint of John Wiley & Sons, formed by the merger of Wiley's global Scientific, Technical, and Medical business with Blackwell Publishing.

All rights reserved (including those of translation into other languages). No part of this book may be reproduced in any form – by photoprinting, microfilm, or any other means – nor transmitted or translated into a machine language without written permission from the publishers. Registered names, trademarks, etc. used in this book, even when not specifically marked as such, are not to be considered unprotected by law.

Composition   Thomson Digital, Noida, India
Printing and Binding   Strauss GmbH, Mörlenbach
Cover Design   Grafik-Design Schulz, Fußgönheim

Printed in the Federal Republic of Germany
Printed on acid-free paper

ISBN: 978-3-527-32585-6

Foreword

The evolution of disease in cancer, metabolic disorders, and immunological disorders is still poorly understood. During the past few decades research has revealed that, in most instances, a complex interaction network of micro-environmental factors including cytokines and cytokine receptors as well as a complex network of signaling pathways and metabolic events contribute to disease evolution and disease progression. In addition, the genetic background, somatic mutations, and epigenetic mechanisms are involved in disease manifestation and disease progression. The heterogeneity of disease points to the complexity of events and factors that may all act together to lead to a frank disorder in the individual patient. Based on this assumption, the evaluation of such complex diseases with respect to the affected cells and cell systems by appropriate biostatistical analysis, including high capacity assays and highly developed multi-parameter evaluation-assays, is a clear medical need.

This book, *Medical Biostatistics for Complex Diseases*, reviews statistical and computational methods for the analysis of high-throughput data and their interpretation with special emphasis on the applicability in biomedical and clinical science. One major aim is to discuss methodologies and assays in order to analyze pathway-specific patterns in various disorders and disease-categories. Such approaches are especially desired because they avoid many problems of methods that focus solely on a single-gene level. For example, detecting differentially expressed genes among experimental conditions or disease stages has received tremendous interest since the introduction of DNA microarrays. However, the inherent problem of a causal connection between a genetic characteristic and a phenotypic trait becomes especially problematic in the context of complex diseases because such diseases involve many factors, externally and internally, and their collective processing. For this reason pathway-approaches form an important step towards a full integration of multilevel factors and interactions to establish a systems biology perspective of physiological processes. From an educational point of view this point cannot be stressed enough because the gene-centric view is still prevalent and dominant in genetics, molecular biology, and medicine. That is why this book can serve as a basis to train a new generation of scientists and to forge their way of thinking.

Medical Biostatistics for Complex Diseases. Edited by Frank Emmert-Streib and Matthias Dehmer
Copyright © 2010 WILEY-VCH Verlag GmbH & Co. KGaA, Weinheim
ISBN: 978-3-527-32585-6

Deciphering complex diseases like cancer is a collaborative endeavor requiring the coordinated effort of an interdisciplinary team and highly developed multivariate methods through which the complexity of disorders can be addressed appropriately. For this reason it is notable that the present book also provides a brief introduction to the molecular biological mechanisms of cancer and cancer stem cells. This will be very helpful for biostatisticians and computational biologists, guiding their interpretations with related projects.

It will be very interesting to observe the development of this field during the next few years and to witness, hopefully, many exciting results that blossom from the methods and concepts presented in this book.

Vienna, February 2010   *Peter Valent*

Acknowledgments

I would like to thank Matthias Dehmer and Frank Emmert-Streib for fruitful discussions.

Contents

Foreword V
Preface XIX
List of Contributors XXIII

Part One General Biological and Statistical Basics 1

1 The Biology of *MYC* in Health and Disease: A High Altitude View 3
Brian C. Turner, Gregory A. Bird, and Yosef Refaeli
1.1 Introduction 3
1.2 *MYC* and Normal Physiology 4
1.3 Regulation of Transcription and Gene Expression 4
1.4 Metabolism 6
1.5 Cell-Cycle Regulation and Differentiation 7
1.6 Protein Synthesis 7
1.7 Cell Adhesion 7
1.8 Apoptosis 8
1.9 MicroRNAs 9
1.10 Physiological Effects of Loss and Gain of *c-myc* Function in Mice 9
1.10.1 Loss of Function 9
1.10.2 Gain of Function: Inducible Transgenic Animals 10
1.11 Contributions of *MYC* to Tumor Biology 11
1.12 Introduction of Hematopoietic Malignancies 12
1.13 Mechanisms of *MYC* Dysregulation in Hematological Malignancies 13
1.14 Mutation(s) in the *MYC* Gene in Hematological Cancers 14
1.15 Role of *MYC* in Cell Cycle Regulation and Differentiation in Hematological Cancers 14
1.16 Role of BCR Signaling in Conjunction with MYC Overexpression in Lymphoid Malignancies 15
1.17 Deregulation of Auxiliary Proteins in Addition to MYC in Hematological Cancers 16

1.18	Conclusion 17
	References 18

2 Cancer Stem Cells – Finding and Capping the Roots of Cancer 25
Eike C. Buss and Anthony D. Ho

2.1	Introduction – Stem Cells and Cancer Stem Cells 25
2.1.1	What are Stem Cells? 25
2.1.2	Concept of Cancer Stem Cells (CSCs) 25
2.2	Hematopoietic Stem Cells as a Paradigm 28
2.2.1	Leukemia as a Paradigmatic Disease for Cancer Research 28
2.2.2	CFUs 29
2.2.3	LTC-ICs 29
2.2.4	*In Vivo* Repopulation 30
2.2.5	Importance of the Bone Marrow Niche 30
2.2.6	Leukemic Stem Cells 31
2.2.6.1	Leukemic Stem Cells in the Bone Marrow Niche 31
2.2.7	CML as a Paradigmatic Entity 32
2.3	Current Technical Approach to the Isolation and Characterization of Cancer Stem Cells 33
2.3.1	Tools for the Detection of Cancer Stem Cells 33
2.3.2	Phenotype of Cancer Stem Cells 34
2.4	Cancer Stem Cells in Solid Tumors 35
2.4.1	Breast Cancer 36
2.4.2	Prostate Cancer 36
2.4.3	Colon Cancer 37
2.4.4	Other Cancers 37
2.5	Open Questions of the Cancer Stem Cell Hypothesis 37
2.6	Clinical Relevance of Cancer Stem Cells 38
2.6.1	Diagnostic Relevance of Cancer Stem Cells 38
2.6.2	Therapeutic Relevance – New Drugs Directed Against Cancer Stem Cells 39
2.7	Outlook 40
	References 40

3 Multiple Testing Methods 45
Alessio Farcomeni

3.1	Introduction 45
3.1.1	A Brief More Focused Introduction 46
3.1.2	Historic Development of the Field 47
3.2	Statistical Background 48
3.2.1	Tests 48
3.2.2	Test Statistics and *p*-Values 49
3.2.3	Resampling Based Testing 49
3.3	Type I Error Rates 50
3.4	Introduction to Multiple Testing Procedures 52

3.4.1	Adjusted *p*-values	52
3.4.2	Categories of Multiple Testing Procedures	52
3.4.3	Estimation of the Proportion of False Nulls	53
3.5	Multiple Testing Procedures	55
3.5.1	Procedures Controlling the FWER	55
3.5.2	Procedures Controlling the FDR	56
3.5.3	Procedures Controlling the FDX	59
3.6	Type I Error Rates Control Under Dependence	61
3.6.1	FWER Control	62
3.6.2	FDR and FDX Control	62
3.7	Multiple Testing Procedures Applied to Gene Discovery in DNA Microarray Cancer Studies	63
3.7.1	Gene identification in Colon Cancer	64
3.7.1.1	Classification of Lymphoblastic and Myeloid Leukemia	64
3.8	Conclusions	67
	References	69

Part Two Statistical and Computational Analysis Methods 73

4 Making Mountains Out of Molehills: Moving from Single Gene to Pathway Based Models of Colon Cancer Progression 75
Elena Edelman, Katherine Garman, Anil Potti, and Sayan Mukherjee

4.1	Introduction	75
4.2	Methods	76
4.2.1	Data Collection and Standardization	76
4.2.2	Stratification and Mapping to Gene Sets	77
4.2.3	Regularized Multi-task Learning	78
4.2.4	Validation via Mann–Whitney Test	79
4.2.5	Leave-One-Out Error	79
4.3	Results	80
4.3.1	Development and Validation of Model Statistics	82
4.3.2	Comparison of Single Gene and Gene Set Models	83
4.3.3	Novel Pathway Findings and Therapeutic Implications	84
4.4	Discussion	85
	References	86

5 Gene-Set Expression Analysis: Challenges and Tools 89
Assaf P. Oron

5.1	The Challenge	89
5.2	Survey of Gene-Set Analysis Methods	91
5.2.1	Motivation for GS Analysis	91
5.2.2	Some Notable GS Analysis Methods	92
5.2.3	Correlations and Permutation Tests	95
5.3	Demonstration with the "ALL" Dataset	97
5.3.1	The Dataset	97

5.3.2	The Gene-Filtering Dilemma	97
5.3.3	Basic Diagnostics: Testing Normalization and Model Fit	99
5.3.4	Pinpointing Aneuploidies via Outlier Identification	102
5.3.5	Signal-to-Noise Evaluation: The Sex Variable	103
5.3.6	Confounding, and Back to Basics: The Age Variable	106
5.3.7	How it all Reflects on the Bottom Line: Inference	107
5.4	Summary and Future Directions	108
	References 111	

6	Multivariate Analysis of Microarray Data Using Hotelling's T^2 Test 113	
	Yan Lu, Peng-Yuan Liu, and Hong-Wen Deng	
6.1	Introduction	113
6.2	Methods	114
6.2.1	Wishart Distribution	114
6.2.2	Hotelling's T^2 Statistic	115
6.2.3	Two-Sample T^2 Statistic	115
6.2.4	Multiple Forward Search (MFS) Algorithm	116
6.2.5	Resampling	117
6.3	Validation of Hotelling's T^2 Statistic	118
6.3.1	Human Genome U95 Spike-In Dataset	118
6.3.2	Identification of DEGs	118
6.4	Application Examples	118
6.4.1	Human Liver Cancers	118
6.4.1.1	Dataset	118
6.4.1.2	Identification of DEGs	120
6.4.1.3	Classification of Human Liver Tissues	122
6.4.2	Human Breast Cancers	124
6.4.2.1	Dataset	124
6.4.2.2	Cluster Analysis	124
6.5	Discussion	124
	References 128	

7	Interpreting Differential Coexpression of Gene Sets 131	
	Ju Han Kim, Sung Bum Cho, and Jihun Kim	
7.1	Coexpression and Differential Expression Analyses	131
7.2	Gene Set-Wise Differential Expression Analysis	133
7.3	Differential Coexpression Analysis	134
7.4	Differential Coexpression Analysis of Paired Gene Sets	135
7.5	Measuring Coexpression of Gene Sets	136
7.6	Measuring Differential Coexpression of Gene Sets	137
7.7	Gene Pair-Wise Differential Coexpression	138
7.8	Datasets and Gene Sets	139
7.8.1	Datasets	139
7.8.2	Gene Sets	139

7.9	Simulation Study *139*
7.10	Lung Cancer Data Analysis Results *140*
7.11	Duchenne's Muscular Dystrophy Data Analysis Results *142*
7.12	Discussion *145*
	References *150*

8	**Multivariate Analysis of Microarray Data: Application of MANOVA** *151*
	Taeyoung Hwang and Taesung Park
8.1	Introduction *151*
8.2	Importance of Correlation in Multiple Gene Approach *152*
8.2.1	Small Effects Coordinate to Make a Big Difference *154*
8.2.2	Significance of the Correlation *155*
8.3	Multivariate ANalysis of VAriance (MANOVA) *155*
8.3.1	ANOVA *156*
8.3.2	MANOVA *157*
8.4	Applying MANOVA to Microarray Data Analysis *159*
8.5	Application of MANOVA: Case Studies *160*
8.5.1	Identifying Disease Specific Genes *160*
8.5.2	Identifying Significant Pathways from Public Pathway Databases *161*
8.5.3	Identification of Subnetworks from Protein–Protein Interaction Data *162*
8.6	Conclusions *163*
	References *165*

9	**Testing Significance of a Class of Genes** *167*
	James J. Chen and Chen-An Tsai
9.1	Introduction *167*
9.2	Competitive versus Self-Contained Tests *169*
9.3	One-Sided and Two-Sided Hypotheses *171*
9.4	Over-Representation Analysis (ORA) *171*
9.5	GCT Statistics *172*
9.5.1	One-Sided Test *174*
9.5.1.1	OLS Global Test *174*
9.5.1.2	GSEA Test *175*
9.5.2	Two-Sided Test *175*
9.5.2.1	MANOVA Test *175*
9.5.2.2	SAM-GS Test *176*
9.5.2.3	ANCOVA Test *177*
9.6	Applications *177*
9.6.1	Diabetes Dataset *177*
9.6.2	p53 Dataset *180*
9.7	Discussion *181*
	References *182*

10	**Differential Dependency Network Analysis to Identify Topological Changes in Biological Networks** *185*	
	Bai Zhang, Huai Li, Robert Clarke, Leena Hilakivi-Clarke, and Yue Wang	
10.1	Introduction *185*	
10.2	Preliminaries *187*	
10.2.1	Probabilistic Graphical Models and Dependency Networks *187*	
10.2.2	Graph Structure Learning and ℓ_1-Regularization *188*	
10.3	Method *188*	
10.3.1	Local Dependency Model in DDN *188*	
10.3.2	Local Structure Learning *189*	
10.3.3	Detection of Statistically Significant Topological Changes *191*	
10.3.4	Identification of "Hot Spots" in the Network and Extraction of the DDN *192*	
10.4	Experiments and Results *192*	
10.4.1	A Simulation Experiment *192*	
10.4.1.1	Experiment Data *193*	
10.4.1.2	Application of DDN Analysis *193*	
10.4.1.3	Algorithm Analysis *195*	
10.4.2	Breast Cancer Dataset Analysis *196*	
10.4.2.1	Experiment Background and Data *196*	
10.4.2.2	Application of DDN Analysis *197*	
10.4.3	*In Utero* Excess E2 Exposed Adult Mammary Glands Analysis *198*	
10.4.3.1	Experiment Background and Data *198*	
10.4.4	Application of DDN Analysis *198*	
10.5	Closing Remarks *199*	
	References *200*	
11	**An Introduction to Time-Varying Connectivity Estimation for Gene Regulatory Networks** *205*	
	André Fujita, João Ricardo Sato, Marcos Angelo Almeida Demasi, Satoru Miyano, Mari Cleide Sogayar, and Carlos Eduardo Ferreira	
11.1	Regulatory Networks and Cancer *205*	
11.2	Statistical Approaches *207*	
11.2.1	Causality and Granger Causality *207*	
11.2.2	Vector Autoregressive Model – VAR *209*	
11.2.2.1	Estimation Procedure *210*	
11.2.2.2	Hypothesis Testing *211*	
11.2.3	Dynamic Vector Autoregressive Model – DVAR *211*	
11.2.3.1	Estimation Procedure *214*	
11.2.3.2	Covariance Matrix Estimation *215*	
11.2.3.3	Hypothesis Testing *215*	
11.3	Simulations *216*	
11.4	Application of the DVAR Method to Actual Data *218*	
11.5	Final Considerations *222*	
11.6	Conclusions *224*	

11.A	Appendix *225*	
	References *227*	
12	**A Systems Biology Approach to Construct A Cancer-Perturbed Protein–Protein Interaction Network for Apoptosis by Means of Microarray and Database Mining** *231*	
	Liang-Hui Chu and Bor-Sen Chen	
12.1	Introduction *231*	
12.2	Methods *233*	
12.2.1	Microarray Experimental Data *233*	
12.2.2	Construction of Initial Protein–Protein Interaction (PPI) Networks *233*	
12.2.3	Nonlinear Stochastic Interaction Model *233*	
12.2.4	Identification of Interactions in the Initial Protein–Protein Interaction Network *236*	
12.2.5	Modification of Initial PPI Networks *238*	
12.3	Results *239*	
12.3.1	Construction of a Cancer-Perturbed PPI Network for Apoptosis *239*	
12.3.2	Prediction of Apoptosis Drug Targets by Means of Cancer-Perturbed PPI Networks for Apoptosis *241*	
12.3.2.1	Common Pathway: CASP3 *244*	
12.3.2.2	Extrinsic Pathway and Cross-Talk: TNF *244*	
12.3.2.3	Intrinsic Pathway: BCL2, BAX, and BCL2L1 *244*	
12.3.2.4	Apoptosis Regulators: TP53, MYC, and EGFR *245*	
12.3.2.5	Stress-Induced Signaling: MAPK1 and MAPK3 *245*	
12.3.2.6	Others: CDKN1A *245*	
12.3.3	Prediction of More Apoptosis Drug Targets by Decreasing the Degree of Perturbation *246*	
12.3.3.1	Prediction of More Cancer Drug Targets by Decreasing the Degree of Perturbation *246*	
12.3.3.2	Prediction of New GO Annotations of the Four Proteins: CDKN1A, CCND, PRKCD, and PCNA *246*	
12.4	Apoptosis Mechanism at the Systems Level *247*	
12.4.1	Caspase Family and Caspase Regulators *247*	
12.4.2	Extrinsic Pathway, Intrinsic Pathway, and Cross-Talk *248*	
12.4.3	Regulation of Apoptosis at the Systems Level *248*	
12.5	Conclusions *248*	
	References *249*	
13	**A New Gene Expression Meta-Analysis Technique and Its Application to Co-Analyze Three Independent Lung Cancer Datasets** *253*	
	Irit Fishel, Alon Kaufman, and Eytan Ruppin	
13.1	Background *253*	
13.1.1	DNA Microarray Technology *253*	
13.1.1.1	cDNA Microarray *253*	

13.1.1.2	Oligonucleotide Microarray	255
13.1.2	Machine Learning Background	255
13.1.2.1	Basic Definitions and Terms in Machine Learning	255
13.1.2.2	Supervised Learning in the Context of Gene Expression Data	256
13.1.3	Support Vector Machines	256
13.1.4	Support Vector Machine Recursive Feature Elimination	258
13.2	Introduction	259
13.3	Methods	260
13.3.1	Overview and Definitions	260
13.3.2	A Toy Example	261
13.3.3	Datasets	263
13.3.4	Data Pre-processing	263
13.3.5	Probe Set Reduction	264
13.3.6	Constructing a Predictive Model	264
13.3.7	Constructing Predictive Gene Sets	264
13.3.8	Estimating the Predictive Performance	266
13.3.9	Constructing a Repeatability-Based Gene List	266
13.3.10	Ranking the Joint Core Genes	267
13.4	Results	267
13.4.1	Unstable Ranked Gene Lists in a Tumor Versus Normal Binary Classification Task	267
13.4.2	Constructing a Consistent Repeatability-Based Gene List	268
13.4.3	Repeatability-Based Gene Lists are Stable	269
13.4.4	Comparing Gene Rankings between Datasets	269
13.4.5	Joint Core Magnitude	270
13.4.6	The Joint Core is Transferable	271
13.4.7	Biological Significance of the Joint Core Genes	272
13.5	Discussion	273
	References	275
14	**Kernel Classification Methods for Cancer Microarray Data**	**279**
	Tsuyoshi Kato and Wataru Fujibuchi	
14.1	Introduction	279
14.1.1	Notation	280
14.2	Support Vector Machines and Kernels	281
14.2.1	Support Vector Machines	281
14.2.2	Kernel Matrix	284
14.2.3	Polynomial Kernel and RBF Kernel	285
14.2.4	Pre-process of Kernels	286
14.2.4.1	Normalization	286
14.2.4.2	SVD Denoising	287
14.3	Metrization Kernels: Kernels for Microarray Data	288
14.3.1	Partial Distance (or kNND)	288
14.3.2	Maximum Entropy Kernel	289
14.3.3	Other Distance-Based Kernels	290

14.4	Applications to Cancer Data *290*	
14.4.1	Leave-One-Out Cross Validation *291*	
14.4.2	Data Normalization and Classification Analysis *291*	
14.4.3	Parameter Selection *292*	
14.4.4	Heterogeneous Kidney Carcinoma Data *292*	
14.4.5	Problems in Training Multiple Support Vector Machines for All Sub-data *293*	
14.4.6	Effects of Partial Distance Denoising in Homogeneous Leukemia Data *293*	
14.4.7	Heterogeneous Squamous Cell Carcinoma Metastasis Data *295*	
14.4.8	Advantages of ME Kernel *296*	
14.5	Conclusion *296*	
14.A	Appendix *298*	
	References *300*	
15	**Predicting Cancer Survival Using Expression Patterns** *305*	
	Anupama Reddy, Louis-Philippe Kronek, A. Rose Brannon, Michael Seiler, Shridar Ganesan, W. Kimryn Rathmell, and Gyan Bhanot	
15.1	Introduction *305*	
15.2	Molecular Subtypes of ccRCC *307*	
15.3	Logical Analysis of Survival Data *308*	
15.4	Bagging LASD Models *311*	
15.5	Results *312*	
15.5.1	Prediction Results are More Accurate after Stratifying Data into Subtypes *313*	
15.5.2	LASD Performs Significantly Better than Cox Regression *313*	
15.5.3	Bagging Improves Robustness of LASD Predictions *314*	
15.5.4	LASD Patterns have Distinct Survival Profiles *314*	
15.5.5	Importance Scores for Patterns and an Optimized Risk Score *314*	
15.5.6	Risk Scores could be used to Classify Patients into Distinct Risk Groups *316*	
15.5.7	LASD Survival Prediction is Highly Predictive When Compared with Clinical Parameters (Stage, Grade, and Performance) *318*	
15.6	Conclusion and Discussion *318*	
	References *322*	
16	**Integration of Microarray Datasets** *325*	
	Ki-Yeol Kim and Sun Young Rha	
16.1	Introduction *325*	
16.2	Integration Methods *325*	
16.2.1	Existing Methods for Adjusting Batch Effects *326*	
16.2.1.1	Singular Value Decomposition (SVD) and Distance Weighted Discrimination (DWD) *326*	
16.2.1.2	ANOVA (Analysis of Variance) Model *327*	
16.2.1.3	Empirical Bayesian Method for Adjusting Batch Effect *327*	

16.2.2	Transformation Method	329
16.2.2.1	Standardization of Expression Data	329
16.2.2.2	Transformation of Datasets Using a Reference Dataset	330
16.2.3	Discretization Methods	332
16.2.3.1	Equal Width and Equal Frequency Discretizations	332
16.2.3.2	ChiMerge Method	333
16.2.3.3	Discretization Based on Recursive Minimal Entropy	333
16.2.3.4	Nonparametric Scoring Method for Microarray Data	333
16.2.3.5	Discretization by Rank of Gene Expression in Microarray Dataset: Proposed Method	335
16.3	Statistical Method for Significant Gene Selection and Classification	336
16.3.1	Chi-Squared Test for Significant Gene Selection	336
16.3.2	Random Forest for Calculating Prediction Accuracy	337
16.4	Example	337
16.4.1	Dataset	338
16.4.2	Prediction Accuracies Using the Combined Dataset	339
16.4.2.1	Data Preprocessing	339
16.4.2.2	Improvement of Prediction Accuracy Using Combined Datasets by the Proposed Method	339
16.4.2.3	Description of Significant Genes Selected from a Combined Dataset by the Proposed Method	340
16.4.2.4	Improvement of Prediction Accuracies by Combining Datasets Performed using Different Platforms	340
16.4.3	Conclusions	341
16.5	Summary	342
	References	342
17	**Model Averaging for Biological Networks with Prior Information**	**347**
	Sach Mukherjee, Terence P. Speed, and Steven M. Hill	
17.1	Introduction	347
17.2	Background	349
17.2.1	Bayesian Networks	349
17.2.2	Model Scoring	350
17.2.3	Model Selection and Model Averaging	351
17.2.4	Markov Chain Monte Carlo on Graphs	354
17.3	Network Priors	356
17.3.1	A Motivating Example	356
17.3.2	General Framework	357
17.3.2.1	Specific Edges	357
17.3.2.2	Classes of Vertices	358
17.3.2.3	Higher-Level Network Features	358
17.3.2.4	Network Sparsity	358
17.3.2.5	Degree Distributions	359
17.3.2.6	Constructing a Prior	359

17.3.3	Prior-Based Proposals	*359*
17.4	Some Results	*360*
17.4.1	Simulated Data	*360*
17.4.1.1	Priors	*361*
17.4.1.2	MCMC	*362*
17.4.1.3	ROC Analysis	*362*
17.4.2	Prior Sensitivity	*362*
17.4.3	A Biological Network	*362*
17.4.3.1	Data	*363*
17.4.3.2	Priors	*364*
17.4.3.3	MCMC	*365*
17.4.3.4	Single Best Graph	*365*
17.4.3.5	Network Features	*365*
17.4.3.6	Prior Sensitivity	*365*
17.5	Conclusions and Future Prospects	*366*
17.6	Appendix	*369*
	References	*370*

Index *373*

Preface

This book, *Medical Biostatistics for Complex Diseases*, presents novel approaches for the statistical and computational analysis of high-throughput data from complex diseases. A complex disease is characterized by an intertwined interplay between several genes that are responsible for the pathological phenotype instead of a single gene. This interplay among genes and their products leads to a bio-complexity that makes a characterization and description of such a disease intricate. For this reason, it has been realized that single-gene-specific methods are less insightful than methods based on groups of genes [1]. A possible explanation for this is that the orchestral behavior of genes in terms of their molecular interactions form gene networks [2, 3] that are composed of functional units (subnetworks) that are called pathways. In this respect, analysis methods based on groups of genes may resemble biological pathways and, hence, functional units of the biological system. This is in the spirit of systems theory [4, 5], which requires that a functional part of a system under investigation has to be studied to gain information about its functioning. The transfer of this conceptual framework to biological problems has been manifested in systems biology [6–8]. For this reason, the methods presented in this book emphasize pathway-based approaches. In contrast to network-based approaches for the analysis of high-throughput data [9] a pathway has a less stringent definition than a network [10] which may correspond to the causal molecular interactions or merely to a set of genes constituting it while neglecting their relational structure. Hence, the methodological analysis methods for both types of approaches vary considerably. Further, the present book emphasizes statistical methods because, for example, the need to test for significance or classify robustly is omnipresent in the context of high-throughput data from complex diseases. In a nutshell, the book focuses on a certain perspective of systems biology for the analysis of high-throughput data to help elucidating aspects of complex diseases that may otherwise remain covered.

The book is organized in the following way. The first part consists of three introductory chapters about basic cancer biology, cancer stem cells, and multiple correction methods for hypotheses testing. These chapters cover topics that recur during the book at various degrees and for this reason should be read first. The provided biological knowledge and the statistical methods are indispensable for a systematic design, analysis, and interpretation of high-throughput data from cancer but also other complex diseases. Despite the fact that the present book has a methodological focus on statistical analysis methods we consider it essential to include also some chapters that provide information about basic biological mechanisms that may be crucial to understand aspects of complex diseases.

The second part of the book presents statistical and computational analysis methods and their application to high-throughput data sets from various complex diseases. Specifically, biological data sets studied are from acute myeloid leukemia (AML), acute lymphoblastic leukemia (ALL), breast cancer, cervical cancer, conventional renal cell carcinoma (cRCC), colorectal cancer, liver cancer, and lung cancer. In addition to these data sets from cancer, also microarray data from diabetes and Duchenne muscular dystrophy (DMD) are used. These biological datasets are complemented by simulated data to study methods theoretically. This part of the book presents chapters that apply and develop methods for identifying differentially expressed genes, integration of data sets, inference of regulatory network, gene set analysis, predicting disease stages or survival times, and pathway analysis. From a methodological point of view the chapters in the second part comprise, for example, analysis of covariance (ANCOVA), bagging, Bayesian networks, dynamic vector autoregressive model, empirical Bayes, false discovery rate (FDR), Granger causality, Hotelling's T^2, kernel methods, least angle regression (LARS), least absolute shrinkage and selection operator (Lasso), Markov chain Monte Carlo (MCMC), model averaging, multiple hypotheses testing, multivariate analysis of variance (MANOVA), random forest, resampling methods, singular-value decomposition (SVD), and support vector machine (SVM).

Regarding the organization of each chapter we decided that the chapters should be presented comprehensively accessible not only to researchers from this field but also to researchers from related fields or even students that have passed already introductory courses. For this reason each chapter presents not only some novel results but also provides some background knowledge necessary to understand, for example, the mathematical method or the biological problem under consideration. In research articles this background information is either completely omitted or the reader is referred to an original article. Hence, this book could also serve as textbook for, e.g., an interdisciplinary seminar for advanced students, not only because of the comprehensiveness of the chapters but also because of its size, which allowing it to fill a complete semester.

The present book is intended for researchers in the interdisciplinary fields of computational biology, biostatistics, bioinformatics, and systems biology studying problems in biomedical sciences. Despite the fact that these fields emerged from traditional disciplines like biology, biochemistry, computer science, electrical engineering, mathematics, medicine, statistics, or physics we want to emphasize that they are now becoming independent. The reasons for this are at least three-fold. First, these fields study problems that cannot be assigned to one of the traditional fields alone, neither biologically nor methodologically. Second, the studied problems are considered of general importance, not only for science itself but society because of their immediate impact on public health. Third, biomedical problems *demand* the development of novel statistical and computational methodology for their problem-oriented and efficient investigation. This implies that none of the traditional quantitative fields provide ready-to-use solutions to many of the urgent problems we are currently facing when studying the basic molecular mechanisms of complex diseases. This explains the eruption of methodological papers that appeared during the last two decades. Triggered by continuing technological developments leading to new or improved high-throughput measurement devices it is expected that this process will continue. The quest for a systematic understanding of complex diseases is intriguing not only because we acquire a precise molecular and cellular "picture" of organizational processes within and among cells but especially because of consequences that may result from this. For example, insights from such studies may translate directly into rational drug design and stem cell research.

Many colleagues, whether consciously or unconsciously, have provided us with input, help, and support before and during the formation of the present book. In particular we would like to thank Andreas Albrecht, Gökmen Altay, Gökhan Bakır, Igor Bass, David Bialy, Danail Bonchev, Ulrike Brandt, Stefan Borgert, Mieczysław Borowiecki, Andrey A. Dobrynin, Michael Drmota, Maria Duca, Dean Fennell, Isabella Fritz, Maria Fonoberova, Boris Furtula, Bernhard Gittenberger, Galina Glazko, Armin Graber, Martin Grabner, Earl Glynn, Ivan Gutman, Arndt von Haeseler, Peter Hamilton, Bernd Haas, Des Higgins, Dirk Husmeier, Wilfried Imrich, Puthen Jithesh, Patrick Johnston, Frank Kee, Jürgen Kilian, Elena Konstantinova, Terry Lappin, D. D. Lozovanu, Dennis McCance, Alexander Mehler, Abbe Mowshowitz, Ken Mills, Arcady Mushegian, Klaus Pawelzik, Andrei Perjan, Marina Popovscaia, William Reeves, Bert Rima, Armindo Salvador, Heinz Georg Schuster, Helmut Schwegler, Chris Seidel, Andre Ribeiro, Ricardo de Matos Simoes, Francesca Shearer, Brigitte Senn-Kircher, Fred Sobik, Doru Stefanescu, John Storey, Robert Tibshirani, Shailesh Tripathi, Kurt Varmuza, Suzanne D. Vernon, Robert Waterston, Bruce Weir, Olaf Wolkenhauer, Bohdan Zelinka, Shu-Dong Zhang, and Dongxiao Zhu, and apologize to all who have not been named mistakenly. We would like also to thank our editors Andreas Sendtko and Gregor Cicchetti from Wiley-VCH who have been always available and helpful. Last but not least we would like to thank our families for support and encouragement during all that time.

Finally, we hope this book helps to spread our enthusiasm and joy we have for this field and inspires people regarding their own practical or theoretical research problems.

Belfast and Hall/Tyrol
January 2010

F. Emmert-Streib and
M. Dehmer

References

1 Emmert-Streib, F. (2007) The chronic fatigue syndrome: a comparative pathway analysis. *J. Comput. Biol.*, **14** (7), 961–972.

2 Barabási, A.L. and Oltvai, Z.N. (2004) Network biology: Understanding the cell's functional organization. *Nat. Rev. Genet.*, **5**, 101–113.

3 Kauffman, S.A. (1969) Metabolic stability and epigenesis in randomly constructed genetic nets. *J. Theor. Biol.*, **22**, 437–467.
4 Bertalanffy, L.v. (1950) An outline of general systems theory. *Br. J. Philos. Sci.*, **1** (2), 134–165.
5 Bertalanffy, L.v. (1976) *General System Theory: Foundations, Development, Applications*, revised edn, George Braziller, New York.
6 Alon, U. (2006) *An Introduction to Systems Biology: Design Principles of Biological Circuits*, Chapman & Hall/CRC.
7 Kitano, H. (ed.) (2001) *Foundations of Systems Biology*, MIT Press.
8 Palsson, B.O. (2006) *Systems Biology: Properties of Reconstructed Networks*, Cambridge University Press, New York.
9 Emmert-Streib, F. and Dehmer, M. (eds) (2008) *Analysis of Microarray Data: A Network-Based Approach*, Wiley-VCH Verlag, Weinheim.
10 Dehmer, M. and Emmert-Streib, F. (eds) (2009) *Analysis of Complex Networks: From Biology to Linguistics*, Wiley-VCH Verlag, Weinheim.

List of Contributors

Gyan Bhanot
Rutgers University
BioMaPs Institute for Quantitative Biology
610 Taylor Road
Piscataway, NJ 08854
USA

Gregory A. Bird
University of Colorado Denver
Department of Dermatology
Charles C. Gates Program in Regenerative Medicine and Stem Cell Biology
12800 E. 19th Avenue
Aurora, CO 80045
USA

A. Rose Brannon
University of North Carolina
Lineberger Comprehensive Cancer Center
CB 7295
Chapel Hill, NC 27599-7295
USA

Eike C. Buss
Heidelberg University
Department of Internal Medicine V
Im Neuenheimer Feld 410
69120 Heidelberg
Germany

Bor-Sen Chen
National Tsing Hua University
Department of Electrical Engineering
101, Section 2, Kuang-Fu Road
Hsinchu 30013
Taiwan

James J. Chen
FDA/National Center for Toxicological Research
Division of Personalized Nutrition and Medicine
3900 NCTR Road
Jefferson, AR 72079
USA

Sung Bum Cho
Seoul National University
College of Medicine
Division of Biomedical and Healthcare Informatics
28 Yongon-dong, Chongno-gu
Seoul 110-799
Korea

Liang-Hui Chu
National Tsing Hua University
Department of Electrical Engineering
101, Section 2, Kuang-Fu Road
Hsinchu 30013
Taiwan

Robert Clarke
Georgetown University Medical Center
Department of Oncology
3970 Reservoir Rd NW
Washington DC, 20057
USA

Marcos Angelo Almeida Demasi
University of Sao Paulo
Institute of Mathematics and Statistics
Av. Prof. Lineu Prestes, 748
Butanta
05508-900 Sao Paulo
Brazil

Hong-Wen Deng
University of Missouri-Kansas City
Departments of Orthopedic Surgery and Basic Medical Sciences
2411 Holmes Street
Kansas City, MO 64108
USA

Elena Edelman
Harvard Medical School
Department of Medicine
185 Cambridge Street
CPZN 4200
Boston, MA 02114
USA

Alessio Farcomeni
Sapienza - University of Rome
Piazzale Aldo Moro, 5
00186 Rome
Italy

Carlos Eduardo Ferreira
University of Sao Paulo
Institute of Mathematics and Statistics
Av. Prof. Lineu Prestes, 748
Butanta
05508-900 Sao Paulo
Brazil

Irit Fishel
Tel Aviv University
School of Computer Sciences and
School of Medicine
Schreiber Building Ramat Aviv
69978 Tel Aviv
Israel

Wataru Fujibuchi
National Institute of Advanced
Industrial Science and Technology
(ASIT)
Computational Biology Research Centre
2-42 Aomi, Koto-ku
Tokyo 135-0064
Japan

André Fujita
University of Sao Paulo
Institute of Mathematics and Statistics
Av. Prof. Lineu Prestes, 748
Butanta
05508-900 Sao Paulo
Brazil

Shridar Ganesan
Cancer Institute of New Jersey
195 Little Albany Street
New Brunswick, NJ 08903
USA

Katherine Garman
Duke University
Institute for Genome Sciences & Policy
Department of Medicine
101 Science Drive
Durham, NC 27708
USA

Leena Hilakivi-Clarke
Georgetown University Medical Center
Department of Oncology
3970 Reservoir Rd NW
Washington, DC 20057
USA

Steven M. Hill
University of Warwick
Centre for Complexity Science
Zeeman Building
Coventry CV4 7AL
UK

Anthony D. Ho
University of Heidelberg
Department of Internal Medicine V
Im Neuenheimer Feld 410
69120 Heidelberg
Germany

Taeyoung Hwang
Seoul National University
Department of Statistics
56-1 Shillim-Dong, Kwang-Gu
Seoul 151-747
Korea

Tsuyoshi Kato
National Institute of Advanced
Industrial Science and Technology
(ASIT)
Computational Biology Research Centre
2-42 Aomi, Koto-ku
Tokyo 135-0064
Japan

Jihun Kim
Seoul National University
College of Medicine
Division of Biomedical and Healthcare
Informatics
28 Yongon-dong, Chongno-gu
Seoul 110-799
Korea

Ju Han Kim
Seoul National University
College of Medicine
Division of Biomedical and Healthcare
Informatics
28 Yongon-dong, Chongno-gu
Seoul 110-799
Korea

Ki-Yeol Kim
Yonsei University College of Dentistry
Oral Cancer Research Institute
250 Seongsanno Seodaemun-gu
Seoul 120-752
Korea

Louis-Philippe Kronek
G-SCOP, Grenoble-Science Conception
Organization and Production
46 Avenue Viallet
38031 Grenoble
France

Huai Li
Bioinformatics Unit
National Institute on Aging
National Institutes of Health
Baltimore, MD 21224
USA

List of Contributors

Peng-Yuan Liu
Washington University School of
Medicine
Department of Surgery and
the Alvin J. Siteman Cancer Center
660 South Euclid Avenue
Campus Box 8109
St. Louis, MO 63110
USA

Yan Lu
Washington University School of
Medicine
Department of Surgery and
the Alvin J. Siteman Cancer Center
660 South Euclid Avenue
Campus Box 8109
St. Louis, MO 63110
USA

Satoru Miyano
University of Sao Paulo
Institute of Mathematics and Statistics
Av. Prof. Lineu Prestes, 748
Butanta
05508-900 Sao Paulo
Brazil

Sach Mukherjee
University of Warwick
Centre for Complexity Science
Zeeman Building
Coventry CV4 7AL
UK

Sayan Mukherjee
Duke University
Institute for Genome Sciences & Policy
Departments of Statistical Science,
Computer Science, and Mathematics
214 Old Chemistry Building
Durham, NC 27708
USA

Assaf P. Oron
University of Washington
Department of Statistics
Box 354322
Seattle, WA 98195
USA

Taesung Park
Seoul National University
Department of Statistics
56-1 Shillim-Dong, Kwang-Gu
Seoul 151-747
Korea

Anil Potti
Duke University
Institute for Genome Sciences & Policy
Department of Medicine
101 Science Drive
Durham, NC 27708
USA

W. Kimryn Rathmell
University of North Carolina
Lineberger Comprehensive Cancer
Center
CB 7295
Chapel Hill, NC 27599
USA

Anupama Reddy
Rutgers University
RUTCOR - Rutgers Center for
Operations Research
640 Bartholomew Rd.
Piscataway, NJ 08854
USA

Yosef Refaeli
University of Colorado Denver
Department of Dermatology
Charles C. Gates Program in
Regenerative Medicine and Stem Cell
Biology
12800 E. 19th Avenue
Aurora, CO 80045
USA

Sun Young Rha
Yonsei University College of Medicine
Yonsei Cancer Center
134 Shinchon-Dong Seodaemun-Ku
Seoul 120-752
Korea

Eytan Ruppin
Tel Aviv University
School of Computer Sciences and
School of Medicine
Schreiber Building Ramat Aviv
69978 Tel Aviv
Israel

João Ricardo Sato
University of Sao Paulo
Institute of Mathematics and Statistics
Av. Prof. Lineu Prestes, 748
Butanta
05508-900 Sao Paulo
Brazil

Michael Seiler
Rutgers University
BioMaPs Institute for Quantitative
Biology
610 Taylor Road
Piscataway, NJ 08854
USA

Mari Cleide Sogayar
University of Sao Paulo
Institute of Mathematics and Statistics
Av. Prof. Lineu Prestes, 748
Butanta
05508-900 Sao Paulo
Brazil

Terence P. Speed
Walter and Eliza Hall Institute of
Medical Research
1G Royal Parade
Parkville Victoria 3052
Australia

Chen-An Tsai
China Medical University
Graduate Institute of Biostatistics &
Biostatistics Center
Taichung
91 Hsueh-Shih Road
Taiwan 40402
R.O.C.

Brian C. Turner
University of Colorado Denver
Department of Dermatology
Charles C. Gates Program in
Regenerative Medicine and Stem Cell
Biology
12800 E. 19th Avenue
Aurora, CO 80045
USA

Yue Wang
Virginia Polytechnic Institute and State
University
Department of Electrical and Computer
Engineering
4300 Wilson Blvd.
Arlington, VA 22203
USA

Bai Zhang
Virginia Polytechnic Institute and State University
Department of Electrical and Computer Engineering
4300 Wilson Blvd., Suite 750
Arlington, VA 22203
USA

Part One
General Biological and Statistical Basics

1
The Biology of *MYC* in Health and Disease: A High Altitude View
Brian C. Turner, Gregory A. Bird, and Yosef Refaeli

1.1
Introduction

The *MYC* oncogene has been intensely studied over the past 25 years, in part due to its extensive involvement in many forms of human cancer. *MYC* appears to be critical for several cellular processes, including cell division (proliferation), cell survival, DNA-replication, transcriptional regulation, energy metabolism, and differentiation. Overall, *MYC* appears to be an important element in a cell's ability to sense and integrate extracellular signals in its environment. This seems to be a feature that arose along with a metazoan lifestyle of organisms. The extensive research that has focused on *MYC* has yet to provide a consensus on the functions of *MYC*, because of its involvement in a large number of cellular functions and the use of systems that provide divergent results. One additional level of complication in the study of *MYC* is that it serves as a regulator of many cellular processes while not being directly involved in those specific pathways. For instance, *MYC* regulates cell division or proliferation, but is not a part of the cell cycle machinery. Likewise, *MYC* has been shown to regulate cell survival, but is not involved in the cellular pathways that regulate apoptosis. Along these lines, *MYC* has also been shown to act as a weak transcriptional activator, but the nature and identity of its target genes are poorly defined. The current view on the role of *MYC* in gene regulation is that it affects the expression of a broad set of genes, perhaps by some greater effects on chromatin modification than a "traditional" transcription factor. In addition, *MYC* appears to be involved in facilitating DNA replication as a means to support cell division. Together, these new ideas may help explain some of the observations regarding roles for *MYC* in stem cell maintenance and differentiation, as well as in transformation. Some of these issues may be clarified with ongoing work in the field, as well as the involvement of additional disciplines in biology, that may be better suited to model some of these enigmas and provide testable hypotheses for experimental biologists. This chapter provides a brief summary of the involvement of *MYC* in many aspects of normal cell physiology, as well as in cancer, with an emphasis on the contributions of *MYC* to hematopoietic malignancies.

The following nomenclature is used in this chapter:

Human gene and protein	MYC
Other human forms of myc	MYCN, L-MYC, S-MYC
	(genes in italics, proteins are not italicized)
Mouse gene	c-myc
Mouse protein	c-Myc

1.2
MYC and Normal Physiology

Pin-pointing precisely the "normal" function, or the mechanism of MYC function, would be a difficult if not impossible task. This is because MYC is involved in the regulation of metabolism, cell-cycle regulation and differentiation, cell adhesion, apoptosis, protein synthesis, and transcription of microRNAs. The involvement of MYC in so many aspects of normal cell physiology has yielded numerous publications concerning its function, but has precluded the formulation of a concerted view of MYCs function. MYC carries out these functions in the cell through various mechanisms, including transcriptional regulation (both activation and repression), control of DNA methylation, and chromatin remodeling [1]. The best way to impart an overall appreciation for the importance of MYC in a normal cells and tissues would be to present a brief overview of each of the areas mentioned above. A more detailed account of the functions of MYC in each of these fields of biology can be found in the various reviews or references cited in the text. An underlying principle that should become evident throughout this chapter is that MYC's powerful role is ultimately defined by the context of its expression (Figure 1.1). Importantly, the expression of MYC is tightly regulated and transient in normal settings. The MYC protein has a very short half-life (roughly 20–30 min) and is a member of a family of loosely associated genes (MYCN, L-MYC, S-MYC). These related genes are expressed at different times and in different tissues and there is some evidence that they have similar or redundant functions. The overexpression of MYC in disease states exaggerates its effects on a particular cellular pathway. These are some of the sources used to ascertain the role of MYC in normal physiology. When drawing conclusions about MYC is it important to consider the experimental design that is being used, keeping in mind the differences between cell lines and whole organisms and possible indirect influences of loss and gain of function.

1.3
Regulation of Transcription and Gene Expression [2]

Transcription regulation and gene expression is a very complicated and highly regulated process. Although various mechanisms for MYC function have been described, the effects MYC exerts on various cell functions described below are

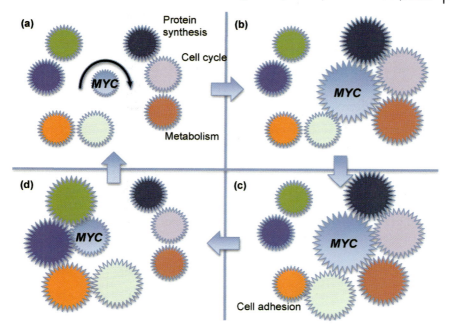

Figure 1.1 The master cog: MYC function is largely determined by the amount and context of gene expression. MYC levels are very low in a normal cell (a); MYC upregulation in a cell powers components of different aspects of the cell machinery (protein, synthesis, cell cycle, and metabolism pictured here) (b); MYC can have many secondary (tertiary, etc.) effects within a cell (cell adhesion pictured here) (c); a critical ability of a normal cell is the downregulation of MYC following its pleiotropic activity (d).

carried out by its ability to regulate transcription. The goal of many biochemical studies looking at MYC's role in transcriptional regulation and gene expression is to discover how MYC controls so many processes and how deregulated MYC can be such a powerful oncogene.

To summarize briefly, MYC belongs to the family of helix-loop-helix leucine zipper proteins that form homo- or heterodimers and bind to DNA sequences. *In vitro* c-Myc can form homodimers or heterodimerize with either Max, Mad1, Mxi1, Mad3, Mad4, or Mnt. *In vivo*, however, c-Myc is only found as a heterodimer with Max. When c-Myc is bound to Max it can both activate and repress transcription of its target genes. Max itself can form homodimers *in vivo*, but neither activate nor repress transcription. Max can also bind Mad family of proteins and they repress transcription. In general, Myc-Max complexes are often the majority of heterodimers found in proliferating cells and Mad-Max/Mnt-Max complexes are the majority in cells that have differentiated or are in a resting phase [3]. Since Max is usually in excess in cells, it is the relative amounts of c-Myc and Mad that ultimately determine whether c-Myc can activate or repress its specific targets and this is probably a reason why the levels of c-Myc inside a cell are tightly regulated and the half-life of this powerful protein is so short. The continuous degradation of MYC and its short half-life suggest that MYC binding to a given site on DNA is transient. The rate of MYC production required to maintain steady-state levels would ensure that all MYC target sequences in a genome may become occupied at some point during the surge of MYC expression. Probably not all of the targets are bound at any one point in time, due to the transient nature of the heterodimers. An additional level of complication is the ability of the complexes that involve MYC to recruit transcriptional coregulators, further increasing the complexity of the transcriptional profile that is affected by MYC. Among these are the TRRAP coactivator, the Tip60 complex, the Pim1-kinase, the Lid/Rpb2 H3-K4 demethylase, and the HectH9 ubiquitin ligase. These factors are involved in histone modification and alteration of chromatin states and nucleosome instability. The absence of a discrete set of gene targets for MYC may come as a result of its ability to induce significant changes at the chromatin level. In addition, the contributions of MYC to reprogramming of somatic cells into induce pluripotent stem cells (iPSs) may result from its ability to induce an open chromatin structure.

1.4
Metabolism [4]

Cell metabolism can be defined as a complex set of chemical reactions that allow the cell to live in a given environment. The types of reactions that take place are set in motion from cues that the cell receives from that particular environment. MYC plays an important role in cell metabolism because it can regulate metabolic processes that enable cells to grow in suboptimal conditions such as hypoxia. Under normal circumstances this is critical for mounting an immune response as specific antigen dependent cells need to hyperproliferate to combat the microbial invader. During the development (and maintenance) of cancer MYC can function to supply the energy for tumor growth when the environment would otherwise tell the cells to stop proliferating in such crowded conditions.

MYC influences cell metabolism by participating in several metabolic pathways, including glucose uptake and glycolysis, which makes sense because a cell that is growing and proliferating needs energy to carry out these activities [5]. MYC specifically upregulates transcripts of important enzymes of glucose metabolism, including glucose transporter, enolase A, lactate dehydrogenase A, phosphofructokinase, and hexokinase II [6–8]. During the process of transformation, MYC has been shown to induce glutaminolysis and glutamine addiction through the upregulation transcripts of glutamine transporters, glutaminase, and lactate dehydrogenase A (LDH-A) [9]. Iron metabolism is also an important cellular function that is driven by MYC as enzymes that catalyze energy metabolism and DNA synthesis require iron. Reports have shown coordinated regulation of iron-controlling gene transcripts by MYC, including cell surface receptors such as the transferring receptor (TFRC1) [10]. MYC also affects transcription of genes involved in generating the building blocks for DNA synthesis, called nucleotides, such as ornithine decarboxylase that functions in the synthesis of polyamines required for nucleotide biosynthesis enzymes [11].

1.5
Cell-Cycle Regulation and Differentiation [12]

The cell-cycle is the process by which one cell divides symmetrically into two daughter cells. This involves a highly-regulated series of events with many checks and balances. It is critical that new cells have all the necessary information (DNA) and machinery (proteins, etc.) to survive as a new cell, respond to physiological cues, and divide as needed.

Expression analysis of *MYC* and cell cycle and growth genes demonstrates that [13] *MYC* influences the transcription of a large number of cell cycle genes and gene products. *MYC* positively regulates expression of proteins that push the cell cycle forward: G1-specific cyclin-dependent kinases (CDKs) by inactivating inhibitors of these kinases. *MYC* also induces activators of specific CDKs. The net result of these activities is that *MYC* prevents cell cycle arrest in the presence of growth-inhibitory signals or after withdrawal of activating signals or under signals to differentiate. If *MYC* is activated, or dysregulated, the cell will be pushing to divide and not differentiate. Hence, many differentiation programs require the downregulation of *MYC* to accomplish terminal differentiation. One recent observation that supports this notion relates to the need for ectopic overexpression of *MYC*, along with three other transcription factors (Oct4, Sox2, and Klf4), to reprogram fibroblasts into iPS cells.

1.6
Protein Synthesis [14]

Protein synthesis is closely tied to cell-cycle because cells need to produce new proteins in order to divide, as one of the check-points in the cell cycle is the determination of whether the cell has reached a large enough mass. As with other processes in a cell, protein synthesis occurs as a result of cues the cell receives from its environment. One of the final effector proteins in this chain of events is *MYC*.

Unsurprisingly, various studies have identified translation initiation (protein synthesis) factors as targets of *c-myc* [14]. As mentioned above, translation initiation directly affects both growth and division in a cell. Ribosomal content and ribosomal genes are affected by *MYC*. In one gene screen with N-myc, it was shown to enhance the expression of a large set of genes functioning in ribosome biogenesis and protein synthesis in neuroblastoma cells [15]. Specific studies have shown the influence of *MYC* on RNA pol I, II, and III activation [15–20].

1.7
Cell Adhesion [4]

Cell adhesion is important for tissues and organisms because for efficient functioning of organs, like heart, lung, and brain, these cells need to remain together. In "organs" such as the immune system, cell adhesion is turned on and off many times during a cell's life because the immune system must patrol the entire body. Cells of the immune system travel through the blood stream and lymph system to receive signals and carry out their effector functions such as antibody production or cell-killing.

Out of 218 differentially expressed genes in keratinocytes from *MYC* transgenic mouse, 30% are downregulated cellular adhesion genes and 11% are cytoskeletal related genes. Specifically, expression analysis in primary human fibroblasts *MYC* was found to repress genes encoding the extracellular matrix proteins fibronectin and collagen, and the cytoskeletal protein tropomyosin [13]. More recently *MYC* has been shown to regulate cell surface adhesion molecules such as N-cadherin on hematopoietic stem cells. Upregulation of *MYC* was associated with downregulation of N-cadherin and mobilization away from the stem cell niche [21].

1.8
Apoptosis [22]

Apoptosis is defined as programmed cell death and is crucial to the homeostasis of many organisms. New cells are created all the time and it is important to have a defined system to remove old cells. Apoptosis is also highly regulated because if cells die when they are not supposed to, or when cells do not die and they are supposed to, there is disease, as in the case of cancer. As mentioned in the introduction *MYC* function is highly dependent on the context of MYC expression. This point is quite clear when the role of *MYC* is considered in the cellular function of apoptosis, or programmed cell death.

c-Myc normally serves as a survival signal under physiological conditions but can contribute to apoptosis under conditions of stress (such as chemotoxic agents, transcription factor inhibitors, etc.). For example, under normal physiological conditions c-Myc can upregulate the glycolysis pathway as a mechanism to regulate cell survival. This is a critical function for the immune system because even if the environment is telling the cell that nutrients are low, an activating signal through c-Myc can supply the energy required to mount an effective immune response. Also, c-Myc has been shown to be critical in the response of activated B-cells to cytokines.

c-Myc is also necessary and sufficient, under stress conditions, for efficient response to transcription/translation inhibitors, hypoxia glucose deprival, chemotoxins, DNA damage, heat shock, and chemotherapeutic agents. This has been shown in work demonstrating the requirement of c-Myc and the function of death receptors [23–25]. Its somewhat paradoxical function of controlling cell fate has been put into a "dual function model" where c-Myc is seen as the ultimate co-ordinate activator of cell proliferation or apoptosis. For example, c-Myc overexpression in cells that are exposed to some form of stress results in continued proliferation until the cells die through the standard p53-dependent forms of apoptosis in the context of genotoxic stress. c-Myc itself, however, is not involved in the death program. In a similar fashion, c-Myc can coordinate proliferation, but is not itself involved in the cell cycle machinery.

1.9
MicroRNAs

MicroRNAs (miRNAs) were only discovered recently and have added another degree of complexity to the study of how cells regulate the content of their particular make-up. Originally, it was believed that proteins were responsible for determining how much of another protein was around, through what are called feedback mechanisms. With the finding of miRNA, it has been shown that nucleic acid sequences can also regulate the amount of protein by directly controlling the amount of message for a particular protein.

Although *MYC*'s role in regulation of MicroRNA is a relatively new field, studies have shown that *MYC* activates a cluster of six microRNAs on human chromosome 13, two of which negatively regulate an important transcription factor E2F1. *MYC* is involved in regulating miRNA transcription, as opposed to their processing or stability. When specific miRNAs that are repressed by c-Myc are forcibly expressed, investigators can reduce tumorigenicity for lymphoma cells [26, 27]. Because the knowledge base of how miRNAs function, how many there are, and what governs their specificities is just beginning, the future will certainly be interesting and challenging for biostatisticians, mathematical modelers, and systems biologists when trying to figure out how a master regulator like *MYC* regulates regulators.

1.10
Physiological Effects of Loss and Gain of c-myc Function in Mice

1.10.1
Loss of Function

Apart from gene array studies in established cell lines, the most informative studies, to date, on the normal function of c-Myc probably come from genetic modification studies where the specific gene of interest can be turned on or off and in specific tissues. Early attempts at reducing the levels of c-Myc showed that there was an increase in cell doubling time in rat fibroblasts that were missing both alleles of *c-myc*. Notably, the rat fibroblasts were generated by chemical mutagenesis and it is unclear what other mutations they might harbor [28]. In addition, the investigators observed decreased cell mass, total mRNA, and protein levels demonstrating the importance of *c-myc* in these processes [29].

To circumvent the problem of embryonic lethality of conventional gene knock-out mice, investigators have injected *c-myc*$-/-$ and *c-myc*$+/-$ cells into blastocysts of wild-type mice to study the requirement of c-Myc in mature immune cells. This approach demonstrated that lymphocytes in *c-myc*$-/-$ have difficulty maturing and they fail to grow and proliferate normally [30]. Importantly, the myc ko animals dies at E14 from severe anemia, implicating c-Myc in Epo signaling. Analysis of cytokines that rely on the gc of the IL-2 receptor in B-cells have shown a critical role for c-Myc in mediating cytokine-dependent signals related to proliferation and survival of activated B-cells [31].

More sophisticated genetic modification methods have been developed for targeted disruption of *c-myc* in mice. One of these systems allows incremental reduction of expression. Because a complete knock out is lethal before birth, fibroblasts from these different mice have been used to show reduced cell proliferation as c-Myc levels are decreased and that cells will exit the cell cycle when no c-Myc is expressed. Reduction of c-Myc levels in the whole organism results in smaller organisms because c-Myc ultimately controls the decision to divide or not to divide. Also, while most organs in the *c-myc* targeted mice were proportionally decreased in size along with the size of the whole animal, the hematopoietic compartment was disproportionally affected. The cellularity of the bone marrow, thymus, spleen, and lymph nodes is highly dependent on endogenous *c-myc* for its homeostasis and maintenance. Such results confirm the role of c-Myc as a critical survival factor in hematopoietic cells.

1.10.2
Gain of Function: Inducible Transgenic Animals

Techniques to study the normal function of c-Myc in specific cell types or tissues often involve the overexpression of *c-myc* by way of tailoring its expression behind a specific tissues promoter. For example, transgenic E beta-myc mice were shown to have abnormal T cell development when c-Myc was overexpressed in thymocytes [32]. Traditional cell lines involving the use of transformed cells that stably overexpress c-Myc have been plagued with problems and shown to provide results that have not held up with more physiologically relevant systems. Two possible reasons for these problems could be the use of already transformed cells as the background for the experiments, and the unregulated, continuous, and high overexpression of a gene whose expression is very transient and tightly regulated and yields a protein with a short half-life. These novel approaches using genetically engineered mice have begun to yield some important information regarding the effects of overexpressing c-Myc in particular cell types and contexts.

Methods to study the effects of turning on *c-myc* at specific time-points in specific tissues began in 1999 with several versions of the tetracycline-transactivating system. One mouse would express *c-myc* in all tissues when a specific drug was given to the mice (doxycycline) and one mouse would express *c-myc* in cells that used the immunoglobulin enhancer element-T-cells and B-cells [33]. Variations on this theme produced results from tissue-specific expression of c-Myc in pancreas and skin. Islet beta-cells that overexpressed c-Myc would proliferate and undergo apoptosis unless exogenous survival signal like Bcl-XL could protect them [34]. In addition, the same group showed that activation of c-Myc in skin causes, proliferation, disruption of differentiation, hyperplasia/dysplasia, and, surprisingly, angiogenesis.

More recently, groups have demonstrated that overexpression of c-Myc in anergic B cells (immune cells that do not respond to antigen) breaks this state of non-responsiveness. Importantly, this work shows c-Myc is downstream of important activating signals and that c-Myc alone can replace for the absence of these signals.

By genetically modifying the context of c-Myc overexpression by way of transgenes, this paper demonstrates that various B cell malignancies can be modeled very precisely in mice when additional signals are provided [35]. The paper demonstrates that if bona fide cooperating transforming events can be determined then a host of new targets suddenly become available for the development of new cancer therapeutics.

1.11
Contributions of MYC to Tumor Biology

Deregulation of MYC expression is one of the most common features in most forms of cancer. The presence of a surfeit of MYC is common in many solid tumors, in addition to hematopoietic malignancies. MYC has been implicated in most breast, gynecological, prostate, and gastrointestinal cancers, among others [36–40]. The role of MYC in these cancers is not fully understood because the actions of MYC are notoriously pleiotropic. Like in hematopoietic malignancies, the deregulation of MYC alone is insufficient for tumorigenesis, but rather the deregulation of MYC must accompany other changes in cell to form a tumor. In fact, MYC overexpression is usually associated with activating mutations in Ras genes, other members of the MAPK signaling pathways, Akt genes, loss of PTEN, or loss of BRCA1. Most of the genetic alterations discussed in this section result in the overexpression of MYC. It is thought that the continuous presence of elevated levels of MYC in the cell alter its physiology by enabling the cell to operate despite physiological control mechanisms. We will next review the various genetic alterations that result in overexpressed MYC that have been reported in hematological malignancies.

Some of these genetic changes are conserved across both hematopoietic cancers and solid tumors, while others are specific to solid tumors, or even certain types of solid tumors. MYC expression promotes progression through the cell cycle and enhances cellular growth in both hematopoietic and non-hematopoietic tumors (discussed above) [36–40]. In addition, MYC promotes increased cell adhesion, metastasis, and vasculogenesis in solid tumors [36, 41]. These are important characteristics of solid tumors, but are dispensable for lymphoid malignancies that are already circulating throughout the body. Finally, in both hematopoietic and non-hematopoietic tumors, increased MYC expression generally correlates to more aggressive tumors and poor patient outcomes.

Deregulation of MYC family genes can occur through several mechanisms. Chromosomal translocations involving MYC figure prominently in lymphoid malignancies, but are uncommon in solid tumors. Instead, MYC overexpression is achieved through either gene amplification, mutations that result in the stabilization of RNA or protein products of MYC family genes, or an increase in MYC transcription through an aberrantly activated signaling pathway and mutations in the transcriptional regulatory sequences of MYC [76]. We focus this part of the chapter on the contributions of MYC to hematopoietic malignancies.

1.12
Introduction of Hematopoietic Malignancies

The cellular components that make up the blood are derived from pluripotent hematopoietic stem cells (HSCs). These HSCs differentiate into mature red and white blood cells through various intermediate cell types before becoming terminally differentiated. HSCs are a heterogonous pool of long-term self-renewing HSC (LT-HSC), transiently self-renewing HSC (short-term HSC), and non-self-renewing multipotent HSC. LT-HSCs have the capacity to develop into lymphoid and myeloid precursors. Lymphoid precursors further differentiate into natural killer cells, B-lymphocytes, and T-lymphocytes whereas myeloid precursors give rise to erythroid (red blood cells), megakaryocytic, or granulocytic/monocytic lineages [42]. The genetic mutations that give rise to cancer can occur at any stage of development and lead to the clonal expansion of cells of a particular developmental stage.

Hematological malignancies are those affecting the blood, bone marrow, and lymph nodes. These diseases include leukemia, lymphoma, and multiple myeloma. Over the past few decades these cancers have been increasingly recognized as a genetic disease accumulating specific genetic mutations that aid in their diagnosis. Characterizing and classifying hematological cancers by taking into account the clinical behavior, morphology, immunophenotype, and cytogenetic data has led to better diagnosis and treatment.

Leukemia consists of several malignancies that originate in the bone marrow and are derived from clonal expansion of myeloid or immature lymphoid cells. Disease occurs when leukemic cells out compete normal bone marrow residents, resulting in a deficiency of blood platelets, white blood cells, and red blood cells. Lymphoma consists of several malignancies that originate from mature lymphoid lineages. Lymphomas commonly originate in lymph nodes and present as an enlarged node. Lymphoma is classified based on the predominant cell type and the degree of differentiation. Malignancies affecting the B cell lineage make up more than 90% of the human non-Hodgkin's lymphomas (NHLs) [43, 44]. Multiple myeloma is a tumor composed of plasma cells. Those are the cells that generate affinity matured antibodies in response to microbial infection. The genetics of multiple myeloma are fairly complex, and have not yet pointed to specific and recurrent genetic abnormalities in several different tumors.

MYC is the most commonly dysregulated genes in the cases of NHL [45–47]. The role of MYC in cellular transformation therefore has remained an area of intense study to better understand tumor biology as well as gain potential insights for the treatment of these life-ending diseases.

1.13
Mechanisms of MYC Dysregulation in Hematological Malignancies

Dysregulated MYC expression in hematological malignancies occurs by several different mechanisms. Cytogenetic and molecular investigations have provided evidence that chromosomal abnormalities such as translocation, gene amplification, and mutations in the MYC open reading frame or promoter/transcriptional regulatory regions can give rise to MYC overexpression. Dysregulated MYC has also been associated with viral infection and dysregulation of auxiliary proteins that stabilize MYC.

In normal cells MYC expression is tightly regulated at both the transcriptional and post-transcriptional levels. One feature common to Burkitt's lymphoma, a prototypic form of NHL, and a small portion of other leukemias is a chromosomal translocation that juxtaposes the MYC proto-oncogene with the regulatory elements of an immunoglobulin gene locus [43, 48–50]. As the heavy and light chain loci are transcriptionally activated during lymphocyte development and thereafter, these translocations lead to MYC overexpression. The continuous transcription of MYC by a powerful immunoglobulin promoter no longer allows for the carefully controlled, and transient, expression of MYC in response to physiological signals. Instead, there are high and consistent levels of MYC throughout.

Three types of MYC translocations have been identified in Burkitt's lymphoma cases. The most common translocation (t8;14) is MYC (chr. 8) to IgH (chr. 14), which is seen in 80% of Burkitt's lymphoma cases. About 15% of Burkitt's lymphoma cases have a t2;8 translocation, where the translocation occurs between MYC and kappa light chain gene, and the remaining 5% have a t8;22 translocation between MYC and lambda light chain gene [43, 49]. In cells that express immunoglobulin genes, these genomic rearrangements result in expression of MYC that would otherwise be tightly regulated [48, 51, 52]. A similar translocation of MYC into the alpha locus of the T cell receptor has also been reported for some T cell leukemias [53].

Amplification of the MYC locus is another genetic abnormality that is observed in some forms of leukemia or lymphomas. These may be observed in about 16% of diffuse large B-cell lymphomas (DLBCL), a common form of NHL that affects adults in North America and Europe [54]. Gene amplification is a cellular process whereby multiple copies of a particular gene accumulate, leading to overexpression of the gene product. Gene amplification can occur by the breakage-fusion-bridge cycle in a cell in which a sister chromatid that has incurred a DNA double strand break fuses to the other sister chromatid forming a bridge. At mitosis, the breakage of this giant inverted repeat leaves each daughter cell with a chromatid lacking one telomere. After replication, the broken sister chromatids fuse again, perpetuating the breakage-fusion-bridge cycle. Amplification occurs when the breakage of the fused sister chromatid is asymmetric and one daughter cell receives both allelic copies of a proto-oncogene [55–57]. Defects in NHEJ component have been observed in human cancers, including leukemia and multiple myeloma [58]. Amplification of the IgH/Myc fusion loci has been reported in some human B cell lymphomas and has been associated with poor prognosis.

1.14
Mutation(s) in the MYC Gene in Hematological Cancers

MYC is rapidly metabolized in cells via the ubiquitin/26s proteasome pathway with a half-life of approximately 30 min [59–62]. When cells enter the cell cycle, MYC can accumulate resulting from stabilization of the MYC protein. The increase in MYC half-life is mediated by two Ras effector pathways, Raf/ERK and PI-3K/AKT that result in MYC phosphorylation at Ser-62 and Thr-58, respectively [63]. MYC levels then return to low basal levels as the cell progresses through the cell cycle. Mutations in MYC that increase the half-life of the protein result in an accumulation of MYC such that these cells continuously expand and do not differentiate [61]. The presence of point mutations in MYC proteins occurs in about 60% of all B cell lymphomas. These mutations occur in two main regions of the open reading frame – those encompassing amino acid 47–62 or amino acids 106–143. Mutations in the amino acids Thr-58 and Ser-62 alter MYC phosphorylation at these residues, resulting in a substantial decrease in MYC degradation [61, 64, 65].

Regulated expression of MYC also occurs at the level of mRNA stability. Mitogens that initiate a proliferative response such as lipopolysaccharide, concanavalin A, or platelet-derived growth factor cause an increase in MYC mRNA concentration and stability [66]. MYC mRNA has a relatively short half-life of approximately 15 min in cells [67]. The 5′ truncated MYC mRNA that results from the chromosomal translocation in B-cell lymphoma was found to be quite stable with a half-life of several hours [68]. Mutations leading to the removal of the 3′ untranslated region (UTR) destabilizing sequences observed in T cell leukemias also result in an accumulation of MYC mRNA [69, 70].

1.15
Role of MYC in Cell Cycle Regulation and Differentiation in Hematological Cancers

MYC is expressed in most proliferating cells and repression of MYC is required for terminal differentiation of many cell types, including hematopoietic cells [71, 72]. Studies investigating conditional *c-myc* knockout alleles demonstrate that loss of *c-myc* stops cellular proliferation and these cells exit the cell cycle [73, 74]. In murine myeloid leukemic cells, overexpression of c-Myc blocks terminal differentiation and its associated growth arrest [75].

Deregulated MYC can maintain cells in a constant state of proliferation; this increases the likelihood that mutations in tumor suppressor, anti-apoptotic, or pro-apoptotic genes accumulate. MYC mediates genomic instability through nucleotide substitutions, double-stranded breaks, gene amplification, and defects in the mitotic spindle checkpoint (reviewed in Reference [76]). Under normal circumstances, these mutations would elicit cell cycle arrest and either correction of the mutation or the cell would be lead down an apoptotic pathway. Overexpression of MYC in cells can lead to a loss of cells cycle arrest and inhibition of apoptosis, allowing cells to accumulate mutations until the cell becomes transformed (Figure 1.2).

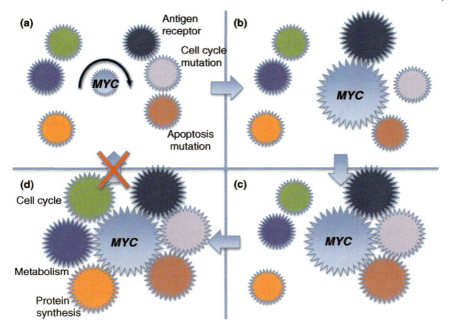

Figure 1.2 How cancer develops: MYC's role in the development of lymphoid cancers is a multistep process: MYC levels are tightly regulated in a normal cell (a); MYC overexpression in a cell can synergize with normal antigen receptor signaling to destabilize normal cell function (b); additional mutations in cell-cycle and/or apoptotic machinery are required for full transformation (c); a tumor cell fails to return to homeostatic levels of MYC but is dependent on antigen receptor signaling and super-physiologic levels of MYC (most likely to drive the internal efforts to meet the increased physiological demands placed on the cell to maintain continuous growth and proliferation) (d).

1.16
Role of BCR Signaling in Conjunction with MYC Overexpression in Lymphoid Malignancies

The notion of a role for chronic inflammation in lymphomagenesis has been with us for many years. Multiple observations suggest that antigenic stimulus can play a role in lymphomagenesis. First, infection with *Helicobacter pylori* is an apparent cause of human lymphomas in mucosal associated lymphoid tissue (MALT) and gut associated lymphoid tissue (GALT) [77]. Treatment with antibiotics to eradicate infection elicits remission of these tumors, as if they might have been sustained by antigenic stimulus from the microbe [78, 79]. Along these lines, a more recent report has shown that cells obtained from MALT lymphoma tumors express a unique, and restricted, antibody repertoire with frequent reactivity to rheumatoid factor [80]. The restriction in the BCR repertoire strongly suggests stringent antigenic selection. Second, mice with graft versus host disease consequent to bone marrow transplantation frequently develop B-cell lymphomas that contain integrations of ecotropic murine leukemia proviruses; these tumors were host-derived, and required histoincompatibility and T-cell help [81]. Third, the gene expression profiles of diffuse large B-cell lymphomas resemble those of B-cells that have mounted a response to antigen [82]. Moreover, the tumor cells obtained from either BL or diffuse large B-cell lymphoma (DLBCL) tumors display high-affinity antigen receptors on their surface, as if they had been subjected to the selective pressure of an antigen [82–87]. These findings prompt the hypothesis that an antigenic stimulus may cooperate with other tumorigenic influences in the genesis of lymphoma [88].

In normal B-cells, the BCR binds antigen and subsequently triggers growth and proliferation of B-cells and production of antigen-specific immunoglobulin. The role of BCR stimulation in conjunction with Myc overexpression in the formation of lymphoid malignancies has been investigated using Eµ–MYC transgenic mice [31]. Transgenic mice were generated that express MYC under a lymphoid specific promoter, B cell receptor to hen egg lysozyme (BCR^{HEL}), and the cognate antigen, soluble HEL (sHEL). The Eµ-MYC/BCR^{HEL}/sHEL mice formed fatal lymphomas as early as five weeks of age. Evidence of tumor in the Eµ-MYC/BCR^{HEL} and the Eµ-MYC/sHEL did not occur until 18 and 22 weeks, respectively [31]. These data provide evidence that BCR stimulation, in conjunction with MYC overexpression, can lead to lymphomagenesis (Figure 1.2).

1.17
Deregulation of Auxiliary Proteins in Addition to MYC in Hematological Cancers

The transformation of normal hematopoietic cells is largely caused by genetic mutations resulting in activated oncogenes and inactivated tumor-suppressors. These mutations give rise to various pathologic features in the neoplasm, including proliferation, immortalization, blocked differentiation, genomic instability, and resistance to apoptosis. The requirement of multiple genetic mutations has been demonstrated for several proto-oncogenes, including MYC, Bcl2, Bcl6, and many more. Cells harboring a single mutation that leads to altered expression of these proto-oncogenes do not give rise to cancer [89]. For example, Eµ–MYC transgenic mouse in which MYC is overexpressed in B-cell progenitors under control of the immunoglobulin heavy chain enhancer develop clonal pre-B and B-cell lymphomas only after acquiring a secondary mutation [89]. Crossing Eµ–MYC transgenic mice with either Eµ-Bcl2 or p53 +/− mice led to accelerated lymphoma development [90–92]. The aggressiveness of hematological malignancies seems to correlate with the accumulation of additional mutations affecting pro-survival, anti-apoptotic, and apoptotic factors. For example, the transformation of an indolent malignancy (follicular lymphoma) to an aggressive malignancy (diffuse large cell lymphoma) has been correlated with secondary mutations involving MYC, p53, Bcl2, or p16/INK4a [93, 94].

Importantly, while alteration to MYC expression and stability can increase the total amount of MYC protein present in the cell at a particular point in time, they do not seem to affect the function of *MYC*, as is the case in activating point mutations for some oncogenes (i.e., Ras). Ras is a proto-oncogene that encodes a GTP-binding protein that plays a role in cell growth and survival [95]. Activated Ras initiates a number of signal transduction pathways that include Raf/MAPK (ERK) and PI3 kinase/AKT that are involved in cell proliferation and survival, respectively [96–98]. Mouse models evaluating Ras, *MYC*, or Ras and *MYC* overexpression show that overexpression of *MYC* alone resulted in tumor formation only after a long latency period of 15–20 weeks while overexpression of Ras led to tumor formation in mice beginning at 4 weeks of age. Mice overexpressing both Ras and *MYC* formed tumors in mice beginning at 3 weeks of age [99].

MYC overexpression accompanied by inactivating mutations for tumor suppressor genes (i.e., p53 and ARF) also lead to a more aggressive malignancy. p53 is a DNA-binding protein that can induce cell-cycle arrest or apoptosis in response to DNA damage and expression of mitogenic oncogenes, such as *MYC* [100, 101]. ARF is upstream of p53 and activates p53 by interfering with its negative regulator, Mdm2 [102–104]. Eµ-*MYC* mouse models evaluating the onset of lymphoma show that the onset of lymphoma mice harboring an additional mutation in ARF or p53 is greatly accelerated relative to Eµ-*MYC* alone [92, 105]. Analyses of many human Burkitt's lymphomas where *MYC* is overexpressed also showed that Arf and p53 mutations occur spontaneously during tumor development [106, 107].

1.18
Conclusion

MYC proteins have important roles in the regulation of a large number of distinct cellular programs that are key for the normal physiological function of a cell. In fact, studies in genetically modified mice suggest that *MYC* is critical in the ability of a cell to respond to extracellular signals and integrate several such signals at any one point in time. The effects of *MYC* on gene expression are still not entirely clear, although this is probably the means by which *MYC* is able to participate and regulate such a distinct number of functions in the cell (Figure 1.1). The mRNA encoding for *MYC* and the protein itself have very short longevity. This is a probably due to its powerful and pleiotropic functions, and the need to tightly control such a factor. The dysregulation of *MYC* expression or turnover has dramatic consequences, as observed in many types of cancer. When *MYC* is overexpressed, the normal functions are extended to confer a competitive advantage to those cells when they meet adverse conditions. Such cells hyperproliferate in a manner that is independent of exogenous growth and survival factors. Those mutant cells can also divide and survive in conditions that would normally counter growth, such as hypoxia. Ultimately, the presence of an excess of *MYC* is likely to foster the development of additional genetic defects through the accumulation of other mutations and large-scale chromosomal abnormalities (Figure 1.2). The different levels of complexity encountered in the studies of *MYC* are quite unique and can tremendously benefit from the influx of additional types of ideas from computational biologists and statisticians. The absence of a consensus on the function of MYC makes this a ripe field for computational modeling and hypothesis generating approaches to biology.

References

1 Menssen, A. and Hermeking, H. (2002) Characterization of the c-MYC-regulated transcriptome by SAGE: identification and analysis of c-MYC target genes. *Proc. Natl. Acad. Sci. USA*, **99** (9), 6274–6279.
2 Adhikary, S. and Eilers, M. (2005) Transcriptional regulation and transformation by Myc proteins. *Nat. Rev. Mol. Cell Biol.*, **6** (8), 635–645. Review.
3 Ayer, D.E. and Eisenman, R.N. (1993) A switch from Myc:Max to Mad:Max heterocomplexes accompanies monocyte/macrophage differentiation. *Genes Dev.*, **7** (11), 2110–2119.
4 Dang, C.V., O'Donnell, K.A., Zeller, K.I., Nguyen, T., Osthus, R.C., and Li, F. (2006) The c-Myc target gene network. *Semin. Cancer Biol.*, **16** (4), 253–264. Epub 2006 Jul. 25. Review.
5 Huang, L.E. (2008) Carrot and stick: HIF-alpha engages c-Myc in hypoxic adaptation. *Cell Death Differ.*, **15** (4), 672–677, Epub 2008 Jan 11, Review.
6 O'Connell, B.C., Cheung, A.F., Simkevich, C.P., Tam, W., Ren, X., Mateyak, M.K., and Sedivy, J.M. (2003) A large scale genetic analysis of c-Myc-regulated gene expression patterns. *J. Biol. Chem.*, **278** (14), 12563–12573.
7 Osthus, R.C., Shim, H., Kim, S., Li, Q., Reddy, R., Mukherjee, M., Xu, Y., Wonsey, D., Lee, L.A., and Dang, C.V. (2000) Deregulation of glucose transporter 1 and glycolytic gene expression by c-Myc. *J. Biol. Chem.*, **275** (29), 21797–21800.
8 Kim, J.W., Zeller, K.I., Wang, Y., Jegga, A.G., Aronow, B.J., O'Donnell, K.A., and Dang, C.V. (2004) Evaluation of myc E-box phylogenetic footprints in glycolytic genes by chromatin immunoprecipitation assays. *Mol. Cell. Biol.*, **24** (13), 5923–5936.
9 Wise, D.R., DeBerardinis, R.J., Mancuso, A., Sayed, N., Zhang, X.Y., Pfeiffer, H.K., Nissim, I., Daikhin, E., Yudkoff, M., McMahon, S.B., and Thompson, C.B. (2008) Myc regulates a transcriptional program that stimulates mitochondrial glutaminolysis and leads to glutamine addiction. *Proc. Natl. Acad. Sci. USA*, **105** (48), 18782–18787.
10 Wu, K.J., Polack, A., and Dalla-Favera, R. (1999) Coordinated regulation of iron-controlling genes, H-ferritin and IRP2, by c-MYC. *Science*, **283** (5402), 676–679.
11 Bello-Fernandez, C., Packham, G., and Cleveland, J.L. (1993) The ornithine decarboxylase gene is a transcriptional target of c-Myc. *Proc. Natl. Acad. Sci. USA*, **90** (16), 7804–7808.
12 Obaya, A.J., Mateyak, M.K., and Sedivy, J.M. (1999) Mysterious liaisons: the relationship between c-Myc and the cell cycle. *Oncogene*, **18** (19), 2934–2941. Review.
13 Coller, H.A., Grandori, C., Tamayo, P., Colbert, T., Lander, E.S., Eisenman, R.N., and Golub, T.R. (2000) Expression analysis with oligonucleotide microarrays reveals that MYC regulates genes involved in growth, cell cycle, signaling, and adhesion. *Proc. Natl. Acad. Sci. USA*, **97** (7), 3260–3265.
14 Schmidt, E.V. (2004) The role of c-myc in regulation of translation initiation. *Oncogene*, **23** (18), 3217–3221. Review.
15 Boon, K., Caron, H.N., van Asperen, R., Valentijn, L., Hermus, M.C., van Sluis, P., Roobeek, I., Weis, I., Voûte, PA., Schwab, M., and Versteeg, R. (2001) N-myc enhances the expression of a large set of genes functioning in ribosome biogenesis and protein synthesis. *EMBO J.*, **20** (6), 1383–1393.
16 Guo, Q.M., Malek, R.L., Kim, S., Chiao, C., He, M., Ruffy, M., Sanka, K., Lee, N.H., Dang, C.V., and Liu, E.T. (2000)

Identification of c-myc responsive genes using rat cDNA microarray. *Cancer Res.*, **60** (21), 5922–5928.

17 Kim, S., Li, Q., Dang, C.V., and Lee, L.A. (2000) Induction of ribosomal genes and hepatocyte hypertrophy by adenovirus-mediated expression of c-Myc *in vivo*. *Proc. Natl. Acad. Sci. USA*, **97** (21), 11198–11202.

18 Gomez-Roman, N., Grandori, C., Eisenman, R.N., and White, R.J. (2003) Direct activation of RNA polymerase III transcription by c-Myc. *Nature*, **421** (6920), 290–294.

19 Grandori, C., Gomez-Roman, N., Felton-Edkins, Z.A., Ngouenet, C., Galloway, D.A., Eisenman, R.N., and White, RJ. (2005) c-Myc binds to human ribosomal DNA and stimulates transcription of rRNA genes by RNA polymerase I. *Nat. Cell Biol.*, **7** (3), 311–318.

20 Arabi, A., Wu, S., Ridderstråle, K., Bierhoff, H., Shiue, C., Fatyol, K., Fahlén, S., Hydbring, P., Söderberg, O., Grummt, I., Larsson, L.G., and Wright, A.P. (2005) c-Myc associates with ribosomal DNA and activates RNA polymerase I transcription. *Nat. Cell Biol.*, **7** (3), 303–310.

21 Wilson, A., Murphy, M.J., Oskarsson, T., Kaloulis, K., Bettess, M.D., Oser, G.M., Pasche, A.C., Knabenhans, C., Macdonald, H.R., and Trumpp, A. (2004) c-Myc controls the balance between hematopoietic stem cell self-renewal and differentiation. *Genes Dev.*, **18** (22), 2747–2763.

22 Prendergast, G.C. (1999) Mechanisms of apoptosis by c-Myc. *Oncogene*, **18** (19), 2967–2987. Review.

23 Hueber, A.O., Zörnig, M., Lyon, D., Suda, T., Nagata, S., and Evan, G.I. (1997) Requirement for the CD95 receptor-ligand pathway in c-Myc-induced apoptosis. *Science*, **278** (5341), 1305–1309.

24 Rohn, J.L., Hueber, A.O., McCarthy, N.J., Lyon, D., Navarro, P., Burgering, B.M., and Evan, G.I. (1998) The opposing roles of the Akt and c-Myc signalling pathways in survival from CD95-mediated apoptosis. *Oncogene*, **17** (22), 2811–2818.

25 Klefstrom, J., Arighi, E., Littlewood, T., Jäättelä, M., Saksela, E., Evan, G.I., and Alitalo, K. (1997) Induction of TNF-sensitive cellular phenotype by c-Myc involves p53 and impaired NF-kappaB activation. *EMBO J.*, **16** (24), 7382–7392.

26 O'Donnell, K.A., Wentzel, E.A., Zeller, K.I., Dang, C.V. and Mendell J.T. (2005) c-Myc-regulated microRNAs modulate E2F1 expression. *Nature*, **435** (7043), 839–843.

27 Chang, T.C., Yu, D., Lee, Y.S., Wentzel, E.A., Arking, D.E., West, K.M., Dang, C.V., Thomas-Tikhonenko, A., and Mendell, J.T. (2008) Widespread microRNA repression by Myc contributes to tumorigenesis. *Nat. Genet.*, **40** (1), 43–50.

28 Sedivy, J.M. and Joyner, A. (1992) *Gene Targeting*, W.H. Freeman Press, New York.

29 Mateyak, M.K., Obaya, A.J., Adachi, S., and Sedivy, J.M. (1997) Phenotypes of c-Myc-deficient rat fibroblasts isolated by targeted homologous recombination. *Cell. Growth Differ.*, **8** (10), 1039–1048.

30 Douglas, N.C., Jacobs, H., Bothwell, A.L., and Hayday, A.C. (2001) Defining the specific physiological requirements for c-Myc in T cell development. *Nat. Immunol.*, **2** (4), 307–315.

31 Refaeli, Y., Field, K.A., Turner, B.C., Trumpp, A., and Bishop, J.M. (2005) The protooncogene MYC can break B cell tolerance. *Proc. Natl. Acad. Sci. USA*, **102** (11), 4097–4102.

32 Broussard-Diehl, C., Bauer, S.R., and Scheuermann, R.H. (1996) A role for c-myc in the regulation of thymocyte differentiation and possibly positive selection. *J. Immunol.*, **156** (9), 3141–3150.

33 Felsher, D.W. and Bishop, J.M. (1999) Reversible tumorigenesis by MYC in hematopoietic lineages. *Mol. Cell.*, **4** (2), 199–207.

34 Pelengaris, S., Khan, M., and Evan, G.I. (2002) Suppression of Myc-induced apoptosis in beta cells exposes multiple oncogenic properties of Myc and triggers carcinogenic progression. *Cell*, **109** (3), 321–334.

35 Refaeli, Y., Young, R.M., Turner, B.C., Duda, J., Field, K.A., and Bishop, J.M. (2008) The B cell antigen receptor and overexpression of MYC can cooperate in the genesis of B cell lymphomas. *PLoS Biol.*, **6** (6), e152.

36 Dang, C.V. (1999) c-Myc target genes involved in cell growth, apoptosis, and metabolism. *Mol. Cell. Biol*, **19** (1), 1–11.

37 Prochownik, E.V. (2004) c-Myc as a therapeutic target in cancer. *Expert Rev. Anticancer Ther.*, **4** (2), 289–302.

38 Nesbit, C.E., Tersak, J.M., and Prochownik, E.V. (1999) MYC oncogenes and human neoplastic disease. *Oncogene*, **18** (19), 3004–3016.

39 Thomas, W.D., Raif, A., and Hansford, L. (2004) N-myc transcription molecule and oncoprotein. *Int. J. Biochem. Cell Biol.*, **36** (5), 771–775.

40 Wu, R., Lin, L., Beer, D.G. et al. (2003) Amplification and overexpression of the L-MYC proto-oncogene in ovarian carcinomas. *Am. J. Pathol.*, **162** (5), 1603–1610.

41 Baudino, T.A., McKay, C., Pendeville-Samain, H., Nilsson, J.A., Maclean, K.H., White, E.L., Davis, A.C., Ihle, J.N., and Cleveland, J.L. (2002) c-Myc is essential for vasculogenesis and angiogenesis during development and tumor progression. *Genes Dev.*, **16** (19), 2530–2543.

42 Blom, B. and Spits, H. (2006) Development of human lymphoid cells. *Annu. Rev. Immunol.*, **24**, 287–320.

43 Boxer, L. and Dang, C. (2001) Translocations involving c-myc and c-myc function. *Oncogene*, **20**, 5595–5610.

44 Morton, L.M., Turner, J.J., Cerhan, J.R., Linet, M.S., Treseler, P.A., Clarke, C.A., Jack, A., Cozen, W., Maynadié, M., Spinelli, J.J., Costantini, A.S., Rüdiger, T., Scarpa, A., Zheng, T., and Weisenburger, D.D. (2007) Proposed classification of lymphoid neoplasms for epidemiologic research from the Pathology Working Group of the International Lymphoma Epidemiology Consortium (InterLymph). *Blood*, **110** (2), 695–708.

45 Pagnano, K.B., Vassallo, J., Lorand-Metze, I., Costa, F.F., and Saad, S.T. (2001) p53, Mdm2, and c-Myc overexpression is associated with a poor prognosis in aggressive non-Hodgkin's lymphomas. *Am. J. Hematol.*, **67** (2), 84–92.

46 Hernandez, L., Hernández, S., Beà, S., Pinyol, M., Ferrer, A., Bosch, F., Nadal, A., Fernández, P.L., Palacín, A., Montserrat, E., and Campo, E. (1999) c-myc mRNA expression and genomic alterations in mantle cell lymphomas and other nodal non-Hodgkin's lymphomas. *Leukemia*, **13** (12), 2087–2093.

47 Chang, C.C., Liu, Y.C., Cleveland, R.P., and Perkins, S.L. (2000) Expression of c-Myc and p53 correlates with clinical outcome in diffuse large B-cell lymphomas. *Am. J. Clin. Pathol.*, **113** (4), 512–518.

48 Cory, S. (1986) Activation of cellular oncogenes in hemopoietic cells by chromosome translocation. *Adv. Cancer Res.*, **47**, 189–234.

49 Dalla-Favera, R., Bregni, M., Erikson, J., Patterson, D., Gallo, R.C., and Croce, C.M. (1982) Human c-myc onc gene is located on the region of chromosome 8 that is translocated in Burkitt lymphoma cells. *Proc. Natl. Acad. Sci. USA*, **79** (24), 7824–7827.

50 Taub, R., Kirsch, I., Morton, C., Lenoir, G., Swan, D., Tronick, S., Aaronson, S., and Leder, P. (1982) Translocation of the c-myc gene into the immunoglobulin heavy chain locus in human Burkitt lymphoma and murine plasmacytoma cells. *Proc. Natl. Acad. Sci. USA*, **79** (24), 7837–7841.

51 Cole, M.D. (1986) The myc oncogene: its role in transformation and differentiation. *Annu. Rev. Genet.*, **20**, 361–384. Review.

52 Cole, M.D. (1986) Activation of the c-myc oncogene. *Basic Life Sci.*, **38**, 399–406.

53 Erikson, J., Finger, L., Sun, L., ar-Rushdi, A., Nishikura, K., Minowada, J., Finan, J., Emanuel, B.S., Nowell, P.C., and Croce, C.M. (1986) Deregulation of c-myc by translocation of the alpha-locus of the T-cell receptor in T-cell leukemias. *Science*, **232** (4752), 884–886.

54 Rao, P.H., Houldsworth, J., Dyomina, K., Parsa, N.Z., Cigudosa, J.C., Louie, D.C.,

Popplewell, L., Offit, K., Jhanwar, S.C., and Chaganti, R.S. (1998) Chromosomal gene amplification in diffuse large B-cell lymphoma. *Blood*, **92** (1), 234–240.

55 Pipiras, E., Coquelle, A., Bieth, A., and Debatisse, M. (1998) Interstitial deletions and intrachromosomal amplification initiated from a double-strand break targeted to a mammalian chromosome. *EMBO J.*, **17** (1), 325–333.

56 Toledo, F., Le Roscouet, D., Buttin, G., and Debatisse, M. (1992) Co-amplified markers alternate in megabase long chromosomal inverted repeats and cluster independently in interphase nuclei at early steps of mammalian gene amplification. *EMBO J.*, **11** (7), 2665–2673.

57 Ma, C., Martin, S., Trask, B., and Hamlin, J.L. (1993) Sister chromatid fusion initiates amplification of the dihydrofolate reductase gene in Chinese hamster cells. *Genes Dev.*, **7** (4), 605–620.

58 Riballo, E., Critchlow, S.E., Teo, S.H., Doherty, A.J., Priestley, A., Broughton, B., Kysela, B., Beamish, H., Plowman, N., Arlett, C.F., Lehmann, A.R., Jackson, S.P., and Jeggo, P.A. (1999) Identification of a defect in DNA ligase IV in a radiosensitive leukaemia patient. *Curr. Biol.*, **9** (13), 699–702.

59 Ciechanover, A., DiGiuseppe, J.A., Schwartz, A.L., and Brodeur, G.M. (1991) Degradation of MYCN oncoprotein by the ubiquitin system. *Prog. Clin. Biol. Res.*, **366**, 37–43.

60 Flinn, E.M., Busch, C.M., and Wright, A.P. (1998) myc boxes, which are conserved in myc family proteins, are signals for protein degradation via the proteasome. *Mol. Cell. Biol.*, **18** (10), 5961–5969.

61 Salghetti, S.E., Kim, S.Y., and Tansey, W.P. (1999) Destruction of Myc by ubiquitin-mediated proteolysis: cancer-associated and transforming mutations stabilize Myc. *EMBO J.*, **18** (3), 717–726.

62 Hann, S.R. and Eisenman, R.N. (1984) Proteins encoded by the human c-myc oncogene: differential expression in neoplastic cells. *Mol. Cell. Biol.*, **4** (11), 2486–2497.

63 Sears, R., Leone, G., DeGregori, J., and Nevins, J.R. (1999) Ras enhances Myc protein stability. *Mol. Cell.*, **3** (2), 169–179.

64 Hoang, A.T., Lutterbach, B., Lewis, B.C., Yano, T., Chou, T.Y., Barrett, J.F., Raffeld, M., Hann, S.R., and Dang, C.V. (1995) A link between increased transforming activity of lymphoma-derived MYC mutant alleles, their defective regulation by p107, and altered phosphorylation of the c-Myc transactivation domain. *Mol. Cell. Biol.*, **15** (8), 4031–4042.

65 Sears, R., Nuckolls, F., Haura, E., Taya, Y., Tamai, K., and Nevins, J.R. (2000) Multiple Ras-dependent phosphorylation pathways regulate Myc protein stability. *Genes Dev.*, **14** (19), 2501–2514.

66 Kelly, K., Cochran, B.H., Stiles, C.D., and Leder, P. (1983) Cell-specific regulation of the c-myc gene by lymphocyte mitogens and platelet-derived growth factor. *Cell*, **35** (3 Pt 2), 603–610.

67 Dani, C., Blanchard, J.M., Piechaczyk, M., El Sabouty, S., Marty, L., and Jeanteur, P. (1984) Extreme instability of myc mRNA in normal and transformed human cells. *Proc. Natl. Acad. Sci. USA*, **81** (22), 7046–7050.

68 Eick, D., Piechaczyk, M., Henglein, B., Blanchard, J.M., Traub, B., Kofler, E., Wiest, S., Lenoir, G.M., and Bornkamm, G.W. (1985) Aberrant c-myc RNAs of Burkitt's lymphoma cells have longer half-lives. *EMBO J.*, **4** (13B), 3717–3725.

69 Aghib, D.F., Bishop, J.M., Ottolenghi, S., Guerrasio, A., Serra, A., and Saglio, G. (1990) A 3′ truncation of MYC caused by chromosomal translocation in a human T-cell leukemia increases mRNA stability. *Oncogene*, **5** (5), 707–711.

70 Jones, T.R. and Cole, M.D. (1987) Rapid cytoplasmic turnover of c-myc mRNA: requirement of the 3′ untranslated sequences. *Mol. Cell. Biol.*, **7** (12), 4513–4521.

71 Freytag, S.O. (1988) Enforced expression of the c-myc oncogene inhibits cell differentiation by precluding entry into a distinct predifferentiation state in G0/G1. *Mol. Cell. Biol.*, **8** (4), 1614–1624.

72 Hoffman, B., Liebermann, D.A., Selvakumaran, M., and Nguyen, H.Q. (1996) Role of c-myc in myeloid

differentiation, growth arrest and apoptosis. *Curr. Top. Microbiol. Immunol.*, **211**, 17–27 Review.

73 de Alboran, I.M., O'Hagan, R.C., Gärtner, F., Malynn, B., Davidson, L., Rickert, R., Rajewsky, K., DePinho, R.A., and Alt, F.W. (2001) Analysis of C-MYC function in normal cells via conditional gene-targeted mutation. *Immunity*, **14** (1), 45–55.

74 Trumpp, A., Refaeli, Y., Oskarsson, T., Gasser, S., Murphy, M., Martin, G.R., and Bishop, J.M. (2001) c-Myc regulates mammalian body size by controlling cell number but not cell size. *Nature*, **414** (6865), 768–773.

75 Amanullah, A., Liebermann, D.A., and Hoffman, B. (2000) p53-independent apoptosis associated with c-Myc-mediated block in myeloid cell differentiation. *Oncogene*, **19** (26), 2967–2977.

76 Meyer, N. and Penn, L.Z. (2008) Reflecting on 25 years with MYC. *Nat. Rev. Cancer*, **8** (12), 976–990. Review.

77 Lee, J.C. and Ihle, J.N. (1981) Chronic immune stimulation is required for Moloney leukaemia virus-induced lymphomas. *Nature*, **289**, 407–409.

78 Jones, R.G., Trowbridge, D.B., and Go, M.F. (2001) Helicobacter pylori infection in peptic ulcer disease and gastric malignancy. *Front. Biosci.*, **6**, E213–E226.

79 Casella, G., Buda, C.A., Maisano, R., Schiavo, M., Perego, D., and Baldini, V. (2001) Complete regression of primary gastric MALT-lymphoma after double eradication Helicobacter pylori therapy: role and importance of endoscopic ultrasonography. *Anticancer Res.*, **21**, 1499–1502.

80 Bende, R.J., Aarts, W.M., Riedl, R.G., de Jong, D., Pals, S.T., and van Noesel, C.J. (2005) Among B cell non-Hodgkin's lymphomas, MALT lymphomas express a unique antibody repertoire with frequent rheumatoid factor reactivity. *J. Exp. Med.*, **201** (8), 1229–1241.

81 Pals, S.T., Zijlstra, M., Radaszkiewicz, T., Quint, W., Cuypers, H.T., Schoenmakers, H.J., Melief, C.J., Berns, A., and Gleichmann, E. (1986) Immunologic induction of malignant lymphoma: graft-vs-host reaction-induced B cell lymphomas contain integrations of predominantly ecotropic murine leukemia proviruses. *J. Immunol.*, **136** (1), 331–339.

82 Chapman, C.J., Mockridge, C.I., Rowe, M., Rickinson, A.B., and Stevenson, F.K. (1995) Analysis of VH genes used by neoplastic B cells in endemic Burkitt lymphoma shows somatic hypermutation and intraclonal heterogeneity. *Blood*, **85**, 2176–2181.

83 Burkitt, D.P. (1971) Epidemiology of Burkitt Lymphoma. *Proc. R. Soc. Med.*, **64**, 909–910.

84 Alizadeh, A.A., Eisen, M.B., Davis, R.E., Ma, C., Lossos, I.S., Rosenwald, A., Boldrick, J.C., Sabet, H., Tran, T., Powell, J.I., Yang, L., Marti, G.E., Moore, T., Hudson, J.J., Lu, L., Lewis, D.B., Tibshirani, R., Sherlock, G., Chan, W.C., Greiner, T.C., Weisenburger, D.D., Armitage, J.O., Warnke, R., Levy, R., Wilson, W., Grever, M.R., Byrd, J.C., Botstein, D., Brown, P.O., and Staudt, L.M. (2000) Distinct types of diffuse large B-cell lymphoma identified by gene expression profiling. *Nature*, **403**, 503–511.

85 Ottesmeier, C.H., Thompsett, A.R., Zhu, D., Wilkins, B.S., Sweetenham, J.W., and Stevenson, F.K. (1998) Analysis of Vh genes in follicular and diffuse lymphoma shows ongoing somatic mutation and multiple isotype transcripts in early disease with changes during disease progression. *Blood*, **91**, 4292–4299.

86 Lossos, I.S., Alizabeth, A.A., Eisen, M.B., Chan, W.C., Brown, P.O., Botstein, D., Staudt, L.M., and Levy, R. (2000) Ongoing immunoglobulin somatic mutation in germinal center B cell-like but not in activated B cell-like diffuse large cell lymphomas. *Proc. Natl. Acad. Sci. USA*, **97**, 10209–10213.

87 Kuppers, R., Rajewski, K., and Hansmann, M.L. (1997) Diffuse large cell lymphomas are derived from mature B cells carrying V region genes with a high load of somatic mutation and evidence of selection for antibody

expression. *Eur. J. Immunol.*, **27**, 1398–1405.

88 Küppers, R. (2005) Mechanisms of B-cell lymphoma pathogenesis. *Nat. Rev. Cancer*, **5** (4), 251–262. Review.

89 Adams, J.M., Harris, A.W., Pinkert, C.A., Corcoran, L.M., Alexander, W.S., Cory, S., Palmiter, R.D., and Brinster, R.L. (1985) The c-myc oncogene driven by immunoglobulin enhancers induces lymphoid malignancy in transgenic mice. *Nature*, **318** (6046), 533–538.

90 Strasser, A., Harris, A.W., Bath, M.L., and Cory, S. (1990) Novel primitive lymphoid tumours induced in transgenic mice by cooperation between myc and bcl-2. *Nature*, **348** (6299), 331–333.

91 Hsu, B., Marin, M.C., el-Naggar, A.K., Stephens, L.C., Brisbay, S., and McDonnell, T.J. (1995) Evidence that c-myc mediated apoptosis does not require wild-type p53 during lymphomagenesis. *Oncogene*, **11** (1), 175–179.

92 Schmitt, C.A., McCurrach, M.E., de Stanchina, E., Wallace-Brodeur, R.R., and Lowe, S.W. (1999) INK4a/ARF mutations accelerate lymphomagenesis and promote chemoresistance by disabling p53. *Genes Dev.*, **13** (20), 2670–2677.

93 Yano, T., Jaffe, E.S., Longo, D.L., and Raffeld, M. (1992) MYC rearrangements in histologically progressed follicular lymphomas. *Blood*, **80** (3), 758–767.

94 Ngan, B.Y., Chen-Levy, Z., Weiss, L.M., Warnke, R.A., and Cleary, M.L. (1988) Expression in non-Hodgkin's lymphoma of the bcl-2 protein associated with the t(14;18) chromosomal translocation. *New Engl. J. Med.*, **318** (25), 1638–1644.

95 White, M.A., Nicolette, C., Minden, A., Polverino, A., Van Aelst, L., Karin, M., and Wigler, M.H. (1995) Multiple Ras functions can contribute to mammalian cell transformation. *Cell*, **80** (4), 533–541.

96 Seger, R. and Krebs, E.G. (1995) The MAPK signaling cascade. *FASEB J.*, **9** (9), 726–735. Review.

97 Lavoie, J.N., L'Allemain, G., Brunet, A., Müller, R., and Pouysségur, J. (1996) Cyclin D1 expression is regulated positively by the p42/p44MAPK and negatively by the p38/HOGMAPK pathway. *J. Biol. Chem.*, **271** (34), 20608–20616.

98 Kauffmann-Zeh, A., Rodriguez-Viciana, P., Ulrich, E., Gilbert, C., Coffer, P., Downward, J., and Evan, G. (1997) Suppression of c-Myc-induced apoptosis by Ras signalling through PI(3)K and PKB. *Nature*, **385** (6616), 544–548.

99 Compere, S.J., Baldacci, P., Sharpe, A.H., Thompson, T., Land, H., and Jaenisch, R. (1989) The ras and myc oncogenes cooperate in tumor induction in many tissues when introduced into midgestation mouse embryos by retroviral vectors. *Proc. Natl. Acad. Sci. USA*, **86** (7), 2224–2228.

100 Kastan, M.B., Onyekwere, O., Sidransky, D., Vogelstein, B., and Craig, R.W. (1991) Participation of p53 protein in the cellular response to DNA damage. *Cancer Res.*, **51** (23 Pt 1), 6304–6311.

101 Hermeking, H. and Eick, D. (1994) Mediation of c-Myc-induced apoptosis by p53. *Science*, **265** (5181), 2091–2093.

102 Kamijo, T., Weber, J.D., Zambetti, G., Zindy, F., Roussel, M.F., and Sherr, C.J. (1998) Functional and physical interactions of the ARF tumor suppressor with p53 and Mdm2. *Proc. Natl. Acad. Sci. USA*, **95** (14), 8292–8297.

103 Pomerantz, J., Schreiber-Agus, N., Liégeois, N.J., Silverman, A., Alland, L., Chin, L., Potes, J., Chen, K., Orlow, I., Lee, H.W., Cordon-Cardo, C., and DePinho, R.A. (1998) The Ink4a tumor suppressor gene product, p19Arf, interacts with MDM2 and neutralizes MDM2's inhibition of p53. *Cell*, **92** (6), 713–723.

104 Zhang, Y., Xiong, Y., and Yarbrough, W.G. (1998) ARF promotes MDM2 degradation and stabilizes p53: ARF-INK4a locus deletion impairs both the Rb and p53 tumor suppression pathways. *Cell*, **92** (6), 725–734.

105 Eischen, C.M., Weber, J.D., Roussel, M.F., Sherr, C.J., and Cleveland, J.L. (1999) Disruption of the ARF-Mdm2-p53 tumor suppressor pathway in Myc-induced lymphomagenesis. *Genes Dev.*, **13** (20), 2658–2669.

106 Wilda, M., Bruch, J., Harder, L., Rawer, D., Reiter, A., Borkhardt, A., and Woessmann, W. (2004) Inactivation of the ARF-MDM-2-p53 pathway in sporadic Burkitt's lymphoma in children. *Leukemia*, **18** (3), 584–588.

107 Lindström, M.S., Klangby, U., and Wiman, K.G. (2001) p14ARF homozygous deletion or MDM2 overexpression in Burkitt lymphoma lines carrying wild type p53. *Oncogene*, **20** (17), 2171–2177.

2
Cancer Stem Cells – Finding and Capping the Roots of Cancer
Eike C. Buss and Anthony D. Ho

2.1
Introduction – Stem Cells and Cancer Stem Cells

2.1.1
What are Stem Cells?

Stem cells are the source for cellular regeneration in all multi-cellular organisms. They exhibit two crucial features: they can (i) renew themselves and (ii) proliferate towards specialized cell types.

In the preferentially studied mammalian system, two types of stem cells are distinguished: embryonic stem cells and adult stem cells. Embryonic stem cells (ESCs) are derived from cells from the inner cell mass of blastocysts. Adult stem cells are found in various adult mammal tissues and can regenerate the cells of this specific organ. The fundamental difference is the potency; ESC can differentiate into all cells of their organism, including adult stem cells – this is called totipotency or pluripotency. Adult stem cells can differentiate only into the differentiated cells of the respective organ – this is called multipotency.

A special, aberrant kind of stem cells are so-called cancer stem cells (CSCs). According to the current popular theory in cancer research, they comprise the origins of a given tumor, that is, they maintain the growth of this tumor and can lead to its re-creation.

2.1.2
Concept of Cancer Stem Cells (CSCs)

The cancer stem cell hypothesis in a nutshell is the idea that within a tumor a privileged population of cells is self-sustaining by cell divisions and can give rise to the bulk of tumor cells. These bulk cells would be considered non-tumorigenic upon metastasis and transplantation. This concept is in analogy to the situation in a healthy organism with "hidden" stem cells maintaining themselves constantly in low

Medical Biostatistics for Complex Diseases. Edited by Frank Emmert-Streib and Matthias Dehmer
Copyright © 2010 WILEY-VCH Verlag GmbH & Co. KGaA, Weinheim
ISBN: 978-3-527-32585-6

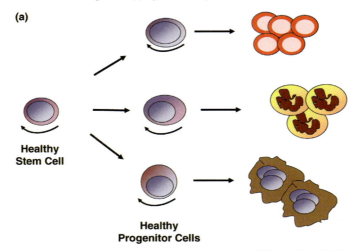
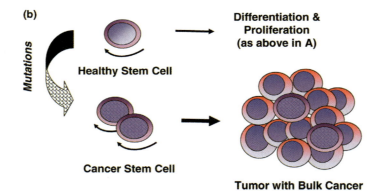
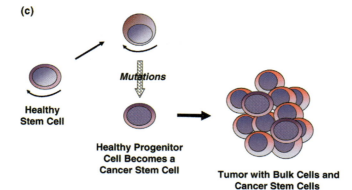

numbers with stem cell features and proliferating and differentiating towards the more "visible" majority of differentiated cells of a given organ [1] (Figure 2.1).

This concept leads to several biological and medical conclusions. The most important practical implication of this concept is the susceptibility to chemotherapy as a therapeutic consequence: It can be expected that these CSCs react differently towards therapeutic drugs compared to the bulk population of tumor cells. If the cancer stem cells differ in their sensitivity towards cytostatic agents from the bulk tumor cells, conventional cytostatic agents might not be able to cure cancer as long as the CSCs are not killed. This in turn would mean that the tumor cannot be permanently cured as long as the stem cells are not eliminated, even if the vast majority of bulk cells are eradicated. The tumor would be poised to regrow again. In contrast, successful eradication of stem cells within a tumor without killing of the bulk cells would lead to slow complete regression of this tumor over time. The difficulty would be that treating solely the stem cells would show now effect of visible tumor reduction in the beginning. Thus, this revolutionary treatment would require patience before success can be expected (Figure 2.2).

The original understanding of tumor growth was that of a uniform growth of all cells of the tumor. This understanding was challenged when it was shown that only a small proportion of the leukemic cells could give rise to leukemic progeny cells in the form of colonies in semisolid cultures [2]. This concept was further refined again by diligent *in vivo* studies (e.g., Reference [3]) that showed not only colony growth, but complete re-constitution of leukemia by very few, specifically selected cells of a prior given leukemia.

This led to the requirement for characterization of cancer stem cells. Only with good characterization can they be easily selected and examined for their molecular signature, and subsequently drug targets can be identified. For successful testing of new anti-CSC drugs meaningful *in vitro* and *in vivo* assays are mandatory. These are the prerequisites for the development of drug screening strategies to selectively target cancer stem cells, which could be resistant to classic treatments while possessing potent tumor-forming capacity. Finally, these drugs can be brought into clinical trials, often in combination with already established drugs. In these trials the current arsenal of technical and laboratory testing on patients and patient samples will be applied to finally identify the new golden bullets against cancer.

Additionally, if the CSC hypothesis holds true, the diagnosis of cancer and the assessment of therapy responses would also change, as the focus would shift from regarding macroscopic tumor size towards assessments of the susceptibility of CSC towards treatment.

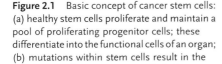

Figure 2.1 Basic concept of cancer stem cells: (a) healthy stem cells proliferate and maintain a pool of proliferating progenitor cells; these differentiate into the functional cells of an organ; (b) mutations within stem cells result in the emergence of a cancer stem cell; their proliferation and partial differentiation leads to the formation of a tumor; (c) alternatively, mutations within a progenitor cell re-induce stem cell features in this cell; together with a malignant transformation, this can also lead to the emergence of a cancer stem cell and subsequent tumor formation.

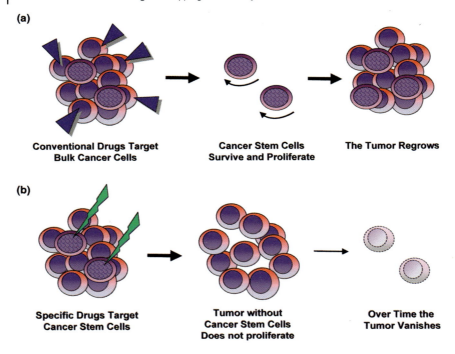

Figure 2.2 Concept of targeted treatment of cancer stem cells: (a) conventional cytostatic drugs target and kill the bulk of tumor cells, but the surviving cancer stem cells can result in the quick reappearance of the tumor; (b) new drugs targeted towards cancer stem cells selectively kill those and so the bulk tumor cells do not proliferate and the tumor eventually vanishes.

The following section highlights some of the different aspects of CSC biology and research to provide a primer for in-depth reading on specific current problems in this hot field of biology and medicine.

2.2
Hematopoietic Stem Cells as a Paradigm

2.2.1
Leukemia as a Paradigmatic Disease for Cancer Research

In medicine, hematology is one of the fields that lead the way towards molecular treatments; at the ASH-conference 2008 it was called the "space program" of medicine. One paramount area is research into hematopoietic stem cells. The beginnings of this field go back to the 1950s with first rarely successful transplantation experiments. In the 1960s the basis for stem cell research was laid with the first detections of colony-forming cells. Further studies led to the discovery of transplants that could re-constitute destroyed bone marrow of experimental animals. With the addition of insights into the immunology of transplantation this concept was applied increasingly successfully in patients in the 1970s.

2.2.2
CFUs

In the early 1960s, Till and McCulloch described how a subpopulation of mouse bone marrow cells can lead to the formation of spleen colony-forming cells in irradiated recipient mice. These were then called accordingly CFU-S (colony forming cells – spleen) and represented in our present understanding a population of progenitor cells [4]. Subsequently, the groups of Sachs and Metcalf developed *in vitro* assays for the detection of colony-forming cells [5, 6]. These assays then also proved to be fundamental for the discovery and functional characterization of cytokines. The basic idea of CFUs is to plant single (selected) cells into a semisolid medium enriched with growth medium and growth factors like cytokines. A progenitor cell under these conditions will form a colony of differentiated progeny cells – at least 20 if it is already very far differentiated and several hundred to thousand if it is immature (Figure 2.3). The colonies can then be enumerated under the microscope and statistically analyzed to provide information about the progenitor cell content of the prior bulk population.

Similarly, the seeding of leukemia cells with progenitor cell capacity into semisolid medium leads to the rise of leukemia colonies [2, 7]. This gave the first hints towards heterogeneity in the leukemic population, because not all seeded leukemic cells gave rise to colonies of daughter cells. In fact, this provided a very strong indication of a hierarchy within the leukemic population in terms of developmental potential of leukemic cells.

2.2.3
LTC-ICs

The next step in the evolution of *in vitro* assays was the development of long-term culture. In these assays, for which a wide variety of protocols exist, first a layer of stroma cells is grown. Stroma cells are large cells of mesenchymal origin in the bone marrow. They provide a mesh between the bones and the blood vessels. The usually

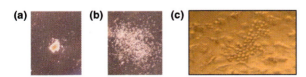

Figure 2.3 Blood cell colonies and leukemia cells in stroma-based cultures. Healthy blood stem and progenitor cells can proliferate *in vitro* in semisolid medium under the stimulation with growth factors towards cell colonies. Each colony represents the offspring of a stem or progenitor cell: (a) burst-forming unit erythroid (BFU-E) – colony of red blood cells (E. Buss); (b) colony-forming unit granulocyte (CFU-G) – colony of white blood cells (here granulocytes) (E. Buss); (c) primary leukemic cells (round cells) with supporting stromal cells in semisolid medium after 7 weeks of *ex vivo* culture (M. Schubert).

smaller and round hematopoietic cells grow in the spaces in between. The close proximity with a special biology of protein interactions leads to the designation as niche, with a special biological meaning of providing support for growth and differentiation of the hematopoietic cells. To replicate this environment *in vitro* stromal cells (often now permanent cell cultures) are cultured *in vitro* as a layer and hematopoietic or leukemic cells are seeded on top and grow in close proximity, receiving signals via direct interaction and via factors secreted by the stromal cells into the medium (Figure 2.3) [8, 9]. In these assays it is possible to grow and maintain healthy and malignant immature progenitor cells for weeks. They can then be read out by CFU assays (see above). True stem cells probably lose their stemness under these conditions.

2.2.4
In Vivo Repopulation

The next consecutive step in the analysis of stem cell function is the injection of putative stem cell populations into animal recipients. The main barrier against transplantations is the immune rejection of the recipient. Initially, these animals were mice of the same inbred strain, so that there would be no rejection. Thereby, it could be shown that certain subpopulations of bone marrow cells could lead to the repopulation of an irradiated recipient. The next step was the development of immunodeficient mouse models to enable the examination of the developmental potential of human cells. The ancestors of mice and men were separated by evolution approximately 60 million years ago. Other mammals are evolutionary closer, namely dogs and monkeys but, as they are large animals, the outlay of experiments is considerably larger than that for mice and also the ethics are more complex, especially for monkeys. It could be shown that there are differences in the biology of blood cells and blood stem cells of men and mice, but, still, most molecular cellular mechanisms of blood cells and blood stem cells are very similar. In addition, the microenvironment of the bone marrow provides all the cues for human and mice blood cells alike to proliferate and grow. Thus the xenotransplantation of human (blood) cells into an animal environment can be used as a surrogate assay for human cell development. Altogether the xenotransplantation experiments are currently the closest possible emulation of human biology and as such are indispensable tools of stem cell and CSC research [10].

2.2.5
Importance of the Bone Marrow Niche

Hematopoietic stem cells reside in the bone marrow. The specific environment is currently under intense research and consists of several cell types and extracellular matrix proteins. As a concept, this environment is called niche. It is vital for feeding and maintaining the HSCs within. The spatial locations of the niche have been identified in the endosteum, at the interface between the bone and BM cavities, as well as around sinusoids and their surrounding reticular cells. The relationship between these niches and the HSPC populations found at each site is under intense investigation [11]. One pivotal molecular interactions is that between the chemokine stromal-derived factor-1 (SDF-1, also named CXCL12) which is produced at high levels by endosteal osteoblasts and endothelial and reticular cells and its surface receptor CXCR4. CXCR4 is expressed by immature and mature stromal and nerve cell and by most hematopoietic cells. The SDF-1/CXCR4 interaction transmits signals for migration, survival, anchorage, and quiescence of hematopoietic stem cells [12].

For normal hematopoietic stem cells (HSCs) the decision between self-renewal or differentiation is vital for maintenance of the stem cell pool as well as sufficient provision of mature cells. This decision is governed by interactions between HSCs and their niche in the marrow. It was demonstrated by us and others that direct contact between adult stem cells and cellular determinants of the microenvironment is essential in regulating asymmetric divisions and promoting stem cell renewal [9, 13, 14]. Examining the interaction between HSCs and mesenchymal stem cells (MSCs), both derived from human marrow as a surrogate model for niche, the role of direct cell–cell contact in self-renewal was defined. The expression of specific genes was shown to regulate long-term hematopoiesis [15]. When HSC lose direct contact with the cellular niche they tend to differentiate and lose their self-renewal capacity; therefore, it protects the HSCs from differentiation and is pivotal for the maintenance of their stem cell features [16].

2.2.6
Leukemic Stem Cells

The colony growth model of HSC was applied also to leukemic cells and it became apparent that there were also subpopulations with varying colony-forming efficiency. The ultimate assessment was the transplantation of selected subpopulations of AML cells into SCID mice [3] and later into the more efficient NOD/SCID model [17]. The disease transplanted into the mice was highly similar to the original patient's leukemia. Experiments to determine the number of leukemic stem cells (LSCs) were performed. They are called limiting-dilution experiments, and essentially involve performing colony or transplantation studies with cell in log-wise reduction of the cell number and subsequent extrapolation of the seeding results. They showed that the leukemia cell capable of initiating an AML in NOD/SCID mice is present at a frequency of 0.2–100 per million mononuclear leukemic cells. Serial transplantations also demonstrated the self-renewal capacity of these cells. These leukemic stem cells were thereby the first proven cancer stem cells and showed the direction of further research in this field.

2.2.6.1 Leukemic Stem Cells in the Bone Marrow Niche
Similar to healthy hematopoietic stem cells, leukemic stem cells interact with their microenvironment, which is one determinant of tumor growth [18]. For LSCs, there are indications that the cellular niche of the marrow also maintains malignant stem cells. They also seem to be dependent on interactions with the cellular environment in the niche [19]. There is evidence that this environment changes with age, as shown

by age dependent modulation of tumorigenicity [20]. Recently, it was also shown that aberrant microenvironment signaling can lead to aberrant hematopoiesis. Deletion of the retinoic acid gamma receptor (RARγ) [21] or retinoblastoma gene (Rb) [22] in mice leads to a condition similar to a myeloproliferative disorder, which can later progress into leukemia. This was caused by altered signaling of the genetically modified microenvironment and not intrinsically by that of the HSCs.

Once LSCs are present they can infiltrate the niche of healthy HSCs and may take control of these normal homeostatic processes. LSCs may also show dysregulated behavior, leading to alternative niche formation [23]. As noted above, one important molecular interaction in the niche is between the chemokine SDF-1 and its receptor CXCR4. This interaction seems to be used by leukemia cells, also. Of prognostic relevance it was shown that high levels of SDF-1 in AML portend a poor prognosis [24]. Thus it is paramount to understand the mechanisms of interaction between the cellular niche and HSC in comparison to that between the niche and LSC to provide a basis for more efficient treatment strategies.

2.2.7
CML as a Paradigmatic Entity

The role of chronic myeloid leukemia (CML) shall be described in detail, as it can be viewed as a milestone in the understanding of cancer pathology, treatment, and, lately, cancer stem cells.

CML is a blood disease with an unrestricted proliferation of blood cells in the bone marrow with consecutive rise of the numbers of white blood cells in the peripheral blood. In some cases the increase can lead to white blood counts a hundred times above the normal count. This led to the term leukemia (white blood) being already in use in the nineteenth century. The designation chronic is derived from the natural slow course of the initial phase over months and years (chronic phase), followed by an accelerated phase and a blast phase with massive production of malignant, immature cells termed blasts. This is then comparable to an acute leukemia with the development of blasts. The natural course of the disease is fatal.

CML became a path-maker for the understanding of leukemia when it was the first cancer for which a chromosomal abnormality was shown – a balanced, reciprocal translocation involving the long arms of chromosomes 9 and 22 termed Philadelphia chromosome after the place of its discovery as early as 1960. The next crucial step was the discovery of the molecular product of this genetic rearrangement, which is the formation of a new gene, termed *bcr-abl*, by the annealing of two formerly unrelated genes, in the late 1980s. The product of this fusion-gene is the abnormally active tyrosine kinase BCR-ABL. This kinase is necessary and sufficient for the malignant transformation of hematopoietic stem cells. The later disease progression towards blast crisis is associated with differentiation arrest, genomic instability and the acquisition of further genetic lesions, telomere shortening and loss of tumor-suppressor function [25]. The knowledge about BCR-ABL was then used to develop a rational treatment with the tyrosine kinase inhibitor imatinib in the late 1990s. As a specific inhibitor for a single causative oncoprotein it was the first truly rational cancer drug. The treatment results in an astonishing hematologic response as it leads to a normalization of the peripheral blood counts in about 95% of the patients and long-lasting responses. Nevertheless, only a fraction of patients reach a molecular remission, when even with highly-sensitive RT-PCR the *bcr-abl* transcript can no longer be detected. In addition, the time course under imatinib treatment shows that a plateau with patients with durable remissions is not reached. All this can be explained by the CSC model. The CML disease contains a clone of stem cells and a bulk of proliferating and differentiating cells. These are effectively suppressed by the treatment with BCR-ABL inhibitors, but not the cancer stem cells inside the tumor. This was evaluated by mathematical modeling of *in vivo* kinetics of response to imatinib, based on analysis of quantitative polymerase chain reaction data, suggesting that imatinib inhibits production of differentiated leukemia cells but does not deplete leukemia stem cells [26].

So the way towards cure of CML is to target the CSCs inside. Important experimental results towards this goal were presented recently by the group of Trumpp and colleagues [27]. They showed in healthy mice a population of dormant blood stem cells that are only recruited by strong stress signals. This can be mimicked by the application of the inflammatory cytokine interferon. Application of interferon-α (IFN-α) in mice in the days before treatment with the cytostatic agent 5-FU led to the activation of dormant stem cells, which were then killed by the 5-FU treatment. This led to a loss of stem cell function, severe anemia, and the death of the mice. 5-FU treatments alone were tolerated well by the animals. It is believed that CML stem cells are biologically very close to healthy blood stem cells, so these findings could be applicable to the CML disease. There is also clinical data available to support this hypothesis. One report is about 12 patients with CML who discontinued imatinib after previous treatment with IFN-α. Six of the 12 patients continued to stay in complete remission with undetectable CML by molecular assays after a median follow-up of 18 months (range 9–24 months) but six relapsed within 6 months [28]. The hypothesis is about to be tested in a trial of the German CML group which will combine imatinib treatment with short courses of IFN-α treatment. There are other candidate drugs with the aim of CSC eradication. Recent *in vitro* and *in vivo* studies showed that the farnesyltransferase inhibitor BMS-214662 selectively induces apoptosis of CML stem/progenitor cells and acts synergistically in combination with imatinib [29].

2.3
Current Technical Approach to the Isolation and Characterization of Cancer Stem Cells

2.3.1
Tools for the Detection of Cancer Stem Cells

The currently favored approach to the identification of cancer stem cells is via the isolation of cancer cell populations by FACS (fluorescence-activated cell sorting) and afterwards characterization of these cells. The methods for characterization include virtually all current biologic tools:

- Broad profiling by chip-based methods of the genome, of the epigenetic features, the transcripted mRNAs, and the proteome. These methods include analysis of large datasets by bioinformatic/biomathematical methods.
- Conventional molecular biology to specifically analyze the role of single molecules.
- Visualization by microscopy and several techniques of fluorescence microscopy.
- *In vitro* functional characterization: culture forming assays, long-term culture initiating cell assays, and other cell culture based techniques.
- *In vivo* functional characterization by injection of isolated cancer stem cells into animal recipients. Usually, these are highly immunodeficient mice that are susceptible for the growth of the foreign cancer cells.
- Genetic modification of cancer cells to prove the role of specific genes in turning cells into cancer stem cells.

2.3.2
Phenotype of Cancer Stem Cells

The standard isolation technique for cancer stem cells is the selection via staining of surface antigen markers with specific monoclonal antibodies. These marked cells can then be selected with several available techniques, namely by magnetic bead selection or by sorting with a FACSort machine. Especially with this latter technique, a cell population can be characterized by staining for several surface markers. Depending on the availability of lasers and detectors in the FACS machine, several colors (= antigens) plus size and granularity of the examined cells can be applied to define a sub-population. The sorting mechanism of FACSort machines allows collection of this population by selecting them cell by cell from the measurement stream, which runs at a rate of up to a several thousand cells per second, and collecting them in test tube for further experimental use.

Defining the antigen profile of a stem cell population is often one of the pivotal aims of research programs themselves. In many cases, profiles of healthy stem cell populations of a tissue is already known and can be used as a starting point to search for a CSC population of tumors of this tissue. Additional hints on the antigen expression profile come from gene expression studies, which help to understand the molecular profile of cancer cell populations.

In addition to surface markers, which are stained by binding of soluble antibodies to the cell surface, several functional stem cell markers have been identified. These rely on the intracellular staining of compartments and organelles and also the activity of cell enzymes. One important example is the substance Hoechst 33 342 (Hoechst), a dye that stains DNA and is actively transported out of the cell by ATP-binding cassette transporter proteins. Stem cells show a low staining with Hoechst and are identified on a double-fluorescence FACS-plot as a so-called side-population (SP). One caveat is that the dye is potentially toxic, so later functional studies might be compromised.

Another functional characterization is staining with the dye Aldefluor, which is cleaved by the enzyme aldehyde dehydrogenase and, therefore, indicates activity of this enzyme [30].

Putative candidate populations are then purified and their CSC potential is examined by the *in vitro* and *in vivo* studies outlined above. If a candidate population leads to tumor growth within transplanted host animals, including secondary and tertiary transplantations, it can be assumed to represent a new CSC population.

There is not "the" CSC antigen, but several antigens and antigen combination are already known for defining CSCs. Current important surface marker combinations are presented below. Notably, these combinations are not fixed; the literature presents more candidate markers and variations. The signature of an individual tumor and its CSC is therefore somewhat unique. The signature of the corresponding healthy stem cell population is often similar; sometimes there are only differences in the level of expression to distinguish them, and sometimes they are undistinguishable with the available marker panels. In addition, fine tuning of the individual staining pattern and the FACS machine and defining the selection gates is a kind of an art.

Surface marker combination for identification (human) leukemic stem cells [31]

Common phenotype: $CD34^+/CD38^-$
- CD34: marker antigen for hematopoietic stem and progenitor cells, should be positive, also reports on $CD34^-$ stem cells.
- CD38: marker of maturation, should be negative.
Additional markers:
- CD33: myeloid lineage marker (for AML);
- CD90: Thy-1, usually stem cells should be $CD90^+$, also reports about $CD34^+CD90^-$ LSC;
- CLL-1: C-type lectin-like molecule-1, a stem cell marker [32];
- Hoechst 33 342: side-population, stem cells are low for this intracellular dye;
- ALDH: high activity of aldehyde dehydrogenase in LSC [30].
See also Figure 2.4.

Surface marker combination for identification (human) stem cells from solid tumors

- CD133: prominin 1, a widely expressed stem cell marker.
- CD44: The receptor for hyaluronic acid, involved in cell–cell interactions, cell adhesion, and migration. Expression on hematopoietic stem cells and on epithelial CSC.
- CD24: cell adhesion molecule, minus or low on several epithelial CSC.

2.4
Cancer Stem Cells in Solid Tumors

Although the healthy stem cells in solid organs were not as well defined as in hematopoiesis, researchers followed the example of leukemia research and managed to identify and isolate populations of tumor cells with stem cell-like features from many solid tumor types. Research into breast cancer showed the first results in this task.

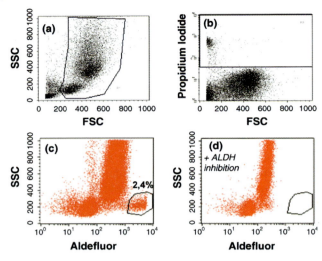

Figure 2.4 Example for the sorting of an ALDH$^+$ leukemia stem cell population. FACS gating of a stained sample of blood or bone marrow cells: (a) gating on a population of intact leukocytes in an FSC/SSC plot (= size/ granularity); (b) gating on propidium iodide (PI) negative cell (= living cells); (c) gating on Aldefluor-positive cells as a marker for ALDH-activity, in fluorescence channel FL1; there are about 2.4% ALDH$^+$ stem cells within the mononuclear cells of this sample; (d) as a control for specificity inhibition of ALDH activity. (D. Ran, M. Schubert and V. Eckstein).

2.4.1
Breast Cancer

Following research on healthy human breast stem cells, Al-Hajj et al. reported a CD24$^{-/low}$/CD44$^+$ fraction of breast cancer cells that showed a high tumorigenic potential when injected into the mammary fat pad of female NOD/SCID mice compared to a low tumorigenicity of the CD24$^+$/CD44$^{+/-}$ cell fraction [33]. These results were further confirmed and refined [34]. Based on recent gene expression studies this model might be more complex, with breast cancer cells switching from a stem-cell like and invasive CD44$^+$ phenotype to a more differentiated CD24$^+$ phenotype and probably also back [35, 36].

2.4.2
Prostate Cancer

Following previous research on healthy prostate stem cells, prostate CSC were isolated and assessed in *in vitro* stroma-based culture [37]. The identified cancer stem cells had a CD44$^+$/α2β1^{hi}/CD133$^+$ phenotype. Approximately 0.1% of cells in all of the examined prostate tumors expressed this phenotype. Later another phenotype with invasive capabilities of NOD/SCID mice upon injection of as little as

100 cells was identified [38]. The CSC population in this study was $CD44^+/CD24^-$. Interestingly, these CSC went into differentiation after *ex vivo* culture in the presence of serum, demonstrating the importance of environmental signals.

2.4.3
Colon Cancer

Several studies could demonstrate the purification of colon cancer initiating cells (CC-IC) in contrast to a larger bulk population, which could not initiate the tumor. In 2007 the group of John Dick described the purification of a CC-IC [39]. Technically, they identified a $CD133^+$ cell from human colon cancers and showed their tumor initiating ability by injection of these cells into the renal capsule of immunodeficient NOD/SCID mice. Conversely, they showed that bulk colon cancer cells that were $CD133^-$ did not initiate tumor growth in these immunodeficient hosts. It was calculated by limiting dilution analysis that there was one CC-IC in 5.7×10^4 unfractionated tumor cells, whereas there was one CC-IC in 262 $CD133^+$ cells, representing a more than 200-fold enrichment. CC-ICs within the $CD133^+$ population were able to maintain themselves as well as differentiate and re-establish tumor heterogeneity upon serial transplantation. These results highlight the fact that a sorting for $CD133^+$ cells purified a population containing the putative cancer stem cell population, but they still represented only 0.38% of the sorted population, leaving the exact phenotype of the CC-IC still elusive.

Further studies at the same time essentially confirmed these results [40, 41]. Conflicting results were presented later by the group of Rafii [42], discussed below.

2.4.4
Other Cancers

These results were rapidly followed by similar findings in a wide variety of different tumors, including brain tumors, pancreatic and hepatic carcinomas, melanoma, and a few other tumor types [43].

2.5
Open Questions of the Cancer Stem Cell Hypothesis

In several studies conflicting results were found concerning the phenotype of CSC populations. One example will be discussed for colon cancer. A $CD133^+$ population had been shown by the group of Dick *et al.* to contain a clear CSC function [39]. The group of Rafii *et al.* [42] tried to reproduce these results but found that both $CD133^+$ and $CD133^-$ colon cancer cells could initiate tumors in immunodeficient NOD/SCID mice. Upon careful analysis of the presented data and the previous publications, it was concluded that the later study focused on metastases whereas the earlier ones looked upon primary tumors. Thus it could be that upon metastasis the colon cancer CSCs change some of their features and also $CD133^-$ offspring become tumorigenic. Furthermore, it seems that in the original publications the CSC population might be the CD133^{high} and not only the CD133$^+$ population [44].

Another important issue is the question which cells are the origin of the CSC. It seems as if it can be transformed healthy stem cells, transformed progenitor cells, or even differentiated cells re-acquiring stem cell capabilities. While there are many similarities, there also are differences between cancer and normal stem cells. Normal stem cells usually represent only a very small population of cells of their host organ, which also remains relatively constant. CSC, on the other hand, can constitute a large part of the total tumor cells. In breast cancer, cells with a CD24$^{-/low}$/CD44$^+$ CSC phenotype could make up to 60% of the tumor cells [33]. In colon cancer, the cancer stem cell population of CD133$^+$ cells constituted up to 24% of total tumor cells [39]. From these results it can be concluded that, in some tumors, cancer stem cells represent the majority of tumor cells, which would render the model considerably less valuable, as fighting the bulk tumor versus the CSC would be the same.

The next question is about the model systems for analyzing the CSC. It has been shown that *in vitro* model systems do not represent a full environment for cellular research. It was also shown that many stem cell types require stromal support to grow. It could be that putative CSC populations are missed in *in vitro* research without stromal support as a biological niche. Establishing stromal support layers *in vitro* is possible and has been demonstrated often.

Another feature of cancer cells is genomic instability and the ability to undergo rapid evolutionary changes. There is also continuous selection for the survival of the fittest. Together this is termed the "clonal evolution" and is somewhat opposed to the CSC hypothesis, which in its strict form views CSC as fairly stable entities. This might not be true, as there is also good evidence that tumor cells and also CSC are dynamic. It is well-established that tumor cells evolve and if more malignant and less differentiated cancer cells have growth advantage then they will be selected and expand within the tumor. Therefore, it could well be that, upon tumor progression, the line between cancer stem cells and the rest of tumor cells might become blurred. As an example, it was recently shown that glioblastoma cancer stem cells can be CD133$^+$ or CD133$^-$ [45]. The previously discussed study about colon cancer CSC [42] points in the same direction. This could mean that either the markers are not good and specific enough or that all tumor cells are tumorigenic but to varying degrees and depending on the environment conditions and that antigen expression profiles can change [36].

2.6
Clinical Relevance of Cancer Stem Cells

2.6.1
Diagnostic Relevance of Cancer Stem Cells

If the CSC is the true culprit for the relapse of a cancer, its biology should be telling about the severity of a given cancer. Along this line several studies have compared clinical response and survival data with the phenotype and/or the amount of the CSC. In several cases these results showed correlations, so this additional diagnostic information on cancer specimens can contribute to assessing the prognosis of a given tumor and help in directing therapy decisions.

In one study the prognostic impact of stem cell frequency in $CD34^+$ AML was investigated. At first the leukemogenic potential of AML blast cells was shown *in vivo* using NOD/SCID mice transplantation experiments. The engraftment correlated with the frequency of $CD34^+CD38^-$ cells of the graft. It was also analyzed whether the frequency of $CD34^+CD38^-$ cells is associated with minimal residual disease (MRD) frequency after chemotherapy and clinical outcome. A high percentage of $CD34^+CD38^-$ stem cells at diagnosis correlated significantly with a high MRD frequency after chemotherapy. Furthermore, the high percentage of $CD34^+CD38^-$ stem cells directly correlated with poor survival. In contrast the total $CD34^+$ percentage alone did not. Together this suggests that the $CD34^+CD38^-$ count at diagnosis could be a new prognostic factor for AML [46]. In a different study, the validity of the ALDH staining was examined. $ALDH^+$ leukemic cells were assessed and their percentage in clinical AML samples determined. It could be shown that a high percentage of these leukemic precursor cells correlates with poor prognostic markers of the examined patients [47].

The profiling of breast tumors cells ($CD24^{-/low}/CD44^+$ and $CD24^+/CD44^{+/-}$) showed that a gene expression signature characteristic of breast cancer stem cells is associated with shorter distant metastasis-free and overall survival [35, 48]. These findings strongly suggest that the presence $CD24^{-/low}/CD44^+$, that is, breast cancer CSC populations also have prognostic relevance.

2.6.2
Therapeutic Relevance – New Drugs Directed Against Cancer Stem Cells

Following the research on biology and clinical relevance of CSC the next step is the exploration of specific drugs to attack these stem cells. Most research advances in this field have been made with antileukemic treatments. Research into drug treatments with small molecules showed *in vitro* and *in vivo* in NOD/SCID mice that the combination of the known anthracycline idarubicin and the proteasome inhibitor MG-132 effectively eradicates leukemia stem cells via a mechanism involving concomitant inhibition of nuclear factor-χB (NF-χB)-mediated survival signals and induction of oxidative stress [49]. Another potential anti-LSC drug was identified with parthenolide, the bioactive chemical component of the medicinal plant feverfew, which was also active as a single agent [50]. The mechanism of action was again through the combined inhibition of NF-χB and induction of oxidative stress. This pointed towards an underlying common biological principle of these agents, although they were chemically very different. To identify further drug candidates, the authors devised an intelligent method by searching databases of gene-expression data for the genetic signature of parthenolide and then used this signature as a template to search for the effect of other drugs with the same expression results. This led to the identification of two new agents, celastrol and 4-hydroxy-2-nonenal (HNE), which effectively eradicate AML cells [51] at the bulk, progenitor, and stem cell level. Celastrol and HNE were examined *in vitro* on sorted $CD34^+CD38^-$ AML cells and led to the cell death of the majority of incubated stem cells. More importantly, engraftment into NOD/SCID mice was reduced strongly by both agents, most remarkably by HNE, after pre-treatment of LSC *in vitro* and subsequent injection.

These results show that it is feasible to target specifically CSC with rationally devised drugs. Nevertheless, determining the optimal treating protocols for patients, also in conjunction with already established substances, remains a major task.

2.7
Outlook

The cancer stem cell hypothesis looks upon cancer development as a disease with disturbed features of healthy tissue cell development. The basic biology of this field is built on all the fancy tools of current biology, including large-scale genomic and post-genomic profiling and *in vivo* experimental approaches. For the interpretation and analysis of the generated data sound biomathematical approaches are indispensable. The clarification of the biology of CSC enables the development of specifically targeted drugs. Together with already established regimens and other innovative approaches like rationally designed inhibitors, immunotherapies, and vaccination strategies this can pave the way to more curative therapies for more cancers.

Acknowledgments

The authors wish to thank Dan Ran, Mario Schubert and Volker Eckstein for providing figures for this chapter.

References

1 Reya, T., Morrison, S.J., Clarke, M.F., and Weissman, I.L. (2001) Stem cells, cancer, and cancer stem cells. *Nature*, **414**, 105–111.

2 Moore, M.A., Williams, N., and Metcalf, D. (1973) In vitro colony formation by normal and leukemic human hematopoietic cells: characterization of the colony-forming cells. *J. Natl. Cancer Inst.*, **50**, 603–623.

3 Lapidot, T., Sirard, C., Vormoor, J., Murdoch, B., Hoang, T., Caceres-Cortes, J., Minden, M., Paterson, B., Caligiuri, M.A., and Dick, J.E. (1994) A cell initiating human acute myeloid leukaemia after transplantation into SCID mice. *Nature*, **367**, 645–648.

4 Till, J.E. and McCulloch, E.A. (1961) A direct measurement of the radiation sensitivity of normal mouse bone marrow cells. *Radiat. Res.*, **14**, 213–222.

5 Pluznik, D.H. and Sachs, L. (1965) The cloning of normal "mast" cells in tissue culture. *J. Cell Physiol.*, **66**, 319–324.

6 Bradley, T.R. and Metcalf, D. (1966) The growth of mouse bone marrow cells in vitro. *Aust. J. Exp. Biol. Med. Sci.*, **44**, 287–299.

7 Minden, M.D., Buick, R.N., and McCulloch, E.A. (1979) Separation of blast

cell and T-lymphocyte progenitors in the blood of patients with acute myeloblastic leukemia. *Blood*, **54**, 186–195.

8 Dexter, T.M., Allen, T.D., and Lajtha, L.G. (1977) Conditions controlling the proliferation of haemopoietic stem cells in vitro. *J. Cell Physiol.*, **91**, 335–344.

9 Punzel, M., Liu, D., Zhang, T., Eckstein, V., Miesala, K., and Ho, A.D. (2003) The symmetry of initial divisions of human hematopoietic progenitors is altered only by the cellular microenvironment. *Exp. Hematol.*, **31**, 339–347.

10 Pearson, T., Greiner, D.L., and Shultz, L.D. (2008) Humanized SCID mouse models for biomedical research. *Curr. Top. Microbiol. Immunol.*, **324**, 25–51.

11 Spiegel, A., Kalinkovich, A., Shivtiel, S., Kollet, O., and Lapidot, T. (2008) Stem cell regulation via dynamic interactions of the nervous and immune systems with the microenvironment. *Cell Stem Cell*, **3**, 484–492.

12 Dar, A., Kollet, O., and Lapidot, T. (2006) Mutual, reciprocal SDF-1/CXCR4 interactions between hematopoietic and bone marrow stromal cells regulate human stem cell migration and development in NOD/SCID chimeric mice. *Exp. Hematol.*, **34**, 967–975.

13 Huang, S., Law, P., Francis, K., Palsson, B.O., and Ho, A.D. (1999) Symmetry of initial cell divisions among primitive hematopoietic progenitors is independent of ontogenic age and regulatory molecules. *Blood*, **94**, 2595–2604.

14 Giebel, B., Zhang, T., Beckmann, J., Spanholtz, J., Wernet, P., Ho, A.D., and Punzel, M. (2006) Primitive human hematopoietic cells give rise to differentially specified daughter cells upon their initial cell division. *Blood*, **107**, 2146–2152.

15 Wagner, W., Ansorge, A., Wirkner, U., Eckstein, V., Schwager, C., Blake, J., Miesala, K., Selig, J., Saffrich, R., Ansorge, W., and Ho, A.D. (2004) Molecular evidence for stem cell function of the slow-dividing fraction among human hematopoietic progenitor cells by genome-wide analysis. *Blood*, **104**, 675–686.

16 Wagner, W., Saffrich, R., Wirkner, U., Eckstein, V., Blake, J., Ansorge, A., Schwager, C., Wein, F., Miesala, K., Ansorge, W., and Ho, A.D. (2005) Hematopoietic progenitor cells and cellular microenvironment: behavioral and molecular changes upon interaction. *Stem Cells*, **23**, 1180–1191.

17 Bonnet, D. and Dick, J.E. (1997) Human acute myeloid leukemia is organized as a hierarchy that originates from a primitive hematopoietic cell. *Nat. Med.*, **3**, 730–737.

18 Mueller, M.M. and Fusenig, N.E. (2004) Friends or foes - bipolar effects of the tumour stroma in cancer. *Nat. Rev. Cancer*, **4**, 839–849.

19 Owens, D.M. and Watt, F.M. (2003) Contribution of stem cells and differentiated cells to epidermal tumours. *Nat. Rev. Cancer*, **3**, 444–451.

20 Campisi, J. (2005) Suppressing cancer: the importance of being senescent. *Science*, **309**, 886–887.

21 Walkley, C.R., Olsen, G.H., Dworkin, S., Fabb, S.A., Swann, J., McArthur, G.A., Westmoreland, S.V., Chambon, P., Scadden, D.T., and Purton, L.E. (2007) A microenvironment-induced myeloproliferative syndrome caused by retinoic acid receptor gamma deficiency. *Cell*, **129**, 1097–1110.

22 Walkley, C.R., Shea, J.M., Sims, N.A., Purton, L.E., and Orkin, S.H. (2007) Rb regulates interactions between hematopoietic stem cells and their bone marrow microenvironment. *Cell*, **129**, 1081–1095.

23 Lane, S.W., Scadden, D.T., and Gilliland, D.G. (2009) The leukemic stem cell niche: current concepts and therapeutic opportunities. *Blood*, **114**, 1150–1157.

24 Spoo, A.C., Lubbert, M., Wierda, W.G., and Burger, J.A. (2007) CXCR4 is a prognostic marker in acute myelogenous leukemia. *Blood*, **109**, 786–791.

25 Melo, J.V. and Barnes, D.J. (2007) Chronic myeloid leukaemia as a model of disease evolution in human cancer. *Nat. Rev. Cancer*, **7**, 441–453.

26 Wodarz, D. (2006) Targeted cancer treatment: resisting arrest. *Nat. Med.*, **12**, 1125–1126.

27 Essers, M.A., Offner, S., Blanco-Bose, W.E., Waibler, Z., Kalinke, U., Duchosal, M.A., and Trumpp, A. (2009) IFNalpha activates dormant haematopoietic stem cells in vivo. *Nature*, **458**, 904–908.

28 Rousselot, P., Huguet, F., Rea, D., Legros, L., Cayuela, J.M., Maarek, O., Blanchet, O., Marit, G., Gluckman, E., Reiffers, J., Gardembas, M., and Mahon, F.X. (2007) Imatinib mesylate discontinuation in patients with chronic myelogenous leukemia in complete molecular remission for more than 2 years. *Blood*, **109**, 58–60.

29 Copland, M., Pellicano, F., Richmond, L., Allan, E.K., Hamilton, A., Lee, F.Y., Weinmann, R., and Holyoake, T.L. (2008) BMS-214662 potently induces apoptosis of chronic myeloid leukemia stem and progenitor cells and synergizes with tyrosine kinase inhibitors. *Blood*, **111**, 2843–2853.

30 Cheung, A.M., Wan, T.S., Leung, J.C., Chan, L.Y., Huang, H., Kwong, Y.L., Liang, R., and Leung, A.Y. (2007) Aldehyde dehydrogenase activity in leukemic blasts defines a subgroup of acute myeloid leukemia with adverse prognosis and superior NOD/SCID engrafting potential. *Leukemia*, **21**, 1423–1430.

31 Warner, J.K., Wang, J.C., Hope, K.J., Jin, L., and Dick, J.E. (2004) Concepts of human leukemic development. *Oncogene*, **23**, 7164–7177.

32 Moshaver, B., van Rhenen, A., Kelder, A., van der Pol, M., Terwijn, M., Bachas, C., Westra, A.H., Ossenkoppele, G.J., Zweegman, S., and Schuurhuis, G.J. (2008) Identification of a small subpopulation of candidate leukemia-initiating cells in the side population of patients with acute myeloid leukemia. *Stem Cells*, **26**, 3059–3067.

33 Al-Hajj, M., Wicha, M.S., Benito-Hernandez, A., Morrison, S.J., and Clarke, M.F. (2003) Prospective identification of tumorigenic breast cancer cells. *Proc. Natl. Acad. Sci. USA*, **100**, 3983–3988.

34 Ponti, D., Costa, A., Zaffaroni, N., Pratesi, G., Petrangolini, G., Coradini, D., Pilotti, S., Pierotti, M.A., and Daidone, M.G. (2005) Isolation and in vitro propagation of tumorigenic breast cancer cells with stem/progenitor cell properties. *Cancer Res.*, **65**, 5506–5511.

35 Shipitsin, M., Campbell, L.L., Argani, P., Weremowicz, S., Bloushtain-Qimron, N., Yao, J., Nikolskaya, T., Serebryiskaya, T., Beroukhim, R., Hu, M., Halushka, M.K., Sukumar, S., Parker, L.M., Anderson, K.S., Harris, L.N., Garber, J.E., Richardson, A.L., Schnitt, S.J., Nikolsky, Y., Gelman, R.S., and Polyak, K. (2007) Molecular definition of breast tumor heterogeneity. *Cancer Cell*, **11**, 259–273.

36 Shipitsin, M. and Polyak, K. (2008) The cancer stem cell hypothesis: in search of definitions, markers, and relevance. *Lab. Invest.*, **88**, 459–463.

37 Collins, A.T., Berry, P.A., Hyde, C., Stower, M.J., and Maitland, N.J. (2005) Prospective identification of tumorigenic prostate cancer stem cells. *Cancer Res.*, **65**, 10946–10951.

38 Hurt, E.M., Kawasaki, B.T., Klarmann, G.J., Thomas, S.B., and Farrar, W.L. (2008) CD44+ CD24(−) prostate cells are early cancer progenitor/stem cells that provide a model for patients with poor prognosis. *Br. J. Cancer*, **98**, 756–765.

39 O'Brien, C.A., Pollett, A., Gallinger, S., and Dick, J.E. (2007) A human colon cancer cell capable of initiating tumour growth in immunodeficient mice. *Nature*, **445**, 106–110.

40 Dalerba, P., Dylla, S.J., Park, I.K., Liu, R., Wang, X., Cho, R.W., Hoey, T., Gurney, A., Huang, E.H., Simeone, D.M., Shelton, A.A., Parmiani, G., Castelli, C., and Clarke, M.F. (2007) Phenotypic characterization of human colorectal cancer stem cells. *Proc. Natl. Acad. Sci. USA*, **104**, 10158–10163.

41 Ricci-Vitiani, L., Lombardi, D.G., Pilozzi, E., Biffoni, M., Todaro, M., Peschle, C., and De Maria, R. (2007) Identification and expansion of human

colon-cancer-initiating cells. *Nature*, **445**, 111–115.

42 Shmelkov, S.V., Butler, J.M., Hooper, A.T., Hormigo, A., Kushner, J., Milde, T., St Clair, R., Baljevic, M., White, I., Jin, D.K., Chadburn, A., Murphy, A.J., Valenzuela, D.M., Gale, N.W., Thurston, G., Yancopoulos, G.D., D'Angelica, M., Kemeny, N., Lyden, D., and Rafii, S. (2008) CD133 expression is not restricted to stem cells, and both CD133+ and CD133- metastatic colon cancer cells initiate tumors. *J. Clin. Invest.*, **118**, 2111–2120.

43 Wicha, M.S., Liu, S., and Dontu, G. (2006) Cancer stem cells: an old idea--a paradigm shift. *Cancer Res.*, **66**, 1883–1890 discussion 1895–1896.

44 LaBarge, M.A. and Bissell, M.J. (2008) Is CD133 a marker of metastatic colon cancer stem cells? *J. Clin. Invest.*, **118**, 2021–2024.

45 Beier, D., Hau, P., Proescholdt, M., Lohmeier, A., Wischhusen, J., Oefner, P.J., Aigner, L., Brawanski, A., Bogdahn, U., and Beier, C.P. (2007) CD133(+) and CD133(−) glioblastoma-derived cancer stem cells show differential growth characteristics and molecular profiles. *Cancer Res.*, **67**, 4010–4015.

46 van Rhenen, A., Feller, N., Kelder, A., Westra, A.H., Rombouts, E., Zweegman, S., van der Pol, M.A., Waisfisz, Q., Ossenkoppele, G.J., and Schuurhuis, G.J. (2005) High stem cell frequency in acute myeloid leukemia at diagnosis predicts high minimal residual disease and poor survival. *Clin. Cancer Res.*, **11**, 6520–6527.

47 Ran, D., Schubert, M., Pietsch, L., Taubert, I., Wuchter, P., Eckstein, V., Bruckner, T., Zoeller, M., and Ho, A.D. (2009) Aldehyde dehydrogenase activity among primary leukemia cells is associated with stem cell features and correlates with adverse clinical outcomes. *Exp. Hematol.*, **37**, 1423–1434

48 Liu, R., Wang, X., Chen, G.Y., Dalerba, P., Gurney, A., Hoey, T., Sherlock, G., Lewicki, J., Shedden, K., and Clarke, M.F. (2007) The prognostic role of a gene signature from tumorigenic breast-cancer cells. *New Engl. J. Med.*, **356**, 217–226.

49 Guzman, M.L., Swiderski, C.F., Howard, D.S., Grimes, B.A., Rossi, R.M., Szilvassy, S.J., and Jordan, C.T. (2002) Preferential induction of apoptosis for primary human leukemic stem cells. *Proc. Natl. Acad. Sci. USA*, **99**, 16220–16225.

50 Guzman, M.L., Rossi, R.M., Karnischky, L., Li, X., Peterson, D.R., Howard, D.S., and Jordan, C.T. (2005) The sesquiterpene lactone parthenolide induces apoptosis of human acute myelogenous leukemia stem and progenitor cells. *Blood*, **105**, 4163–4169.

51 Hassane, D.C., Guzman, M.L., Corbett, C., Li, X., Abboud, R., Young, F., Liesveld, J.L., Carroll, M., and Jordan, C.T. (2008) Discovery of agents that eradicate leukemia stem cells using an in silico screen of public gene expression data. *Blood*, **111**, 5654–5662.

3
Multiple Testing Methods

Alessio Farcomeni

3.1
Introduction

Statistical hypothesis testing questions whether a null hypothesis, which could be approximately true at population level, can be safely rejected to drive some conclusion of interest. The conclusions, which are based on the evidence provided by the data, will necessarily be uncertain. This uncertainty grows very rapidly when more and more hypotheses are simultaneously tested, and one can be practically sure of making one or more errors if suitable corrections are not used. This chapter reviews in detail this rationale, the set up, and some of the numerous approaches that have been developed in the literature.

To give a practical and simple motivation, we can readily look at some numbers, provided in Table 3.1. We repeatedly simulated the case of a number m of simultaneous tests, each time with 10% false hypotheses, and report in the table the number of rejected hypotheses together with the number of erroneously rejected hypotheses when single tests are performed at the level $\alpha = 0.05$. It can be seen that while when $m = 1$ the expected number of false rejections is correctly below α, as m increases the number of false rejections increases as well, more or less keeping a ratio of 1-to-3 of the total rejections. The list of rejected hypotheses, evaluated as a whole, is hence polluted by a number of false rejections that is proportional to the number of tests. Such lists are of no practical use in many applications.

A very early solution dates back to Bonferroni [1], and consists simply in dividing the desired significance level by the number of tests, thus ideally equally splitting among the m hypotheses the α error probability one is prepared to spend. Table 3.2 gives the outcome of the toy introductory simulation. The expected number of false rejections is now under control regardless of the number of tests.

Bonferroni's approach, despite being easy and effective, is not satisfactory in contexts in which the number of tests is high: of the 1000 false hypotheses that could be detected when $m = 10000$, in Table 3.2 we were able to detect only approximately 150.

Medical Biostatistics for Complex Diseases. Edited by Frank Emmert-Streib and Matthias Dehmer
Copyright © 2010 WILEY-VCH Verlag GmbH & Co. KGaA, Weinheim
ISBN: 978-3-527-32585-6

Table 3.1 Average number of rejections plus number of false rejections for different multiple testing procedures; uncorrected testing; testing is at level $\alpha = 0.05$.

m	Rejections	False rejections
1	0.11	0.04
10	1.14	0.48
50	5.57	2.24
200	22.40	8.94
1000	112.13	45.26
10 000	1121.33	448.69

Table 3.2 Average number of rejections plus number false rejections for different multiple testing procedures; Bonferroni correction; testing is at level $\alpha = 0.05$.

m	Rejections	False rejections
1	0.10	0.04
10	0.54	0.05
50	2.05	0.05
200	6.18	0.05
1000	23.44	0.04
10 000	150.68	0.04

A number of tests in the order of thousands are not rare in applications nowadays. In recent years, advances in technology have made it possible to simultaneously measure expression levels of tens of thousands of genes from a single biological sample. The aim is to screen a large number of genes for effects linked to a particular biological condition. In such applications, m is very large and the Bonferroni solution may not be appropriate. In this chapter we introduce multiple testing in generality, but with a focus on cases in which the number of tests is large.

In the rest of this section we restate some concepts from this short general introduction in a more focused way, together with a brief review of the historic development of the field. In Section 3.2 we provide part of the necessary background on statistical inference and testing. In Section 3.3 we discuss type I error rates. Multiple testing procedures are categorized in Section 3.4 and described in Section 3.5. In Section 3.6 we discuss how the procedures should be applied in many real situations in which the test statistics are dependent. Examples related to gene discovery in cancer are developed in Section 3.7, and Section 3.8 provides a conclusion.

3.1.1
A Brief More Focused Introduction

The problem of simultaneous inference in testing is usually referred to as multiple testing. Other reviews of multiple testing methods can be found in References [2, 3], the latter being focused on the context of DNA microarrays.

Recall the genomic example of the previous section. The measurements on genes are collected in a data matrix of n rows (samples, from individuals in each of two or more biological conditions) with m columns (one for each gene); plus one column for each group indicator, covariate, and so on.

After data cleaning, a significance test is often applied to each gene to test for difference among biological conditions leading to m simultaneous tests. The n observations for each gene are combined to compute test statistics, obtaining a vector of mp-values. One could then declare significance for all the genes for which the corresponding p-value is below a threshold α, say $\alpha = 0.05$.

In any event, even though each test would be in this way stringent enough to avoid false rejections, when the number of tests is large it is very likely that at least one hypothesis is rejected erroneously. When a null hypothesis is erroneously rejected, a gene with no link with the disease is declared to be differentially expressed among biological conditions.

The number of falsely selected genes would then be greater than zero with high probability. For instance, if $m = 10000$ true null hypotheses are simultaneously tested at the level $\alpha = 0.05$, around 500 false discoveries are expected. The consequences of so high a number of false discoveries in real applications would usually be deleterious.

The list of significant genes should be selected based on a threshold smaller than $\alpha = 0.05$, which is fixed using a multiple testing procedure (MTP) that controls a sensibly chosen type I error rate. Type I error rates are discussed in Section 3.3, and procedures in Section 3.5.

Using a suitable multiple testing procedure allows the researcher to build a list of genes with a low enough number of false discoveries, while still having a high number of true discoveries. The final list is often validated using low-throughput procedures like polymerase chain reaction (PCR), which leads to discarding of the false positives. Finally, selected genes can be used to explain the genetic causes of differences among biological conditions and/or for building predictive models.

3.1.2
Historic Development of the Field

One of the first instances of a multiple testing problem was raised in Reference [4], where the multiplicity issues arising from the exploration of effects within subpopulations was pointed out. It is noted that if one goes on and on splitting the population according to (possibly irrelevant) criteria any null hypothesis can be proved false just by chance at least in one subpopulation. To fix the ideas, the chance of a male birth is mentioned: the population can be split according to age, profession, region, and so on; and as one increases the number of such splits one of them will soon become significant. Interestingly, the problem was deemed to be insoluble [4]. The issue of dichotomous splits has been tackled much more recently [5].

After an early proposal [1] and a few other papers before and after Bonferroni, the modern field of multiple testing in practice started its developments after the Second World War [6, 7]. A general approach for multiple comparisons in the ANOVA setting was developed [8] and stimulated the famous work by Scheffé [9]. The same author developed the first Bayesian approaches [10, 11], along the lines of the decision-theoretic (frequentist) approach of Lehmann [12, 13].

The first book was published in 1961, with a later edition in 1981 [14]. This book was soon followed by many others, among which References [15, 16] are widely cited.

Later developments regard improvements in terms of power [17, 18], the problem of dependence, Reference [19] and many other works, graphical methods [20], optimality [21] and many other works (see Reference [22] for a review).

Further reading on the historic development of the field of multiple testing is available [15, 23].

The breakthrough paper of Benjamini and Hochberg [24], following early work by Seeger [25], introduced the concept of false discovery proportion. After that work much research has been devoted to casting multiple testing in a framework in which the number of tests can be massive.

3.2
Statistical Background

3.2.1
Tests

Let $X_j, j = 1, \ldots, m$ be a random vector based on n replicates from the same random variable. Each random vector, for $j = 1, \ldots, m$, can be drawn from a different distribution depending on unknown parameters. Parameters typically include means, differences in means, variances, ratios of variances, regression coefficients, and so on.

For each distribution a *null hypothesis* is then formulated, which summarizes an absence of effect for a specific parameter. For instance, when comparing two biological conditions, the null hypothesis is usually fixed as $H_0(j) : \mu_{1j} = \mu_{2j}$, where μ_{1j} indicates the mean of the measured expression for the j-th variable under the first condition, and μ_{2j} under the second. We thereby have m null hypotheses.

We then perform m tests to verify if and for which j the data are sufficiently in disagreement with the null hypothesis of no differential effect at population level.

Each null hypothesis can be rejected (having a discovery) or not. When a null hypothesis is erroneously rejected there is a type I error, meaning that $H_0(j)$ is (approximately) true but the data were in (a small) disagreement due to chance. This situation is also referred to as false discovery. When a large number of false discoveries occur the conclusions of the analysis may be misleading.

When the null hypothesis is actually false but it is not rejected, a type II error occurs. Type II errors imply a failure in discovering a significant effect. A large number of type II errors may lead to inconclusive results.

The *level* of the test is the probability of a type I error (before seeing the data), and it can be interpreted as the proportion of type I errors among all the tests performed on data generated from true null hypotheses. Tests are designed to yield a nominal level bounded above by a small α, usually set as 5, 1 or 10%. In this case, there is control of the type I error. Analogously, in multiple testing there is type I error rate control when the multiple testing procedure is known to yield a nominal type I error rate smaller than or equal to α.

The power of a test can be loosely defined as 1 minus the probability of the type II error, and relates to the ability of the test to detect true departures from the null hypothesis.

3.2.2
Test Statistics and *p*-Values

Each vector X_j of observations is used to compute a test statistic $T_n(j)$. Test statistics are defined on the basis of the problem and data (see below), such that higher values indicate a larger discrepancy between the data and the null hypothesis.

We define the *j*-th *p*-value to be:

$$p_j = \Pr(T_n(j) > t_n(j) | H_0(j) \text{ is true}) \tag{3.1}$$

where $t_n(j)$ is the observed value of the test statistic $T_n(j)$. Throughout we adopt the notation $p_{(j)}$ to denote the *j*-th smallest *p*-value, with $p_{(0)} = 0$ and $p_{(m+1)} = 1$.

Commonly used test statistics include *T*-statistics for testing on the mean of a single population or comparing the means of two populations, *F*-statistics for comparing the means of three or more populations, χ^2-statistics for tests on categorical data. The *T* and *F* statistics rely on the assumption of normality for X_j. When this assumption may not be met or tested, it is better to use nonparametric rank-based methods, like the Mann–Whitney and Kruskal–Wallis test statistics. See for instance References [26, 27] for details on an application in cancer research. The probability in Equation (3.1) is then computed based on the asymptotic distribution under the null hypothesis of each statistic, which is known or in many cases approximately normal for large samples. In other cases, a permutation or bootstrap can be applied and the *p*-values estimated by resampling, as we briefly describe in next section.

3.2.3
Resampling Based Testing

Suppose the null hypothesis is $H_0(j) : \mu_{1j} = \mu_{2j}$. Under the null hypothesis, the group labels can be thought of as being randomly assigned. The observations can then be resampled and actually randomly assigned to one of the two groups, and the operation can be repeated many times. It can be shown that a *p*-value that gives the desired level for the test is given by the proportion of times the test statistic computed on the resampled and randomly assigned data is at least as extreme as the original observed test statistic.

Ad hoc resampling strategies have been developed for multiple testing, a few of which will be described below. The main aim is to preserve and use information from the dependence in the data. A detailed discussion on resampling in multiple testing has been published [16].

In general, the observations can be resampled by permutation or by bootstrap.

In permutation testing [28] the data is simply randomly shuffled, while in bootstrap the data is sampled with replacement and in each resampled vector the same observation may appear more than one time. Permutation methods are usually quicker and lead to the desired level in finite samples, while in certain cases the type I error rate may be inflated if using bootstrap, and only asymptotic control is guaranteed. However, permutation methods cannot be always used since they require the assumption of exchangeability under the null hypothesis, which is called subset pivotality in this context. Subset pivotality means that the multivariate distribution of any subset of p-values is dependent only on the size of the subset and not on the specific choice of the subset. This condition is often satisfied, for instance when all combinations of null and false hypotheses are possible. A situation in which subset pivotality fails is when testing on the elements of a correlation matrix.

Resampling can be applied when the distribution of the test statistics under the null hypothesis is not known, but it often is time consuming and computationally intensive, and it often leads to high p-values (hence, low power) when n is small.

Ge et al. [29] have reviewed resampling based multiple testing in the setting of microarray data analysis.

3.3
Type I Error Rates

The setting of multiple testing can be formalized as summarized in Table 3.3. We let M_0 denote the number true nulls, and M_1 the number of false nulls, with $M_0 + M_1 = m$. The term R denotes the number of rejected null hypotheses. $N_{0|1}$ and $N_{1|0}$ are the exact (unknown) number of errors made after testing; $N_{1|1}$ and $N_{0|0}$ are the number of correctly rejected and correctly retained null hypotheses.

Generalizations of the type I error in the single testing situation must be functions of the counts of false positives $N_{1|0}$.

The classical type I error rate is the family-wise error rate (FWER), which is the probability of having one or more type I errors:

$$\text{FWER} = \Pr(N_{1|0} \geq 1) \tag{3.2}$$

Table 3.3 Outcomes in testing m hypotheses.

	H_0 not rejected	H_0 rejected	Total
H_0 true	$N_{0|0}$	$N_{1|0}$	M_0
H_0 false	$N_{0|1}$	$N_{1|1}$	M_1
Total	$m-R$	R	m

Many modern type I error rates are based on the false discovery proportion (FDP); defined as the proportion of erroneously rejected hypotheses, if any:

$$\text{FDP} = \begin{cases} \dfrac{N_{1|0}}{R} & \text{if } R > 0 \\ 0 & \text{if } R = 0 \end{cases} \quad (3.3)$$

Benjamini and Hochberg [24] propose to control the expectation of the FDP, commonly referred to as the false discovery rate (FDR). Dudoit et al. [30] and independently Genovese and Wasserman [31] along similar lines propose to control the tail probability of the FDP. This error measure is sometimes referred to as false discovery exceedance (FDX):

- FDR, expected proportion of type I errors:

$$\text{FDR} = E\,[\text{FDP}] \quad (3.4)$$

- FDX, tail probability of the FDP:

$$\text{FDX} = \Pr\,(\text{FDP} > c). \quad (3.5)$$

Typical choices are $c = 0.1, c = 0.05$, and $c = 0.5$. We set $c = 0.1$ in all the examples.

Control (in expectation or in the tail) of the FDP is justified by the idea that any researcher is prepared to bear a higher number of type I errors when a higher number of rejections are made, from which we have the use of the *proportion* of type I errors rather than their actual number. FWER control when the number of tests is large may lead to very low power, while FDR/FDX controlling procedures usually yield a high number of rejections while still keeping under control the number of type I errors. FWER control is, on the other hand, more desirable when the number of tests is small, and when moderate or large effect sizes are expected, so that a good number of rejections can be made, and all can be trusted to be true findings.

There are further generalizations of the FWER and FDR in References [32–34] and in a few other papers.

A general comparison is given by the inequalities:

$$E[N_{1|0}]/m \le \min(\text{FDR}, \text{FDX}) \le \max(\text{FDR}, \text{FDX}) \le \text{FWE} \le E[N_{1|0}].$$

Procedures controlling error rates from left to right are increasingly stringent. The last term $E[N_{1|0}]$ is sometimes referred to as *per family* type I error rate, and the first $E[N_{1|0}]/m$ as *per comparison* error rate; in fact, $E[N_{1|0}]$ is the expected number of type I errors and $E[N_{1|0}]/m$ is the expected marginal probability of erroneously rejecting a given hypothesis.

Genovese and Wasserman [35] and Sarkar [36] generalize the concept of type II error in the single test setting with the false negatives rate (FNR), defined as:

$$E\left[\frac{N_{0|1}}{m - R + 1_{(m-R)=0}}\right], \quad (3.6)$$

where 1_C is the indicator function of condition C. If two procedures control the same error rate, the one with lowest FNR is, loosely speaking, more powerful.

3.4
Introduction to Multiple Testing Procedures

A multiple testing procedure is simply an algorithm for choosing $T \in (0, 1)$ such that all hypotheses corresponding to $p_j \leq T$ can be rejected while still keeping under control a type I error rate.

The cut-off T is set small enough so that the error rate is at most equal to a pre-specified $\alpha \in [0, 1]$. On the other hand, T should be as high as possible to provide as many rejections as possible.

3.4.1
Adjusted p-values

Since T is data dependent, a p-value of say 0.0001 may or may not lead to rejection, depending on the other p-values, the number of tests m, the chosen error rate, and so on.

To provide interpretable evidence it is better to report the adjusted p-values. Adjusted p-values $\tilde{p}_j$ are a function of ordinary p-values p_j, and are defined as:

$$\tilde{p}_j = \inf\{\alpha : \text{The } j\text{-th hypothesis is rejected with nominal error rate } \alpha\}$$

In certain cases adjusted p-values are easily computed: if one controls the FWER with the Bonferroni correction, thereby setting $T = \alpha/m$, then $\tilde{p}_j = \min(mp_j, 1)$. A different strategy of computation for the adjusted p-values is needed for each multiple testing procedure. A general discussion is given in Reference [37].

It can be shown that, for each procedure, it is perfectly equivalent to consider adjustment of threshold $T = \alpha$ or of p-values, since it is equivalent to reject hypotheses corresponding to $p_j \leq T$ or to $\tilde{p}_j \leq \alpha$.

3.4.2
Categories of Multiple Testing Procedures

MTPs are usually categorized as:

- **One-step** in one-step procedures, all p-values are compared to a predetermined cut-off, usually only a function of α and m.
- **Step-down** In step-down procedures, each $p_{(j)}$ is compared with a step-down constant α_j. The p-values are examined in order, from smallest to largest. At each step, the null hypothesis is rejected if its corresponding p-value is smaller than its cut-off. Once a p-value is found to be larger than its cut-off, the corresponding test is not rejected together with all the remaining (even if one or more is corresponding to a p-value below the cut-off).

- **Step-up** Step-up procedures are similar to step-down procedures. The *p*-values are examined from the largest to the smallest. At each step, the test is not rejected if its *p*-value is larger than its step-up constant α_j. Once a *p*-value is found to be significant, the corresponding null hypothesis is rejected together with all the remaining.

If a step-up and a step-down procedure are based on the same constants, the step-up version will reject at least the same number of hypotheses, thus being at least as powerful as the step-down method. If we denote with J the index of the largest *p*-value corresponding to a rejected hypothesis, we can set $T = p_{(J)}$ (and $T = 0$ if there are no rejected hypotheses).

Much work has been devoted to a general theoretical analysis of stepwise procedures, see for instance Reference [38] for an early approach. Much work has also been devoted to admissibility and optimality of stepwise methods.

Multiple testing procedures may also be *augmentation* based. Augmentation procedures proceed iteratively, first rejecting a certain number of hypotheses and then rejecting an additional number chosen as function of the number rejected at the first step. Simulations comparing some of the multiple testing procedures that will be reviewed can be found in Reference [2].

3.4.3
Estimation of the Proportion of False Nulls

Here we review some estimators for $a = M_1/m$, the proportion of false nulls. The estimates can be used to increase the power of some multiple testing procedures as described in Section 3.5. Estimation of the number of true/false null hypotheses may be of interest *per se*; see, for example, Reference [39] for applications in functional magnetic resonance imaging.

The basis for estimating a is the t_0-estimator: fix $0 < t_0 < 1$, and let:

$$\hat{a} = \max\left(\frac{\left(\sum 1_{p_j < t_0}\right) - mt_0}{m - mt_0}, 0\right) \tag{3.7}$$

The t_0-estimator in (3.7) was originally proposed by Schweder and Spjøtvoll [20], and is based on the idea that *p*-values corresponding to false null hypotheses cluster towards zero. Hence, the difference between the count of *p*-values below a (small) threshold t_0 and the expected number of *p*-values below t_0 if all the null hypotheses were true gives a rough estimate of the number of false null hypotheses that give *p*-values in the interval $(0, t_0)$. Figure 3.1 provides an illustration, with histograms of *p*-values generated for different values of a, together with their cumulative density functions. Notably, these graphs may not be so clear (i.e., estimators for a may have higher variance) with smaller number of tests or, as often happens, values of $a > 0$ closer to zero.

Different strategies have been proposed for fixing t_0, which give rise to different estimators.

A common choice is $t_0 = 0.5$, or smaller [20].

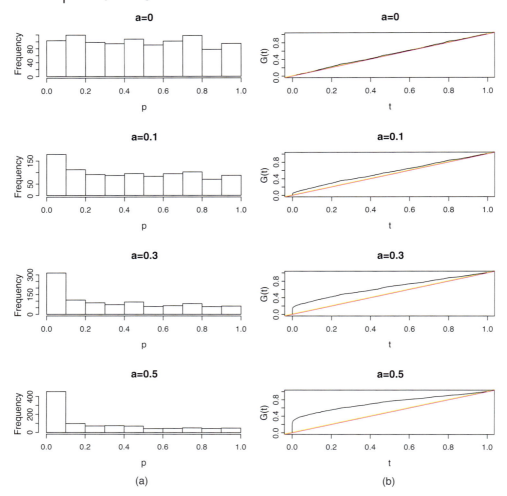

Figure 3.1 Histogram (a) and CDF (b) of p-values for $m = 1000$ and $a = 0, 0.1, 0.3, 0.5$. The red line indicates, for each t, the expected number of p-values below the threshold under the complete null hypothesis.

Storey [32] suggests choosing t_0 by minimizing the mean square error (MSE), estimated with bootstrap. Data are resampled and the estimates computed for different values of t_0 on a grid of values in the interval $(0, 1)$. The MSE for each t_0 is estimated as the average squared difference between the resampled estimates and the original estimates. Finally, t_0 is set as the one leading to the smallest estimated MSE.

Another possibility is to apply any FWER controlling procedure and set t_0 as the smallest not rejected p-value [39].

More recently, Meinshausen and Rice [40] have noted that an important property of estimators for a is conservativeness: $\hat{a} \leq a$ with high probability. In fact, whenever $\hat{a} > a$ and the estimator is used for controlling a type I error rate, there is a risk for loss of control. Estimators in Reference [40] are based on bounding sequences of the weighted empirical distribution of p-values. One of those estimators that is strictly related to FDR control and uses on optimal bounding sequence is given by:

$$\hat{a} = \sup_{t \in (0,1)} \max \left(\frac{\sum 1_{p_j \leq r} - t/\alpha}{1-t} \right) \quad (3.8)$$

With the same aim of proposing conservative estimators Reference [41] suggests the use of a proportion of rejected hypotheses from any FWER controlling procedure as an estimate for a, and shows how to take into account the uncertainty brought about by estimation.

3.5 Multiple Testing Procedures

3.5.1 Procedures Controlling the FWER

In this subsection we briefly review procedures to control the family-wise error rate, as defined in (3.2). More details can be found elsewhere [14–16, 42].

- **Bonferroni:** The Bonferroni correction is a one-step method at level $T = \alpha/m$. It has been proposed in Reference [1].
- **Step-down Holm** [17]: propose to improve on Bonferroni by using the step-down constant $\alpha_j = \alpha/(m-j+1)$.
- **Step-up Hochberg** [43]: proves the same constant of Holm can be used in a (more powerful) step-up method.
- **Step-down minP:** Let $F_{r,\alpha}(\cdot)$ indicate the α percentile of the distribution of the minimum of the last r p-values. The "Step-down minP" procedure fixes a step-down constant $\alpha_j = F_{j,\alpha}(p_{(m-j+1)}, \ldots, p_{(m)})$.
- **One-step Sidak** [44]: sets $T = 1 - \sqrt[m]{1-\alpha}$.
- **Step-down Sidak:** a step-down version of the Sidak correction is given in Reference [45], and uses the step-down constant $\alpha_j = 1 - {}^{m-j+1}\sqrt{1-\alpha}$.

A further improvement of Bonferroni is given by the use of an estimate of the proportion of false nulls for computation of the one-step constant $\alpha/m(1-\hat{a})$. Similarly, in one-step Sidak the one-step constant $1 - {}^{m(1-\hat{a})}\sqrt{1-\alpha}$ can be used.

For the minP procedure the step-down constants arise from distribution of the minima of the last p-values. Pesarin [28] suggests a permutation algorithm to estimate this distribution and hence the constants:

1) set $j = m$;
2) for the hypothesis corresponding to the j-th ordered p-value, compute B permutation p-values $p_{j,1}, \ldots, p_{j,B}$;

3) enforce monotonicity by setting $q_{j,b} = \min(q_{j+1,b}, p_{j,b})$, with $q_{m+1,b} = 1$, and estimate the j-th adjusted p-value as $\tilde{p}_j = \sum_b \mathbf{1}_{q_{j,b} \leq p_{(j)}} / B :=$ set $j : j-1$;
4) if $j > 0$, go to Step 2. If $j = 0$, enforce monotonicity of the estimated p-values: $\tilde{p}_j = \max(\tilde{p}_{j-1}, \tilde{p}_j)$, $j = 2, \ldots, m$;
5) reject the hypotheses for which $\tilde{p}_j \leq \alpha$.

The procedure starts by permuting and estimating the least significant p-value as the proportion of resampled maxima above the observed $p_{(m)}$. Permutation is then repeated for the second least significant p-value, and each permuted p-value is forced to be below the permuted p-value for the least significant hypothesis, that is, $p_{(m-1),b} \leq p_{(m),b}$ for each $b = 1, \ldots, B$. After this, the second least significant adjusted p-value can be estimated as the proportion of successive minima below the observed $p_{(m-1)}$, and the procedure iterated until the most significant p-value $p_{(1)}$ is used. Finally, monotonicity of the estimated adjusted p-values is enforced to preserve the ordering implied by the observed p-values.

The maxT method is a dual of the minP procedure that makes use only of the test statistics (thus not needing the computation of p-values). Suppose without loss of generality that the test statistics are ordered. Let $F'_{r,1-\alpha}(\cdot)$ indicate the $1-\alpha$ percentile of the distribution of the maximum of the last r ordered test statistics. The maxT procedure fixes $C_j = F'^{-1}_{j,1-\alpha}(T_n(m-j+1), \ldots, T_n(m))$, and proceeds in a step-down fashion stopping the first time $T_n(j) \leq C_j$, and rejecting the hypotheses corresponding to $T_n(1), \ldots, T_n(j-1)$. The functions $F'_{r,\alpha}(\cdot)$ can be estimated through permutation with a straightforward extension of the algorithm described above.

The minP and maxT are equivalent when the test statistics are identically distributed under the null hypothesis; otherwise they may lead to different results.

Among the reviewed FWER controlling procedures, step-down Sidak is the most powerful under independence of the test statistics. In that case, the minP approach is approximately equivalent since $F_{j,\alpha}(p_{(m-j+1)}, \ldots, p_{(m)})$ exactly coincide with the Sidak step-down constants.

Dunnet and Tamhane [46] propose a step-up multiple testing procedure, optimal in terms of power, when the test statistics are distributed like a Student's T.

Note that in general, the higher the stepwise constants the more powerful is the procedure. To provide a theoretical comparison between some FWER controlling procedures, we provide in Figure 3.2 a general comparison of such constants for $m = 10$.

3.5.2
Procedures Controlling the FDR

In this subsection we briefly review procedures controlling the FDR, as defined in (3.4). While the idea dates back at least to [24], FDR was popularized in the seminal paper [24].

FDR is now probably the most popular error measure for high-throughput data since it provides a better balance between false positives and false negatives than FWER control when the number of tests m is large.

3.5 Multiple Testing Procedures

The following procedures control the FDR:

1) **BH:** this procedure consists in fixing a step-up constant equal to $\alpha_j = j\alpha/m$.
2) **Plug in** [47]: suggest using the step-up constant $\alpha_j = j\alpha/m(1-\hat{a})$, where $\hat{a}$ is any estimator of the proportion of false hypotheses M_1/m.
3) **Resampling-based YB** [48]: suggests the following procedure:

   a) bootstrap the data to obtain B vectors of resampled p-values;
   b) without loss of generality let the ordered p-values $p_{(k)}$ be the possible thresholds; for each sample let $r(p_{(k)})$ be the number of resampled p-values below $p_{(k)}$, and let $r_\beta(p_{(k)})$ be the $1-\beta$ quantile of $r(p_{(k)})$ for a small β (say $\beta = 0.05$); then, for each threshold compute $Q^*(p_{(k)})$ as the resampling based mean of the function:

   $$Q(p_{(k)}) = \begin{cases} \dfrac{r(p_{(k)})}{r(p_{(k)}) + k - mp_{(k)}} & \text{If } mp_{(k)} \leq k - r_\beta(p_{(k)}) \\ 1 & \text{Otherwise} \end{cases}$$

   c) Let $k_\alpha = \max_k \{Q^*(p_{(k)}) \leq \alpha\}$ and set threshold $T = p_{(k_\alpha)}$.

The BH procedure was originally proposed in Reference [49], but it did not receive much attention at that time. Benjamini and Hochberg [24] prove it controls the FDR at level $(1-a)\alpha$, and hence at level α. BH stepwise constants are plotted in Figure 3.2. The higher power of FDR control can be appreciated from the comparison with FWER constants in the same figure.

The plug-in procedure is a direct improvement of BH and makes use of an estimator for the proportion of false nulls. If $\hat{a}$ is consistent, it controls the FDR

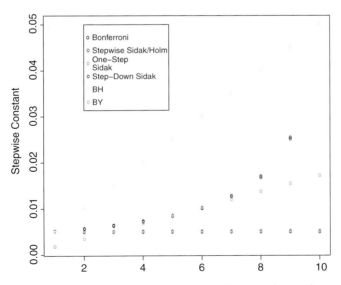

Figure 3.2 Stepwise constants of FWER controlling procedures with $m = 10$ and $\alpha = 0.05$.

at level α and hence it is less conservative than the BH procedure. The only problems are linked with uncertainty related to estimation of the proportion of false nulls, which may lead to loss of control of the FDR in small samples. A discussion on how to incorporate uncertainty caused by the estimation of M_1/m in certain cases has been published [41]. A further improvement of the plug-in method has been made [50], in which plug-in is used iteratively, and at each iteration an estimator of the number of false nulls is given by the number of rejections at the previous step.

The YB resampling approach was introduced to improve on BH by taking into account the possible dependence among the test statistics. A different resampling method is proposed in Reference [51]. Significance analysis for microarrays (SAMs) is especially devised for DNA microarray data, and does not actually control the FDR but another functional of the FDP that is approximately equal to the FDR. For further discussion on SAM, see Reference [3]. As noted before, resampling methods may not yield type I error rate control with small sample sizes relative to the number of tests.

Example 3.1 (Multiple endpoints in clinical trials)

To fix the ideas, consider the data about myocardial infarction of Reference [52], which were used [24] to support the use of FDR.

In a randomized multicenter trial of 421 patients with acute myocardial infarction, a new front-loaded administration of rt-PA (thrombolysis with recombinant tissue-type plasminogen activator) has been compared with APSAC (anisoylated plasminogen streptokinase activator complex). The treatments are deemed to reduce in-hospital mortality.

There are 15 endpoints of interest, related to cardiac and other events after the start of the thrombolytic treatment; hence $m = 15$.

The ordered p-values are computed as: 0.0001, 0.0004, 0.0019, 0.0095, 0.0201, 0.0278, 0.0298, 0.0344, 0.0459, 0.3240, 0.4262, 0.5719, 0.6528, 0.7590, and 1.000; and the comparison with respect to in-hospital mortality rate corresponds to $p_{(4)}$. If a value of $p_j = 0.0095$ can be declared statistically significant, then rt-PA is to be preferred for reducing the in-hospital mortality rate, otherwise the study does not provide convincing evidence for the use of the new therapy. All the FWER controlling procedures considered would lead to the rejection of 3 p-values, thus not supporting a statement about different mortality rate. On the other hand, FDR controlling procedures lead to different conclusions: it can be seen that BH leads to rejection of four hypotheses, plug-in (with t_0-estimator and $t_0 = 0.5$) to 9, and so YB.

To detail further the rationale behind stepwise procedures, we show in Figure 3.3 p-values and BH step-down constants. A close look at the figure reveals why we are led to reject four hypotheses.

We stress that the error measure and the controlling procedure must be chosen before actually seeing the data, otherwise having a data-snooping (see for instance Reference [53]) may lead to more false rejections than actually expected.

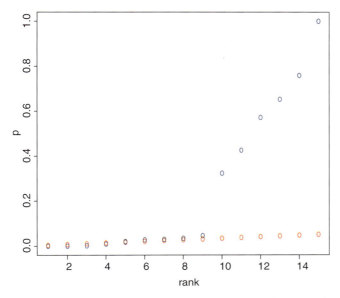

Figure 3.3 p-Values (blue) and stepwise constants (red) of BH procedure for APSAC data.

3.5.3
Procedures Controlling the FDX

In this subsection we briefly review procedures to control the FDX, as defined in Equation (3.5).

When controlling the FDR, the expectation of the FDP is bounded above by α. Hence one "expects" the realized proportion of false positives in the specific experiment to be more or less around its expectation α, and hopefully below. The realized FDP can be way above its expectation, even if concentration inequalities can be used to show that this happens with small probability. FDX control is a direct control for the realized FDP to be below a threshold, c, with high probability.

This is particularly useful in cases in which the FDP may not be concentrated around its mean, for instance in presence of strong dependence among the test statistics [54], many small effects, and small sample sizes.

Some of the procedures that can be used to control the FDX are:

Augmentation

The algorithm is as follows:

```
Reject S hypotheses with any FWER controlling
procedure
if S > 0 then
    k(c, α) = max{j ∈ {0,..., m−S} : j/(j+S) ≤ c}
```

Reject the $S+k(c,\alpha)$ **most significant hypotheses.**
end if

Generalized Augmentation (GAUGE)

The algorithm is as follows:

Reject the S hypotheses corresponding to p-values smaller than a certain $q \in (0,1)$.
if $S > 0$ **then**

$$i^* = \max_{m_0=1,\ldots,m} \min\left\{i : \sum_{k=i}^{m_0} \binom{m_0}{k} q^k(1-q)^{m_0-k} \leq \alpha\right\} \quad (3.9)$$

if $\frac{(i^*-1)}{S} \leq c$ **then**

$$k(c,\alpha) = \max\left\{j \in \{0,\ldots,m-S\} : \frac{j+i^*-1}{j+S} \leq c\right\}$$

Reject the $S+k(c,\alpha)$ **most significant hypotheses.**
end if
if $\frac{(i^*-1)}{S} > c$ **or** i^* **does not exist then**
$k'(c,\alpha) =$

$$\max_{m_0=1,\ldots,m} \min_{k=0,\ldots,S}\left\{k : 1_{\{S-k>0\}} \left[\sum_{i=0}^{m_0} \sum_{j=0}^{\min(k,i)} 1_{\{\frac{i-j}{S-k}>c\}} \binom{m_0}{i} q^i(1-q)^{m_0-i} \frac{\binom{i}{j}\binom{m-i}{k-j}}{\binom{m}{k}}\right] < \alpha\right\}$$
$$(3.10)$$

Reject only the $S-k'(c,\alpha)$ **most significant hypotheses.**
end if
end if

Step-down LR

The authors of Reference [33] propose to use the step-down constant $\alpha_j = (\lceil cj \rceil + 1)\alpha/(m + \lceil cj \rceil + 1 - j)$.

Resampling-based LBH

A resampling-based procedure is proposed in Reference [55]:
1) Bootstrap the data, compute the resampled test statistics, and center each vector of test statistics by its own mean.
2) Estimate the density of the test centered statistics, for instance by bootstrapping again, and call it $q_0(\cdot)$. Estimate the density of the non-centered test statistics and call it $g(\cdot)$. Sample the indicator of each null hypothesis to be false from a Bernoulli with parameter given by an estimated ratio of the null and marginal density $q_0(T_n(j))/g(T_n(j))$.
3) Estimate the realized FDX for each possible cut-off $p_{(1)}, \ldots, p_{(k)}$.

4) Repeat steps 1–3 B times, where B is large.
5) Estimate the FDX for each cut-off as the average of the realized FDX at each iteration. Set the cut-off for the p-values as the highest cut-off giving estimated FDX below α.

Step-down LR arises mainly from combinatorial and probabilistic reasoning. It is powerful and can be easily extended to dependence (Section 3.6). Improvements have been developed [56, 57].

Augmentation is a clever method proposed in Reference [30]. Any procedure controlling a type I error rate less stringent than FWER should result in the rejection of at least the same hypotheses. Hence, one can control the FWER and then add an opportune additional number. Advantages of augmentation are its generality and flexibility, and the robustness with respect to dependence inherited by the FWER controlling procedure used at the first step. The main drawback is that the power may be low for large number of tests, since FWER controlling procedures used at the first step get more and more conservative as the number of tests grows. The fewer hypotheses are rejected at the first stage, the fewer at the second.

For this reason Reference [58] replaces FWER control at the first step with uncorrected testing, providing generalized augmentation (GAUGE). After the first step, if augmentation is possible an appropriate number of rejections are added; while if too many hypotheses are rejected at the first stage, some are removed. Since uncorrected testing is used at the first stage, the number of hypotheses tentatively rejected is usually high, even when the number of tests is large. GAUGE may then be more suitable than augmentation in high-dimensional problems, even if it does not share the same robustness with respect to dependence (Section 3.6). A known drawback is that the number of rejections may not vary smoothly with respect to the choice of the parameter q, which must be made in advance. A suggested choice for the parameter q is $q = 0.05/100$ (for further discussion and other strategies see Reference [58]).

The resampling-based method in Reference [55] is another possibility to enhance power. The main drawback is the high computational cost: it is a double-resampling (there is a bootstrap within each bootstrap iteration).

3.6
Type I Error Rates Control Under Dependence

While independence among observations is often taken for granted, in real data applications almost always there is dependence among the test statistics. Use of multiple testing procedures must be considered with attention to the particular assumptions on dependence that can be made on the data at hand. There are extensions of many procedures that can deal with arbitrary dependence, that is, with no assumption on the dependency structure. These are the safest choices, but often at the price of a loss of power.

High-throughput data almost always show dependence. For instance, test statistics arising from DNA microarrays should almost always be considered as dependent. Genes measured with the same technology in the same laboratory are subject to common sources of noise. Moreover, changes in expression are part of the same biological mechanism, and hence the expression of each gene is not unrelated to the expression of the other genes.

A general positive result on multiple testing under dependence is given in a recent breakthrough paper [59], whose authors show that if the distributions of the test statistics under the null hypotheses are not heavy-tailed and dependence does not increase with the number of tests then procedures devised for the independence case are asymptotically valid also under dependence. According to their results, in many real situations with large m, the procedures reviewed in Section 3.5 can be safely applied.

Another general positive result is given in Reference [60], whose authors have derived a strategy to remove dependence, resulting in independent parameter estimates, test statistics, and p-values. After this sort of filter, one can apply any procedure derived under dependence to the new p-values. The authors assume the existence of a dependence kernel, a low-dimensional subspace driving dependence. This sort of scenario is applicable in latent variable models and other cases. In practice, in most situations the dependence kernel will not be known and will be estimated, so that the resulting p-values will only be closer to independence, but not exactly independent.

Given below are considerations and modifications of the procedures that could be used in different settings, many of which provide exact control of the error rate under arbitrary dependence or under special assumptions.

3.6.1
FWER Control

Dependence is not a problem in FWER control, since Bonferroni and step-down Holm are valid under arbitrary dependence. Step-up Hochberg requires assumptions of positive dependence. Precise definitions of such assumptions [precisely, multivariate totally positive of order two (MTP$_2$) test statistics are needed] can be found in Reference [61]. Step-up Hochberg can then be applied under assumption of multivariate normality with non-negative correlations among all the test statistics, and other situations that can be found also in Reference [62]. A similar condition (positive orthant dependence) is needed for Sidak procedures. Again, assumption of multivariate normality with all non-negative correlations suffices. See also Reference [63] for other examples.

3.6.2
FDR and FDX Control

Benjamini and Yekutieli [64] provide a procedure that can be used to control the FDR under general dependence, by setting the step-up constant:

$$a_j = j\alpha / \left(m \sum_{i=1}^{m} 1/i \right)$$

We call this method BY. Even if applicable under arbitrary dependence, this approach is very conservative and usually leads to much lower power with respect to BH. This is illustrated by comparing the BY stepwise constants in Figure 3.2.

The same paper shows that some positive dependence assumptions [precisely, Positive Regression Dependency on the Subset of true null hypotheses (PRDS)] can be used to extend the applicability of BH. For instance, as before, BH can be used under assumptions of multivariate normality with all non-negative correlations. See also Reference [65] for other examples. Further, Reference [66] shows that under conditions of weak dependence both plug-in and BH procedures control the FDR when the number of tests is moderate to large, and suggests robust estimators for the proportion of false nulls a. Weak dependence can be assumed whenever a permutation of the p-values can be assumed to show decreasing dependence as the number of tests grows. It is argued in Reference [66] hence that BH and plug-in can be used for the analysis of DNA microarray data (especially with observations repeated over time), change-point detection in time series, and a few other applications.

Augmentation procedures that control the FDX are valid under arbitrary dependence, provided the FWER controlling procedure at the first step is valid under arbitrary dependence. Moreover, the resampling based procedure in Reference [55] is adaptive and provides control also under dependence.

Lehmann and Romano [33] prove their procedure controls the FDX under the same assumptions needed for step-up Hochberg. Finally, they suggest a more conservative procedure controlling the FDX under general dependence that involves simply dividing their step-up constants by a factor of:

$$\sum_{i=1}^{\lceil cm \rceil + 1} 1/i$$

Finally, GAUGE is argued to be valid under assumptions of positive or negative dependence (precisely, positive or negative association); for instance, in the case of multivariate normality with all non-negative or all non-positive correlations. For moderate and large m, GAUGE is valid also under the same weak dependence assumptions needed for the BH procedure. A version valid under arbitrary dependence, which we denote with $\text{GAUGE}_{\text{dep}}$, can be obtained by replacing i^* in (3.9) with $i^* = \lceil mq/\alpha \rceil$, and $k'(c, \alpha)$ in (3.10) with:

$$k'(c,\alpha) = \min_{k=0,\ldots,S} \left\{ k : 1_{\{S-k>0\}} \left(\sum_{i=0}^{m} \sum_{j=0}^{\min(k,i)} 1_{\{\frac{i-j}{S-k}>c\}} \min(mq/i, 1) \frac{\binom{i}{j}\binom{m-i}{k-j}}{\binom{m}{k}} \right) < \alpha \right\}$$

This version, as could be expected, is seen to be more conservative than GAUGE.

3.7 Multiple Testing Procedures Applied to Gene Discovery in DNA Microarray Cancer Studies

In microarray studies a list of significant genes is produced, often with the aim of a first screening before a validation phase with low-throughput procedures.

Hence, a small proportion of false positives is allowed, while too many false positives would make the validation expensive and time consuming: control of FDR or FDX is then naturally desirable in the microarray setting. On the other hand, FWER controlling procedures may prove to be too strict and end up in too small a list of prospective differentially expressed genes.

The FDP was popularized in the bioinformatics literature mainly for this reason (see for instance Reference [67]).

Two examples on benchmark data sets are shown below.

3.7.1
Gene identification in Colon Cancer

Alon *et al.* [68] have recorded expression of genes from 40 tumoral and 22 normal samples from the colon of a total of 62 patients. The gene expression levels are normalized to remove systematic bias due to slide, dye effects, and similar sources of error. The normalized expression levels are used to compute a two-sample t statistic for each gene for testing the null hypothesis $H_0(j) : \mu_{1j} = \mu_{2j}$, where μ_{1j} indicates the mean expression of the j-th gene in the population of normal colon tissues, and μ_{2j} the mean expression of the j-th gene in the population of tumoral colon tissues. We have a total of $m = 2000$ null hypotheses and corresponding test statistics.

Figure 3.4 shows a histogram of the 2000 t-statistics. Colon cancer is well known to be related to genetic variations, and in fact the histogram itself suggests the presence of a few significant genes.

The p-values are easily computed as $p_j = \Pr(T_{60} > |t_n(j)|)$, where T_{60} denotes a Student's T random variable with 60 degrees of freedom and $t_n(j)$ is the j-th test statistic.

Figure 3.5 shows the empirical CDF of the 2000 p-values, with a red line indicating the complete null CDF. The divergence between the two lines, which starts for very small values of p, denotes an excess of small p-values, which is likely to be associated with false null hypotheses clustering towards zero.

For a comparison, we apply different multiple testing procedures to the vector of p-values. Table 3.4 reports the number of rejections. The number of selected genes depends heavily on the chosen error rate, with a large difference between FWER and FDR/FDX controlling procedures.

3.7.1.1 Classification of Lymphoblastic and Myeloid Leukemia

While an important task in microarray studies is to identify significantly differentially expressed genes, a second stage may involve the use of gene expressions for classification of patients (mainly diagnostic, but also prognostic).

While it would be too expensive to classify patients based on their entire genome, often a small significant subset of genes can be used for accurate and less expensive classification. Use of the list of genes identified as significant with a multiple testing procedure has been seen to be convenient in many applications.

3.7 Multiple Testing Procedures Applied to Gene Discovery in DNA Microarray Cancer Studies

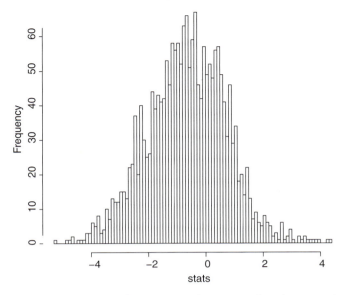

Figure 3.4 Histogram of 2000 two-sample t-statistics for colon cancer data.

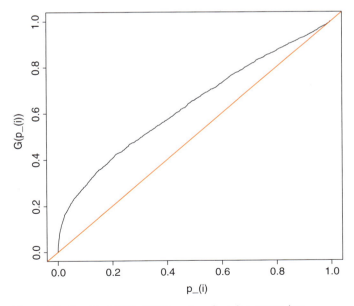

Figure 3.5 Empirical CDF of 2000 p-values for colon cancer data.

Table 3.4 Colon cancer data: number of selected genes.

FWER controlling procedures	
Bonferroni	11
Step-down Holm	11
One-step Sidak	11
Step-down Sidak	11
Step-up Hochberg	11
Step-down MinP	11
FDR controlling procedures	
BH	190
BY	38
Plug-in	217
FDX controlling procedures	
Augmentation with step-down Sidak at first step	12
Augmentation with Bonferroni at first step	12
LR	33
GAUGE	41
GAUGE$_{dep}$	20

As an example, consider the microarray data from Reference [69] on human acute leukemia. The goal is to distinguish between patients with acute lymphoblastic leukemia (ALL) and patients with acute myeloid leukemia (AML). A set of genes can be selected and profiled for classification of the variant of leukemia for future patients.

We have $m = 3051$ genes whose expression is repeatedly measured on a total of 38 samples (27 ALL, 11 AML).

After selecting genes with a multiple testing procedure, we classify the samples using k-nearest neighbors [70], with $k = 3$. The 3-NN approach classifies a new sample by selecting the three closest samples (with respect to sum of Euclidean distances between expressions on the selected genes). The new sample is assigned label (ALL/AML) of the majority of the three closest samples.

To evaluate the performance of the classifier we split the data into a training set of 15 samples, nine chosen at random from the ALL samples and six chosen at random from the AML samples. The p-values are computed again from two-sample t-tests. For each set of selected genes the remaining test set of 34 samples, (18 ALL, 5 AML), was used to estimate the classification error, that is, the proportion of samples in the test set that were misclassified by the 3-NN classifier. The operation is repeated 1000 times and the average number of selected genes recorded with the average classification error. Table 3.5 gives the results for different multiple testing procedures.

In this example FWER controlling procedures end up by selecting a list of genes that is too small and leads to a high classification error when compared to the other procedures. FDR controlling procedures achieve the lowest classification errors, but at the price of larger lists of selected genes. FDX controlling procedures lead to slightly higher classification errors, but with smaller lists of selected genes.

Table 3.5 Leukemia data: average number of selected genes and estimated classification error.

FWER controlling procedures		
Bonferroni	15.68	0.0684
Step-down Holm	15.73	0.0683
One-step Sidak	15.88	0.0673
Step-down Sidak	15.93	0.0669
Step-up Hochberg	15.73	0.0682
Step-down MinP	15.92	0.0669
FDR controlling procedures		
BH	240.46	0.0251
BY	33.66	0.0571
Plug-in	368.45	0.0248
FDX controlling procedures		
Augmentation with step-down Sidak at first step	17.11	0.0663
Augmentation with Bonferroni at first step	16.84	0.0666
LR	35.18	0.0521
GAUGE	97.13	0.0275
$GAUGE_{dep}$	32.86	0.0510

3.8 Conclusions

Clearly, multiple hypothesis testing is concerned with probabilistically controlling the number of false positives, so that conclusions of an analysis (i.e., at the coarsest stage, a list of rejections) can be trusted. Procedures should control the chosen type I error rate, possibly maximizing the number of rejections, and hence the ability of discovering true departures from any of the null hypotheses.

A multiple testing situation presents many substantial differences from the single hypothesis setting, primarily in the need for a correction on the significance level, arising from a chosen error rate. In our opinion the researchers should carefully (a priori) ponder which error rate, and which controlling procedure, is best for the application, and the data, at hand. Many methodological developments have been devised since the early 1940s, and many will be developed, due to the fact that a single solution cannot be suitable for all problems.

There are now available different methodologies for dealing with multiplicity problems when applying testing to high-throughput data. Table 3.6 summarizes the reviewed approaches.

The researcher must choose the *type I error rate*, how to compute *p*-values, and then one of the corrections that is known to control the chosen error rate. We did not focus on how to compute *p*-values, while we gave few guidelines on how to choose the error rate. The multiple testing procedure should then be chosen based on the known properties with respect the specific data situation (number of tests, dependence, proportion of false nulls, strength of the signal, etc.).

Table 3.6 Multiple testing procedures and their characteristics.

Name	Type	Dependence
Control of FWER		
Bonferroni	One-step	Arbitrary
Step-down Holm	Step-down	Arbitrary
One-step Sidak	One-step	Positive orthant
Step-down Sidak	Step-down	Positive orthant
Step-up Hochberg	Step-up	MTP_2
Step-down MinP	Step-down (permutation)	Arbitrary
Control of FDR		
Benjamini and Hochberg (BH)	Step-up	PRDS, weak dependence
Plug-in	Step-up	PRDS
Yekutieli and Benjamini (BY)	Step-up (bootstrap)	Arbitrary
Benjamini and Yekutieli (BY)	Step-up	Arbitrary
Control of FDX		
Augmentation with step-down Sidak at first step	Augmentation/step-down	Positive orthant
Augmentation with Bonferroni at first step	Augmentation	Arbitrary
Lehmann and Romano (LR)	Step-down	MTP_2
Lehmann and Romano conservative version	Step-down	Arbitrary
LBH	Bootstrap	Arbitrary
GAUGE	Augmentation	Positive/negative association, weak dependence
$GAUGE_{dep}$	Augmentation	Arbitrary

There is a plethora of research that has not been reviewed in this chapter. The reader interested in weighted procedures is referred to the literature [71–73]. Multiple comparisons arising from interim analysis pose very different problems, and the reader can refer for instance to Reference [74]; while for multiple testing specifically arising from multiple endpoints we refer to References [75–78]. Some research has been also devoted to estimation, rather than control, of the FDP, and the possible uses of this estimates; for example, References [79–82] and many others. It is acknowledged that controlling an estimate of the FDR does not imply that the FDR is controlled, so that estimation approaches can be deemed to be inherently different from the probabilitistically controlling approaches described here. Finally, the problem of choosing the sample size in multiple testing has not been developed much, with a few notable exceptions [83, 84].

The field is open for much further research. Much attention has been devoted recently on new error rates, which mainly generalize FWER and FDR. An open problem for the practitioner is how to set parameters for the error rates. While it is clear in statistics that the 1-5-10% levels for α are not a dogma, they are widely accepted and comfortably chosen. On the other hand, clear guidelines on how to choose c for the FDX are not yet found. Another example is given by k-FWER of Reference [33], where it is not easy to practically choose the parameter k.

Another open problem relates to dealing with dependent test statistics, a case of special interest for applications in genomics and in many other fields. Two routes have been followed: one route developed more stringent procedures under sufficient conditions on the dependence. Assuming conditions on the dependence of the test statistics is often hard, because it is hard to evaluate the degree and direction of dependence. Further, usually, the weaker the conditions the less powerful the extended procedure, with a lower bound given by procedures for arbitrarily dependent test statistics. The second route tries to use information arising from dependence, for instance through resampling. The problem with such methods is that they are often computationally demanding, and further can guarantee error control only approximately or with (seldom available) large samples.

References

1 Bonferroni, C.E. (1935) Il calcolo delle assicurazioni su gruppi di teste, in *Studi in Onore del Professore Salvatore Ortu Carboni*, Rome, pp. 13–60.

2 Farcomeni, A. (2008) A review of modern multiple hypothesis testing with particular attention to the false discovery proportion. *Stat. Methods Med. Res.*, **17**, 347–388.

3 Dudoit, S., Shaffer, P.J., and Boldrick, J.C. (2003) Multiple hypothesis testing in microarray experiments. *Stat. Sci.*, **18**, 71–103.

4 Cournot, A.A. (1843) *Exposition de la Théorie des Chances et des Probabilités*, Hachette, Paris.

5 Shafer, G. and Olkin, I. (1983) Adjusting p-value to account for selection over dichotomies. *J. Am. Stat. Assoc.*, **78**, 674–678.

6 Tukey, J.W. (1949) Comparing individual means in the analysis of variance. *Biometrics*, **5**, 99–114.

7 Paulson, E. (1949) A multiple decision procedure for certain problems in the analysis of variance. *Ann. Math. Stat.*, **20**, 95–98.

8 Duncan, D.B. (1951) A significance test for differences between ranked treatments in an analysis of variance. *Virginia J. Sci.*, **2**, 172–189.

9 Scheffé, H. (1953) A method for judging all contrasts in the analysis of variance. *Biometrika*, **40**, 87–104.

10 Duncan, D.B. (1961) Bayes rules for a common multiple comparisons problem and related Student-t problems. *Ann. Math. Stat.*, **32**, 1013–1033.

11 Duncan, D.B. (1965) A Bayesian approach to multiple comparisons. *Technometrics*, **7**, 171–222.

12 Lehmann, E.L. (1957) A theory of some multiple decision problems, I. *Ann. Math. Stat.*, **28**, 1–25.

13 Lehmann, E.L. (1957) A theory of some multiple decision problems, II. *Ann. Math. Stat.*, **28**, 547–572.

14 Miller, R.G. (1981) *Simultaneous Statistical Inference*, John Wiley & Sons, Inc. New York.

15 Hochberg, Y. and Tamhane, A.C. (1987) *Multiple Comparisons Procedures*, John Wiley & Sons, Inc. New York.

16 Westfall, P.H. and Young, S.S. (1993) *Resampling-based Multiple Testing: Examples and Methods for p-value Adjustment*, John Wiley & Sons, Inc. New York.

17 Holm, S. (1979) A simple sequentially rejective multiple test procedure. *Scand. J. Stat.*, **6**, 65–70.

18 Holland, B.S. and Copenhaver, M.D. (1987) An improved sequentially rejective Bonferroni test procedure. *Biometrics*, **43**, 417–423, Corr: **43**, 737.

19 Hommel, G. (1983) Tests of the overall hypothesis for arbitrary dependence structures. *Biomet. J.*, **25**, 423–430.

20 Schweder, T. and Spjøtvoll, E. (1982) Plots of p-values to evaluate many hypotheses simultaneously. *Biometrika*, **69**, 493–502.

21 Spjøtvoll, E. (1972) On the optimality of some multiple comparison procedures. *Ann. Math. Stat.*, **43**, 398–411.

22 Shaffer, J.P. (2006) Recent developments towards optimality in multiple hypothesis testing, *Optimality: The 2nd Erich L. Lehmann Symposium* (ed. J. Rojo), IMS Lecture Notes–Monograph Series, vol. **49**, Institute of Mathematical Statistics, Beachwood, Ohio, pp. 16–32.

23 Harter, H.L. (1980) Early history of multiple comparison tests, in *Handbook of Statistics*, vol. **1** (ed. P.R. Krishnaiah), North-Holland, Amsterdam, pp. 617–622.

24 Benjamini, Y. and Hochberg, Y. (1995) Controlling the false discovery rate: A practical and powerful approach to multiple testing. *J. R. Stat. Soc. B Method.*, **57**, 289–300.

25 Seeger, P. (1968) A note on a method for the analysis of significance en masse. *Technometrics*, **10**, 586–593.

26 Farcomeni, A. (2008) Parametric assumptions in single and multiple testing: when should we rely on them? *Biomed. Stat. Clin. Epidemio.*, **2**, 57–69.

27 Ferretti, E., De Smaele, E., Po, A., Di Marcotullio, L., Tosi, E., Espinola, M.S.B. *et al.* (2009) MicroRNA profiling in human medulloblastoma. *Int. J. Cancer*, **124**, 568–577.

28 Pesarin, F. (2001) *Multivariate Permutation Tests with Applications to Biostatistics*, John Wiley and Sons, Ltd, Chichester.

29 Ge, Y., Dudoit, S., and Speed, T.P. (2003) Resampling-based multiple testing for microarray data analysis. *Test*, **12**, 1–77.

30 van der Laan, M.J., Dudoit, S., and Pollard, K.S. (2004) Augmentation procedures for control of the generalized family-wise error rate and tail probabilities for the proportion of false positives. *Stat. Appl. Genet. Mol. Biol.*, **3** (1).

31 Genovese, C.R. and Wasserman, L. (2006) Exceedance control of the false discovery proportion. *J. Am. Stat. Assoc.*, **101**, 1408–1417.

32 Storey, J.D. (2002) A direct approach to false discovery rates. *J. R. Stat. Soc. B Method.*, **64**, 479–498.

33 Lehmann, E.L. and Romano, J.P. (2005) Generalizations of the familywise error rate. *Ann. Stat.*, **33**, 1138–1154.

34 Sarkar, S.K. (2007) Stepup procedures controlling generalized FWER and generalized FDR. *Ann. Stat.*, **35**, 2405–2420.

35 Genovese, C.R. and Wasserman, L. (2002) Operating characteristics and extensions of the FDR procedure. *J. R. Stat. Soc. B Method.*, **64**, 499–518.

36 Sarkar, S.K. (2004) FDR-controlling stepwise procedures and their false negatives rates. *J. Stat. Plan. Infer.*, **125**, 119–137.

37 Wright, S.P. (1992) Adjusted p-values for simultaneous inference. *Biometrics*, **48**, 1005–1010.

38 Welsch, R.E. (1977) Stepwise multiple comparison procedures. *J. Am. Stat. Assoc.*, **72**, 566–575.

39 Turkheimer, F.E., Smith, C.B., and Schmidt, K. (2001) Estimation of the number of "true" null hypotheses in multivariate analysis of neuroimaging data. *NeuroImage*, **13**, 920–930.

40 Meinshausen, N. and Rice, J. (2006) Estimating the proportion of false null hypotheses among a large number of independently tested hypotheses. *Ann. Statis.*, **34**, 373–393.

41 Farcomeni, A. (2006) More powerful control of the false discovery rate under dependence. *Stat. Method Appl.*, **15**, 43–73.

42 Shaffer, J. (1995) Multiple hypothesis testing. *Ann. Rev. Psychol.*, **46**, 561–584.

43 Hochberg, Y. (1988) A sharper Bonferroni procedure for multiple tests of significance. *Biometrika*, **75**, 800–802.

44 Sidak, Z. (1967) Rectangular confidence regions for the means of multivariate normal distributions. *J. Am. Stat. Assoc.*, **62**, 626–633.

45 Sidak, Z. (1971) On probabilities of rectangles in multivariate Student distributions: their dependence on correlations. *Ann. Math. Stat.*, **42**, 169–175.

46 Dunnet, C.W. and Tamhane, A.C. (1992) A step-up multiple test procedure. *J. Am. Stat. Assoc.*, **87**, 162–170.

47 Benjamini, Y. and Hochberg, Y. (2000) The adaptive control of the false discovery rate in multiple hypothesis testing with independent test statistics. *J. Educ. Behav. Stat.*, **25**, 60–83.

48 Yekutieli, D. and Benjamini, Y. (1999) Resampling-based false discovery rate controlling multiple test procedures for correlated test statistics. *J. Stat. Plan. Infer.*, **82**, 171–196.

49 Simes, R.J. (1986) An improved Bonferroni procedure for multiple tests of significance. *Biometrika*, **73**, 751–754.

50 Benjamini, Y., Krieger, A.M., and Yekutieli, D. (2006) Adaptive linear step up procedures that control the false discovery rate. *Biometrika*, **93**, 491–507.

51 Tusher, V.G., Tibshirani, R., and Chu, G. (2001) Significance analysis of microarrays applied to the ionizing radiation response. *Proc. Natl. Acad. Sci. USA*, **98**, 5116–5121.

52 Neuhaus, K.L., Von Essen, R., Tebbe, U., Vogt, A., Roth, M., Riess, M. *et al.* (1992) Improved thrombolysis in acute myocardial infarction front-loaded administration of Alteplase: results of the rt-PA-APSAC patency study (TAPS). *J. Am. Coll. Cardiol.*, **19**, 885–891.

53 Romano, J.P. and Wolf, M. (2005) Stepwise multiple testing as formalized data snooping. *Econometrica*, **73**, 1237–1282.

54 Owen, A.B. (2005) Variance of the number of false discoveries. *J. R. Stat. Soc. B Method.*, **67**, 411–426.

55 van der Laan, M.J., Birkner, M.D., and Hubbard, A.E. (2005) Empirical Bayes and resampling based multiple testing procedure controlling tail probability of the proportion of false positives. *Stat Appl. Genet. Mol. Biol.*, **4** (1).

56 Guo, W. and Romano, J. (2007) A Generalized Sidak-Holm procedure and control of generalized error rates under independence. *Stat. Appl. Genet. Mol. Biol.*, **6** (1).

57 Romano, J.P. and Wolf, M. (2007) Control of generalized error rates in multiple testing. *Ann. Stat.*, **35**, 1378–1408.

58 Farcomeni, A. (2009) Generalized augmentation to control the false discovery exceedance in multiple testing. *Scand. J. Stat.*, **36**, 501–517.

59 Clarke, S. and Hall, P. (2009) Robustness of multiple testing procedures against dependence. *Ann. Stat.*, **37**, 332–358.

60 Leek, J.T. and Storey, J.D. (2008) A general framework for multiple testing dependence. *Proc. Natl. Acad. Sci. USA*, **105**, 18718–18723.

61 Sarkar, S.K. (1998) Some probability inequalities for ordered $MTP2$ random variables: a proof of the Simes conjecture. *Ann. Stat.*, **26**, 494–504.

62 Sarkar, S.K. and Chang, C.K. (1997) The Simes method for multiple hypothesis testing with positively dependent test statistics. *J. Am. Stat. Assoc.*, **92**, 1601–1608.

63 Jogdeo, K. (1977) Association and probability inequalities. *Ann. Stat.*, **5**, 495–504.

64 Benjamini, Y. and Yekutieli, D. (2001) The control of the false discovery rate in multiple testing under dependency. *Ann. Stat.*, **29**, 1165–1188.

65 Sarkar, S.K. (2002) Some results on false discovery rate in stepwise multiple testing procedures. *Ann. Stat.*, **30**, 239–257.

66 Farcomeni, A. (2007) Some results on the control of the false discovery rate under dependence. *Scand. J. Stat.*, **34**, 275–297.

67 Reiner, A., Yekutieli, D., and Benjamini, Y. (2003) Identifying differentially expressed genes using false discovery rate controlling procedures. *Bioinformatics*, **19**, 368–375.

68 Alon, U., Barkai, N., Notterman, D.A., Gish, K., Ybarra, S., Mack, D. *et al.* (1999) Broad patterns of gene expression revealed by clustering analysis of tumor and normal colon tissue probed by oligonucleotide arrays. *Proc. Natl. Acad. Sci. USA*, **96**, 6745–6750.

69 Golub, T.R., Slonim, D.K., Tamayo, P., Huard, C., Gaasenbeek, M., Mesirov, J.P., Coller, H. *et al.* (1999) Molecular classification of cancer: class discovery and class prediction by gene expression monitoring. *Science*, **286**, 531–537.

70 Cover, T. and Hart, P. (1967) Nearest neighbor pattern classification. *IEEE T. Inform. Theory*, **IT-13**, 21–27.

71 Genovese, C.R., Roeder, K., and Wasserman, L. (2006) False discovery control with *p*-value weighting. *Biometrika*, **93**, 509–524.

72 Westfall, P.H., Kropf, S., and Finos, L. (2004) Weighted FWE-controlling methods in high-dimensional situations, in *Recent Developments in Multiple Comparison Procedures*, (eds Y. Benjamini, F. Bretz, and S. Sarkar), IMS Lecture Notes–Monograph Series, vol. **47**, Institute of Mathematical Statistics, Beachwood, Ohio, pp. 143–154.

73 Benjamini, Y. and Hochberg, Y. (1997) Multiple hypothesis testing with weights. *Scand. J. Stat.*, **24**, 407–418.

74 Moyé, L.A. (1998) P-value interpretation and alpha allocation in clinical trials. *Ann. Epidemiol.*, **8**, 351–357.

75 Pocock, S.J., Geller, N.L., and Tsiatis, A.A. (1987) The analysis of multiple endpoints in clinical trials. *Biometrics*, **43**, 487–498.

76 Lehmacher, W., Wassmer, G., and Reitmeir, P. (1991) Procedures for two-sample comparisons with multiple endpoints controlling the experiment-wise error rate. *Biometrics*, **47**, 511–521.

77 Follmann, D. (1995) Multivariate tests for multiple endpoints in clinical trials. *Stat. Med.*, **14**, 1163–1175.

78 Chi, G.Y.H. (1998) Multiple testings: multiple comparisons and multiple endpoints. *Drug Inf. J.*, **32**, 1347S–1362S.

79 Storey, J.D. and Tibshirani, R. (2001) Estimating false discovery rates under dependence, with applications to DNA microarrays. Department of Statistics, Stanford University, pp. 2001–2028.

80 Newton, M.A., Noueiry, A., Sarkar, D., and Ahlquist, P. (2004) Detecting differential gene expression with a semiparametric hierarchical mixture method. *Biostatistics*, **5**, 155–176.

81 Pawitan, Y., Calza, S., and Ploner, A. (2006) Estimation of false discovery proportion under general dependence. *Bioinformatics*, **22**, 3025–3031.

82 Alfo, M., Farcomeni, A., and Tardella, L. (2007) Robust semiparametric mixing for detecting differentially expressed genes in microarray experiments. *Comput. Stat. Data Anal.*, **51** (11), 5253–5265.

83 Müller, P., Parmigiani, G., Robert, C., and Rousseau, J. (2004) Optimal sample size for multiple testing: the case of gene expression microarrays. *J. Am. Stat. Assoc.*, **99**, 990–1001.

84 Tibshirani, R. (2006) A simple method for assessing sample sizes in microarray experiments. *BMC Bioinformatics*, **7**, 106.

Part Two
Statistical and Computational Analysis Methods

4
Making Mountains Out of Molehills: Moving from Single Gene to Pathway Based Models of Colon Cancer Progression

Elena Edelman, Katherine Garman, Anil Potti, and Sayan Mukherjee

4.1
Introduction

Cancer is a heterogeneous disease requiring the accumulation of mutations to proceed through tumorigenesis. The genetic heterogeneity of the disease is caused by two main sources: time or stage of disease progression and variability across individuals. Building separate models for different disease stages addresses heterogeneity across time and selecting genes that are consistently mutated addresses variation across individuals. The problem with this stratification approach is loss of power due to smaller sample sizes in each separate model. A classic paradigm in addressing this problem is to borrow strength by building models jointly across all of the data. We applied this paradigm both across genes and stages of progression.

In modeling tumor progression it is vital to both analyze the transitions between individual stages and learn what is common to progression in general. The analysis of specific transitions would shed light on the molecular mechanism driving a particular stage of tumorigenesis. The analysis of progression in general would shed light on shared mechanisms. We use a machine learning algorithm called regularized multi-task learning (RMTL) that allows us to model a tumor's progression through advancing disease stages.

In addition to genetic heterogeneity acquired over time, there is a great deal of heterogeneity across individuals. An indication of this is that typically about 15 mutated genes drive cancer; however, these genes differ greatly from individual to individual [1]. In fact, most genes are mutated in less than 5% of tumors. Wood *et al.* describe the genomic landscape of cancer as having a few "gene mountains" and many "gene hills." The gene mountains refer to the genes found to be mutated in almost all tumors of a given type. The gene hills are mutated less frequently and likely comprise a smaller number of pathways or functional sets since numerous gene mutations can result in the same phenotypic alteration [1, 2]. This variability in the gene hills makes it difficult to understand which genes are acting as drivers of tumorigenesis. The idea of pathway analysis is to borrow strength across genes by considering a priori defined sets of genes rather than individual genes. Modeling tumor progression at the pathway level can help bring structure to the complicated landscape of cancer. Pathway analysis has proven to be useful in providing insight about the underlying biologic processes governing tumor development and has provided a means for better functional and mechanistic insight into the cause of phenotypic differences [3–9]. Pathway analysis is particularly important for studying cancer development because of the degree of variability in mutations at the single gene level, highlighting the idea that disease development can follow various courses. We believe that studying tumorigenesis on the pathway level will provide finer structure in modeling cancer progression by organizing the variability seen in single genes into underlying functional occurrences.

In this chapter we advance the colorectal cancer progression model presented by Fearon and Vogelstein [10] from the single gene level to the pathway level. Fearon and Vogelstein [10] presented a model of colorectal cancer progression, identifying times at which specific genes or chromosomal regions tend to experience perturbations during the course of the disease. Vital to the progression model is the idea that multiple mutations must occur for the disease to develop and it is not the specific order in which these mutations arise but the general accumulation that is necessary. The main genomic alterations in the Fearon and Vogelstein model are KRAS activation, TP53 inactivation, and APC inactivation [10]. Subsequent studies have supported these findings, including the recent report by Wood *et al.* [1] that describes KRAS, TP53, and APC as the gene mountains of colorectal cancer.

The KRAS, TP53, and APC gene mountains are difficult to target by drug treatments and using these genes as a basis for new treatments has proven unsuccessful. Analyses on the single gene level have not been able to isolate any of the gene hills as significant in colorectal cancer. Gaining a deeper understanding of the composition of gene hills into biological pathways that are relevant to colon cancer initiation and progression may lead to identification of novel targets for drug treatment. We investigated regulatory pathways that become perturbed at different stages of colorectal cancer development in order to identify new "pathway mountains," pathways that become deregulated in most colorectal cancer samples. The result is the identification of biological pathways predicted to be not only important in colon tumorigenesis but also represent rational targets for therapeutic strategies.

4.2
Methods

The steps involved in the data collection and analysis in this chapter are provided. Further details on RMTL and modeling tumor progression can be found in the literature [23, 24].

4.2.1
Data Collection and Standardization

The data consisted of 32 samples of normal colon epithelium (n), 32 samples of colon adenoma (a), 35 samples of stage 1 carcinoma (c_1), 82 samples of stage 2 carcinoma

(c_2), 70 samples of stage 3 carcinoma (c_3), and 43 samples of stage 4 carcinoma (c_4), all collected from NCBIs Gene Expression Omnibus (GEO, http://www.ncbi.nlm.nih.gov/geo). The reference series for the data are GSE5206, GSE2138, GSE2109, GSE2461, and GSE4107. All samples were assayed on the Affymetrix Human Genome U133 Plus 2.0 Array.

These samples are a collection from studies that used various normalization methods and processing. For this reason we preprocessed the data using quantile normalization so that the distribution of expression measurements over the probes on the array is comparable across samples. The normalized samples and their corresponding stages are provided in Supplemental Table 5.

4.2.2
Stratification and Mapping to Gene Sets

Each dataset was initially split in half where the first half was used to build the model (training data) and the second half was used to validate the model (testing data). The first two steps in the analysis are stratifying the data and mapping the data into a representation based on pathways. These steps were applied to both the training and testing datasets.

The data can be represented as a set of pairs $D = \{(x_i, y_i)\}_{i=1}^{n}$ where $x_i \in \mathbb{R}^p$ is the expression over p genes and y_i is the disease stage of the patient. Assume that there are six stages, $y \in \{n, a, c_1, c_2, c_3, c_4\}$ with $n_1, n_2, n_3, n_4, n_5, n_6$ samples in each stage of the training data and $n_7, n_8, n_9, n_{10}, n_{11} n_{12}$ samples in each stage of the testing data. The progression is $\{n \rightarrow a \rightarrow c_1 \rightarrow c_2 \rightarrow c_3 \rightarrow c_4\}$. There are five steps in this progression, $T = 5$.

We first stratify the train and test datasets with respect to these five steps. The first dataset $D_1 = \{(x_1, y_1)\}_{i=1}^{n_1+n_2}$ consists of the n_1 training samples corresponding to stage n followed by the n_2 training samples corresponding to stage a with the label of the first n_1 samples labeled as 0 (less serious) and the remaining n_2 labeled as 1 (more serious). D_2 is constructed similarly, consisting of training samples corresponding to stage a followed by stage c_1 and again labeled as 0 and 1, respectively, for less and more serious. Likewise D_3 consists of the c_1 and c_2 training samples, D_4 consists of the c_2 and c_3 training samples, and D_5 consists of the c_3 and c_4 training samples. The same procedure was applied to the testing samples to create $D_6, \ldots, D_{10}$.

Each dataset D_t is then mapped into a representation with respect to sets of genes or pathways. This is achieved using the pathway annotation tool ASSESS [25], which assays pathway variation in individuals. Given phenotypic label data $Y_n = \{y_1, \ldots, y_n\}$, expression data $X_n = \{x_1, \ldots, x_n\}$, and gene sets $\Gamma = \{\gamma_1, \ldots, \gamma_m\}$ defined a priori, ASSESS provides the summary statistic $S_n = S(X_n, Y_n, \Gamma)$. The summary statistic S_n is a matrix with n columns corresponding to samples and m rows corresponding to gene sets with each element S_{ij} as the enrichment of gene expression differences in the j-th sample with respect to phenotype for genes in the i-th gene set. The application of ASSESS to the stratified datasets $D_1, \ldots, D_{10}$ results in ten datasets $S_1, \ldots, S_{10}$. The functional and positional gene sets used in our analysis were those annotated in the MSigDB [9] and are listed in Supplemental Tables 1 and 2 respectively. The analysis was preformed twice, once using the gene sets in Supplemental Table 1 to find relevant functional gene sets and then again using the gene sets in Supplemental Table 2 to find relevant positional gene sets.

4.2.3
Regularized Multi-task Learning

The idea behind the methodologies called multi-task learning [24] in the machine learning literature and hierarchical models with mixed effects in the statistics literature is that given T classification problems the conditional distributions of the response variable Y given the explanatory variable X of these T problems – $Y_t|X_t$ for $t = 1, \ldots, T$ – are related. Here we restrict ourselves to linear models and classification. The basic idea is that we have T classification problems in our case assigning a sample x_i to labels 0 (less serious) or 1 (more serious). We assume that the classification tasks are related so the conditional distributions of the phenotype given the summary statistics $\mu_t(Y|S)$ are also related. The tasks in our case are the different steps in tumor progression and the data over all tasks is $S = \{S_1, \ldots, S_T\}$ where $S_j = \{(y_{1j}, s_{1j}), \ldots, (y_{n_jj}, s_{n_jj})\}$ and n_j is the number of samples in the j-th task. We assume the generalized linear model:

$$y_{it} = g[s_{it} \cdot (w_0 + v_t) + b] = g[s_{it} \cdot w_t + b] \qquad (4.1)$$

where

$w_t = w_0 + v_t$, y_{it} is the i-th sample in task t,
s_{it} are the summary statistics of the i-th sample in task t,
w_0 is the baseline term over all tasks,
v_t are the task specific corrections,
b is an offset.

The vectors w_t correspond to the linear model for each task.

We used the RML framework developed in Reference [24] to estimate the model parameters w_0, v_t, b:

$$\min_{w_0, v_t, b} \sum_{t=1}^{T} \sum_{i=1}^{n_T} (1 - y_{it} \cdot f(s_{it}))_+ + \lambda_1 ||w_0||^2 + \lambda_2 \sum_{t=1}^{T} ||v_t||^2 \qquad (4.2)$$

where $(u)_+ = \min(u, 0)$ is the hinge loss, $f(s_{it}) = s_{it} \cdot (w_0 + v_t) + b$, and λ_1, and λ_2 are positive regularization parameters that trade-off between fitting the data and the smoothness or robustness of the estimates. See Supplementary Methods for how lambdas were chosen.

Given the vectors w_t we simply use a threshold, τ, to select gene sets corresponding to coordinates of the vectors with $|w_{ti}| > \tau$ to find pathways relevant to the t-th step in progression. In this chapter τ is selected such that we obtain a specific number of pathways.

We use regularized multi-task learning (RMTL) to find gene sets relevant to progression. The RMTL algorithm was first applied to $\{S_1, S_2\}$ to find the gene sets relevant in early progression, from $\{n \rightarrow a \rightarrow c_1\}$ in the training sets. RMTL was then applied to $\{S_3, S_4, S_5\}$ to find the gene sets relevant during carcinoma progression, $\{c_1 \rightarrow c_2 \rightarrow c_3 \rightarrow c_4\}$ in the training sets. The same procedure was carried out for the test datasets. For both the early progression and the carcinoma progression analyses, the RMTL algorithm output a set vectors $\{w_0, w_t\}$ where the elements of w_0 correspond to the relevance of a gene set over all stages of the particular analysis and the elements of w_t correspond to the relevance of a gene set with respect to the t-th step in progression of the particular analysis. Therefore, the result is a list of gene sets ordered by relevance to $\{n \rightarrow a \rightarrow c_1\}$, a list of gene sets ordered by relevance to $\{c_1 \rightarrow c_2 \rightarrow c_3 \rightarrow c_4\}$, and lists of gene sets ordered by relevance to each stage transition. These lists were created for both the training and testing datasets.

4.2.4
Validation via Mann–Whitney Test

We selected the top 50 functional gene sets from each list from the training data. We tested the significance of these lists of 50 gene sets by applying the Mann–Whitney test on the lists generated from the testing datasets. The 50 top gene sets from the training data were labeled as class 1 and the remaining gene sets were labeled as class 2. The Mann–Whitney test was used to assess whether class 1 and class 2 had the same distribution in the testing data. A p-value of ≤ 0.05 validated that the top 50 gene sets from the training data were also relevant in the testing data.

As mentioned early, the same procedure was used for both the functional and positional gene sets. The only difference at this step was that the top 50 functional gene sets were selected and the top 40 positional gene sets were selected. We selected these numbers as they were the smallest numbers that returned p-values ≤ 0.05 for each stage transition (Table 4.1).

We further tested for significance by randomly selecting a list of 50 gene sets for the functional gene set analysis and 40 gene sets for the positional gene set analysis, labeling them as class 1 and the remainders as class 2, and performed the Mann–Whitney test on the same test data as described above. We repeated this randomization 1000 times and calculated the p-value from the Mann–Whitney test for each randomization. These p-values were considered the null distribution of p-values from the Mann–Whitney test and we found where the true p-value fell within this null distribution. In all cases, the p-values gave confidence in the significance of the results (see Supplemental Table 6 for these results).

4.2.5
Leave-One-Out Error

We applied the leave-one-out procedure for classification accuracy. The dataset $\{S_t\}_{t=1}^{T}$ is split into s_i (the i-th data sample) and $S^{/i}$ (the data without the i-th sample). RMTL is applied to the training set, $S^{/i}$ to build a classifier based on $\{w_0, w_t\}_{t=1}^{T}$ which

Table 4.1 Significance of the gene sets identified in the analysis. The top 40 positional (chromosomal region) gene sets and the top 50 functional (pathway) gene sets were identified from the first half of the data for each stage and p-values were calculated using the Mann–Whitney rank test on the second half of the data; 286 positional gene sets and 511 functional gene sets were used in the analysis. Rows indicate the p-values and Bonferroni corrected FWER p-values of the sets identified over multiple stage transitions or individual stage transitions. Samples are classified as normal (n), adenoma (a), stage 1 carcinoma (c_1), stage 2 carcinoma (c_2), stage 3 carcinoma (c_3), and stage 4 carcinoma (c_4).

Stages	Positional	Functional
$n \to a \to c_1$	5.31×10^{-6} (0.0015)	2.11×10^{-16} (1.08×10^{-13})
$c_1 \to c_2 \to c_3 \to c_4$	0.038 (>1)	0.031 (>1)
$n \to a$	5.80×10^{-9} (1.66×10^{-6})	1.18×10^{-25} (6.03×10^{-23})
$a \to c_1$	1.67×10^{-8} (4.77×10^{-6})	5.05×10^{-21} (2.58×10^{-18})
$c_1 \to c_2$	0.046 (>1)	0.011 (>1)
$c_2 \to c_3$	0.0043 (>1)	0.049 (>1)
$c_3 \to c_4$	4.01×10^{-8} (1.15×10^{-5})	2.34×10^{-9} (1.20×10^{-6})

is applied to s_i to obtain a prediction $\hat{y}_i$. Prediction accuracy is computed by applying the leave-one-out procedure to all samples in the dataset.

4.3 Results

Previous studies have shown that there is a genetic basis for the differences between normal, adenoma, and carcinoma colon cancer samples [1, 2, 11]. We preformed hierarchical clustering single linkage clustering [12] on a dataset of normal, adenoma, and stage 1 carcinoma samples; see Section 4.2 for details on the samples. The results confirm that these three classes can be differentiated based on expression profiles (Figure 4.1). This separation suggests that different biological processes may be relevant in different stages of progression and provides a logical basis for stratifying the samples into the categories of normal (n), adenoma (a), stage 1 carcinoma (c_1), stage 2 carcinoma (c_2), stage 3 carcinoma (c_3), and stage 4 carcinoma (c_4) [see Section 4.2 (Methods) for details of sample collection].

The a priori defined gene sets used in our model consist of 511 functional pathway gene sets and 286 chromosome position gene sets as defined by Reference [9]; see Section 4.2 (Methods) for details regarding the gene sets. Regularized multi-task learning was used to infer a list of functional pathways and positional gene sets relevant across all stages of progression and those relevant to specific stages. We first state summary statistics of gene sets enriched across stages of colorectal cancer and show that our model is robust and predictive. Gene sets found to be significant in our analysis are then compared to the Fearon and Vogelstein model [10]. In this part of the analysis we found that their single gene model could be recapitulated on the pathway level through the identification of alterations in the KRAS, P53, and WNT pathways (Figure 4.2). The final results relate novel findings from our model to possible new

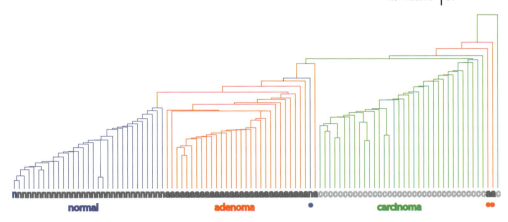

Figure 4.1 Hierarchical clustering on the gene expression of 32 normal (labeled "n", colored blue), 32 adenoma (labeled "a", colored red), and 35 stage 1 carcinoma (labeled "c", colored green) samples. With the exception of one normal sample and two adenoma samples (indicated with asterisks), all samples cluster with their respective cell type, validating that there is indeed a genetic basis for the difference between the cell types.

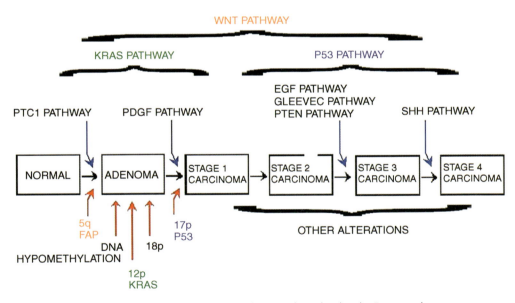

Figure 4.2 Model of the deregulation in colorectal cancer progression. Pathways are indicated at the top of the figure. Pathways identified to be relevant at specific points in progression are indicated with blue arrows. The KRAS, P53, and WNT pathways are shown to be relevant over multiple stages in progression. Single genes deregulated in the Fearon and Vogelstein model [10] are shown on the bottom of the figure with red arrows indicating the times in colorectal cancer progression when they tend to be mutated. The three gene mountains and corresponding pathways are color-coded in green, purple, and orange.

drug treatments for colorectal cancer. Here, we infer the relationship of pathways such as SHH, PDGF, and Gleevec to colorectal cancer and discuss the therapeutic potential and optimal times to target these pathways.

4.3.1
Development and Validation of Model Statistics

We identified pathways and chromosomal regions deregulated at specific transitions in colorectal cancer as well as pathways and chromosomal regions deregulated over multiple stages of progression. These gene sets were identified using half of the samples in each class and their significance was then validated on the second half of the data using a Mann–Whitney test [see Section 4.2 (Methods) for details]. The resulting *p*-values and Bonferroni corrected family-wise error rates (FWER) are displayed in Table 4.1. The gene sets selected are significant at the 0.05 level for all transitions.

The robustness of the inference was measured using two metrics. First, we tested the accuracy in predicting disease stage phenotype. A leave-one-out cross validation analysis resulted in 100% accuracy in the prediction of the normal, adenoma, and stage 1 carcinomas and 81.5% for prediction of carcinoma stages 2 through 4. For the second metric we tested the variability in the pathways selected as significant in each stage and across stages. We split the data in half and applied our procedure to both splits and computed the overlap between gene sets found to be significant at the 0.05 level in the two splits respectively. The number of overlapping gene sets was found to be significant for both individual stages and across all stages of progression for both positional and functional gene sets; see Table 4.2 for *p*-values. The *p*-values were computed from the hypergeometric distribution.

A confounding factor in pathway level analyses is the fact that since genes may appear in multiple pathways it is difficult to attribute relations between pathways to mechanism or function rather than how many genes overlap between pathways. This confound is typically not an issue. For example, we found that the KRAS and EGF pathways are both significant in progression of colorectal cancer without any genes

Table 4.2 *p*-Values corresponding to significance of the overlap between the gene sets determined to be significant in two independent splits of the data. For each stage, the data is split in half and the overlap of the significant gene sets in both splits is computed. The *p*-value is computed using a hypergeometric distribution.

Stages	Chromosomal regions	Pathways
$n \to a \to c_1$	0.0069	2.00×10^{-4}
$c_1 \to c_2 \to c_3 \to c_4$	0.019	0.018
$n \to a$	8.23×10^{-6}	7.18×10^{-6}
$a \to c_1$	0.012	2.50×10^{-4}
$c_1 \to c_2$	0.025	0.017
$c_2 \to c_3$	0.032	0.016
$c_3 \to c_4$	0.011	0.0024

overlapping. In fact of all the pathways involved in our model of progression the only ones that shared more than two genes in common were the Gleevec, PTEN, and PDGF pathways, which consisted of 22, 18, and 27 genes respectively. The overlap between the EGF pathway and the Gleevec pathway was six genes, as was the overlap with the EGF pathway and the PDGF pathway. The Gleevec and PDGF pathways have 15 genes in common.

4.3.2
Comparison of Single Gene and Gene Set Models

Our gene set based model is compared to the single gene model of colorectal cancer progression proposed by Fearon and Vogelstein [10]. There is strong agreement between our gene set based model and the Fearon and Vogelstein model, as shown in Figure 4.2.

The first component of the single gene model is a mutation in the KRAS gene, located on chromosome 12p12. It had been previously reported that approximately 50% of colorectal tumors show a RAS mutation by the time they reach the carcinoma stage [11] and the mutation can potentially act as an initiating event or a driver of an adenoma into a carcinoma [10]. Likewise, we found that the KRAS pathway gene set is increasingly expressed from $\{n \to a \to c_1\}$. Additionally, gene sets representing the chromosomal region of KRAS, along with surrounding regions were found to be deregulated. Both 12p11 and 12p13 are found to be overexpressed early in progression, $\{n \to a \to c_1\}$, followed by 12p12 over-expression as the tumor progresses during carcinoma, $\{c_2 \to c_3\}$. We also found the deregulation of pathways that are closely associated with RAS. For instance, the EGF pathway is upregulated during the transition from $\{c_2 \to c_3\}$. Similarly associated with the RAS pathway is the PTDINS gene set which is upregulated from $\{c_3 \to c_4\}$. This gene set describes PI3-kinases and their downstream targets. Members of the PTDINS gene set are known to act as activators of the AKT pathway, an effector pathway of RAS. Genes in the PTDINS gene set also signal the PTEN pathway. The PTEN pathway normally functions in tumor suppression but is shown to be downregulated from $\{c_2 \to c_3\}$, allowing for cell proliferation.

Vogelstein et al. [11] observed that chromosome 17p, where TP53 is located, is deleted in 75% of colorectal cancer cases. The Fearon and Vogelstein model [10] includes a mutation to 17p in late adenoma to early carcinoma. In our analysis, we found that a P53 gene set is inactivated throughout the progression from $\{c_1 \to c_2 \to c_3 \to c_4\}$. We also found the chromosome 17p gene set to be lost in early carcinoma, $\{c_1 \to c_2\}$.

Another tumor suppressor gene included in the Fearon and Vogelstein model [10] was the APC gene, located on chromosome 5q. APC is the most commonly acquired mutation in sporadic colon cancer, occurring in 60% of colorectal carcinomas [13]. We found the gene set for chromosome 5q21 was lost at the tumor initiation stage, $\{n \to a\}$, which is consistent with previous studies [10]. At the pathway level we identified regulatory pathways that associated with allelic loss of 5q and APC. APC is a tumor suppressor gene that suppresses the oncogene β-catenin (CTNNB1).

APC and β-catenin are components of the WNT signaling pathway, which we found upregulated during the entire course of progression, $\{n \rightarrow a \rightarrow c1\}$ and $\{c1 \rightarrow c2 \rightarrow c3 \rightarrow c4\}$. When this pathway is activated, the APC complex, which normally degrades β-catenin, is inhibited, allowing for β-catenin build up and uncontrolled cell proliferation.

The final major component of the Fearon and Vogelstein model was a mutation in 18q in the late adenoma stage. Although there is not a regulatory pathway associated with this chromosomal region, we found the allelic loss of the chromosome 18q gene set in the $\{a \rightarrow c_1\}$ transition. This region is found to be lost in more than 70% of colorectal cancers by the time they reach the carcinoma stage [10].

In addition to reiterating the Fearon and Vogelstein model on the pathway level, the predictions of our analysis agree strongly with the gene mountains described by Wood et al. [1], who observed that KRAS, TP53, and APC had at least one non-synonymous mutation in each of 131 colorectal tumors in the study, with APC showing the most mutations per sample.

4.3.3
Novel Pathway Findings and Therapeutic Implications

One hypothesis for modeling tumorigenesis [1, 2] is that the heterogeneity of the disease cannot be captured by single gene models since there are very few gene mountains and the vast majority of genes implicated in tumor progression, the gene hills, are mutated in only a fraction of individuals. It is essential to understand these mutations as they make up the greatest part of the genomic landscape of colorectal cancer. By integrating the gene hills into functional pathways or positional gene sets our objective is to identify new mountains on the pathway level, or "pathway mountains." Another strong motivation of our analysis was to find novel pathways that can be targeted with current drug therapies. The genes strongly implicated in single gene models such as KRAS, TP53, and APC have been difficult to target with current drug therapies. For these reasons we focused in greater detail on gene sets found in our analysis that have not typically been associated with colorectal cancer in order to identify new pathways as potential targets for novel therapy.

The sonic hedgehog (SHH) pathway was found to be upregulated from $\{c_3 \rightarrow c_4\}$. The SHH pathway has been implicated in the development of several cancer types such as specific brain and skin carcinomas [14, 15], but rarely with colorectal cancer. In a more recent study [16], colorectal cancer cells were treated with cyclopamine, an inhibitor of SHH signaling. Both adenomas and carcinomas experienced apoptosis. Additionally, our analysis has shown the PTC1 pathway to be deregulated in the $\{n \rightarrow a\}$ transition. The PTC1 pathway describes the genes involved as PTCH1, a receptor in the SHH pathway, regulates the cell cycle. The WNT, SHH, and PCT1 pathways often act together in controlling cell growth. Our analysis identified these pathways to be deregulated, suggesting that targeting these pathways may be beneficial for colorectal cancer treatment. Our inference that the PTC1 pathway is deregulated before the SHH pathway suggests a basis for the order of events during tumorigenesis.

The Gleevec pathway – genes that respond to treatment by imatinib mesylate – was found to be deregulated in the $\{c_2 \to c_3\}$ transition. Further evidence supporting the use of imatinib mesylate as therapeutic agent was the deregulation of the PDGF pathway, a target for imatinib mesylate, in the $\{a \to c_1\}$ transition. Imatinib mesylate has been used to treat chronic myeloid leukemia [17–19] as well as gastrointestinal stromal tumors [20, 21]. The affects of imatinib mesylate in colorectal cancer has been less well studied. However, a study of imatinib mesylate on human colorectal cancer cells [22] found that the treatment of human colorectal cancer cells with imatinib suppressed cell proliferation. The mechanism for this seemed to be inhibition of β-catenin signaling by tyrosine phosphorylation.

4.4 Discussion

Colorectal tumorigenesis is an example of a complex trait as it is controlled by many genes that do not interact additively and the relationship between genetic and phenotypic variation is nonlinear. Standard genetic models of tumor progression are based on a multi-step process formulated as mutations and interactions of single genes – a framework common to many models of complex traits. In this chapter we use an approach that integrates variation both across genes as well as across stages of progression using the concepts of pathway analysis and multi-task learning. We believe this is a promising general approach to model tumor progression.

Using this approach the colorectal cancer progression model presented by Fearon and Vogelstein [10] was extended from the single gene level to the pathway level. Many of the findings in the Fearon and Vogelstein model such as mutation of the "gene mountains" KRAS, TP53, and APC were recapitulated at the pathway level. In addition, we inferred the stage in progression that these pathways drive tumorigenesis: KRAS pathway was upregulated across early progression, P53 pathway was downregulated across carcinoma progression, and APC was implicated throughout all of progression through WNT signaling upregulation.

The ability of our approach to identify a small number of pathways important to a majority of tumors resulted in the novel association of pathways to progression in colorectal cancer. An implication of our approach is that although single genes may be greatly variable across tumors, groups of genes corresponding to pathways integrate the gene hills into pathway mountains that become deregulated in most colorectal cancer samples. Some of the novel pathways we identify suggest both drug agents and at what stages of progression the agents would be most efficacious.

Supporting Information

All supplemental tables can be found at: http://people.genome.duke.edu/~eje2/supplemental/.

Acknowledgments

S.M. and A.P. would like to acknowledge the IGSP for funds. S.M. would like to acknowledge NSF DMS 0732260 and NIH (P50 GM 081883) for funding. A.P. would like to acknowledge the American Cancer Society and the Emilene Brown Cancer Research Fund for funding.

References

1 Wood, L.D., Parsons, D.W., Jones, S., Lin, J., Sjoblom, T. et al. (2007) The genomic landscapes of human breast and colorectal cancers. *Science*, **318**, 1108–1113.

2 Sjoblom, T., Jones, S., Wood, L.D., Parsons, D.W., Lin, J. et al. (2006) The consensus coding sequences of human breast and colorectal cancers. *Science*, **314**, 268–274.

3 Huang, E., Ishida, S., Pittman, J., Dressman, H., Bild, A. et al. (2003) Gene expression phenotypic models that predict the activity of oncogenic pathways. *Nat. Genet.*, **34**, 226–230.

4 Black, E.P., Huang, E., Dressman, H., Rempel, R., Laakso, N. et al. (2003) Distinct gene expression phenotypes of cells lacking Rb and Rb family members 1,2. *Proc. Am. Assoc. Cancer Res.*, **63**, 3716–3723.

5 Mootha, V.K., Lindgren, C.M., Eriksson, K.F., Subramanian, A., Sihag, S. et al. (2003) PGC-1 a-responsive genes involved in oxidative phosphorylation are coordinately downregulated in human diabetes. *Nat. Genet.*, **34**, 267–273.

6 Sweet-Cordero, A., Mukherjee, S., Subramanian, A., You, H., Roix, J.J. et al. (2005) An oncogenic KRAS2 expression signature identified by cross-species gene-expression analysis. *Nat. Genet.*, **37**, 48–55.

7 Alvarez, J.V., Febbo, P.G., Ramaswamy, S., Loda, M., Richardson, A. et al. (2005) Identification of a genetic signature of activated signal transducer and activator of transcription 3 in human tumors. *Proc. Am. Assoc. Cancer Res.*, **65**, 5054–5062.

8 Febbo, P.G., Richie, J.P., George, D.J., Loda, M., Manola, J. et al. (2005) Neoadjuvant docetaxel before radical prostatectomy in patients with high-risk localized prostate cancer. *Clin. Cancer Res.*, **11**, 5233.

9 Subramanian, A., Tamayo, P., Mootha, V.K., Mukherjee, S., Ebert, B.L. et al. (2005) Gene set enrichment analysis: A knowledge-based approach for interpreting genome-wide expression profiles. *Proc. Natl. Acad. Sci. USA*, **102**, 15545–15550.

10 Fearon, E.R. and Vogelstein, B. (1990) A genetic model for colorectal tumorigenesis. *Cell*, **61**, 759–767.

11 Vogelstein, B., Fearon, E.R., Hamilton, S.R., Kern, S.E., Preisinger, A.C. et al. (1988) Genetic alterations during colorectal-tumor development. *New Engl. J. Med.*, **319**, 525–532.

12 Eisen, M., Spellman, P.T., Brown, P.O., and Botstein, D. (1998) Cluster analysis and display of genome-wide expression patterns. *Proc. Natl. Acad. Sci. USA*, **95** (25), 14863–14868.

13 Powell, S., Zilz, N., Beazer-Barclay, Y., Bryan, T., Hamilton, S. et al. (1992) APC mutations occur early during colorectal tumorigenesis. *Nature*, **395**, 235–237.

14 Berman, D.M., Desai, N., Wang, X., Karhadkar, S.S., Reynon, M. et al. (2004) Roles for hedgehog signaling in androgen production and prostate ductal morphogenesis. *Dev. Biol.*, **267**, 387–398.

15 Dahmane, N., Lee, J., Robins, P., Heller, P., and Ruiz i Altaba, A. (1997) Activation of the transcription factor Gli1 and the Sonic hedgehog signalling pathway in skin tumours. *Nature*, **389**, 876–881.

16 Qualtrough, D., Buda, A., Gaffield, W., Williams, A.C., and Paraskeva, C. (2004) Hedgehog signalling in colorectal tumour

cells: Induction of apoptosis with cyclopamine treatment. *Int. J. Cancer,* **110**, 831–837.

17 Sattler, M. and Griffin, J.D. (2001) Mechanisms of transformation by the BCR/ABL oncogene. *Int. J. Hematol.,* **73**, 278–291.

18 Pestell, K. (2001) Anti-cancer drug success emerges from molecular biology origins. *Trends Pharmacol. Sci.,* **22**, 342.

19 Mauro, M.J. and Druker, B.J. (2001) STI571: Targeting BCR-ABL as therapy for CML. *The Oncol.,* **6**, 233.

20 Heinrich, M.C., Corless, C.L., Von Mehren, M., Joensuu, H., Demetri, G.D. et al. (2003) PDGFRA and KIT mutations correlate with the clinical responses to imatinib mesylate in patients with advanced gastrointestinal stromal tumors (gist). *Proc. Am. Soc. Clin. Oncol.,* **22**, A3274.

21 Demetri, G.D. (2001) Targeting c-kit mutations in solid tumors: scientific rationale and novel therapeutic options. *Semin. Oncol.,* **28**, 19–26.

22 Zhou, L., An, N., Haydon, R.C., Zhou, Q., Cheng, H. et al. (2003) Tyrosine kinase inhibitor STI-571/Gleevec down-regulates the β-catenin signaling activity. *Cancer Lett.,* **193**, 161–170.

23 Edelman, E., Guinney, J., Chi, J., Febbo, P., and Mukherjee, S. (2008) Modeling cancer progression via pathway dependencies. *PLoS Comput. Biol.,* **4**, e28.

24 Evgeniou, T., Micchelli, C., and Pontil, M. (2005) Learning multiple tasks with kernel methods. *J. Mach. Learn. Res.,* **6**, 615–637.

25 Edelman, E., Porrello, A., Guinney, J., Balakumaran, B., Bild, A. et al. (2006) Analysis of sample set enrichment scores: assaying the enrichment of sets of genes for individual samples in genome-wide expression profiles. *Bioinformatics,* **22**, e108–e116.

5
Gene-Set Expression Analysis: Challenges and Tools
Assaf P. Oron

5.1
The Challenge

This chapter focuses on gene-set (GS) expression analysis, which is hailed as a new and promising direction in the microarray field. It is often taken for granted, and sometimes overlooked, that microarray analysis in general and gene-set (GS) signal detection in particular is a sequence of successive data-reduction steps:

1) a tissue sample is biochemically prepared for analysis;
2) the prepared sample is hybridized to a microarray chip containing a selection of cDNA oligonucleotide probes;
3) through optical detection of tagged molecules, hybridization information is reduced to a set of pixel images (typically several per sample);
4) images are pre-processed to produce probe-level summaries;
5) from these summaries, average expression estimates are calculated for each set of replicate probes, producing a $G \times n$ matrix (G genes, n samples, hereafter the expression matrix);
6) the expression matrix is normalized and transformed to make it more "well-behaved";
7) the normalized expression matrix is filtered to remove "redundant" or otherwise "uninformative" probe-sets;
8) dataset-wide expression statistics are calculated for each gene;
9) gene-level statistics are used to calculate GS-level statistics, helping identify differentially expressed or otherwise interesting gene-sets.

The list is not comprehensive: the biochemical steps were described in less detail, due to this chapter's data-analysis focus. In any case, each step in the sequence involves information loss, and introduces potential errors and distortions. One might shrug at this; such sequences are common with modern technology. A useful analogy is the electron microscope, which – just like microarrays – can provide information about organisms at the subcellular level. The interaction between electron beams and the imaging sample's surfaces produces the original signal, which is then translated and converted several times before reaching the viewer. But with electron microscopy, the laws of physics enabling its design and optimization have been known with high precision for quite a while.

Microarray analysis, too, relies upon solid scientific principles, such as the very high binding specificity between matching DNA and RNA strands, and the optical properties of the tagging molecules which enable image scanning. However, other aspects, such as batch and time effects or the degree of nonspecific binding and its dependence on sequence, are poorly understood. As a result, microarray image files (produced by step 3) are already a rather noisy representation of expression patterns. At this point (from step 4 onwards) statisticians and other data analysts are called in to further refine and decipher the picture. This is also where the gap between microarray technology and microscopy is at its starkest. With microscopy, we do have a general notion about how a surface *should* look like; therefore, image calibration and noise removal are fairly straightforward. In contrast, in microarray research settings there is almost no clear, a priori understood expression pattern to work towards. What microarray data analysis is often expected to deliver, therefore, is insight about the very processes whose knowledge could have enabled the technology to produce coherent signals in the first place!

After an initial burst of excitement, the microarray field has recently turned to search for a solid performance baseline, most prominently via the Microarray Quality Control (MAQC) consortium. In 2006 this project declared initial success, because microarrays produced similar, albeit definitely noisier, signals to more precise methods on a selected set of artificial comparisons and were generally in rough agreement with each other after discarding outlier arrays and sites [1]. This announcement was doubted by others [2], but, in general, it seems that when the original expression picture is known (and it was with the MAQC tests) one can extract a useful product from microarrays. Yet, since gene-set analysis lies at the very end of a tortuous and partially understood data-reduction process, caution is advised.

This chapter presents GS expression analysis from a statistical perspective. A GS is any group of genes sharing some common biological property, such as lying in the same chromosomal locus, being associated with the same metabolic pathway, and so on. It is important to keep in mind that statistical models are not, generally speaking, an alternative to scientific laws governing the production of biological signals. Rather, statistical models are pragmatic tools to detect such signals in a responsible manner. In particular, statistical inference procedures facilitate the incorporation of healthy skepticism into the signal-detection process. The next section presents a brief survey of notable GS methods. Section 5.3 walks through a GS data analysis example, starting at step 7 – that is, with a normalized expression matrix. All software used for the analysis was coded in the R statistical language, and is available via the open-source Bioconductor repository (http://bioconductor.org). The chapter concludes with a short summary.

5.2
Survey of Gene-Set Analysis Methods

5.2.1
Motivation for GS Analysis

The individual-gene level (step 8) has been the dominant approach to microarray analysis: to identify a list of differentially expressed (DE) genes. Quite often the list of a priori suspected genes is very short or nonexistent, and the analysis arguably becomes a "fishing expedition" for signals from among thousands, or even tens of thousands, of potential candidates. According to statistical theory, gene-level analysis is a venture deep into the quagmire of *multiple testing*: even in the absence of any true DE gene, spurious signals are inevitably produced in a random manner. Statistical solutions to this problem abound, with the false discovery rate (FDR) [3, 4] becoming a de-facto standard. This method, interestingly developed just before the advent of microarrays, controls the expected false-positive fraction in the DE gene list (under certain statistical assumptions).

However, FDR does not address the scientific and engineering questions of *signal meaning and quality*. Figure 5.1a shows the most commonly used gene-level DE statistic: a *t*-test comparing two phenotype groups of acute lymphoblastic leukemia

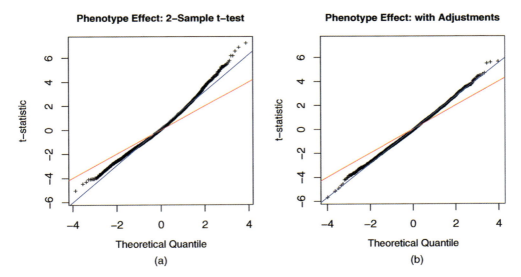

Figure 5.1 (a) Gene-specific *t*-statistics from a test for the phenotype effect in the ALL dataset; 4500 genes were tested; the red line denotes the standard *t*-distribution with 77 degrees of freedom (DF) and the blue line a best-fit *t*-curve; (b) the analogous statistics and fitted curves, but after re-normalizing expression levels by sample, removing samples from teenage subjects, and adjusting for the effects of age and hyperdiploidy. Here the *t*-distribution curve has 50 DF.

(ALL) patients. According to the null hypothesis of no real expression difference, these statistics should be t-distributed with 77 degrees of freedom (shown as a straight red line). The true t-statistic distribution is more disperse and skewed upward. This indicates the existence of unaccounted-for sources of variability in the dataset. These sources may be asymmetrically associated with phenotype-group membership – that is, they are a source for confounding. Confounding may lead to spurious DE signals that cannot be corrected by FDR. Figure 5.1b plots phenotype effect t-statistics for the same dataset, calculated via gene-specific regression models simultaneously adjusting for age and hyperdiploidy. Additionally, expression levels were re-normalized and samples from teenage patients (who belong overwhelmingly to one of the groups) were removed. The curve is much more well-behaved, albeit still more disperse than the theoretical curve. A simple correction of the theoretical curve to reflect the true mean and variance of the t-statistics (straight blue line) seems to suggest there are almost no DE genes, since practically all points are very close to the line. However, in fact we do have scientific knowledge that at least a handful of specific genes should definitely be DE, especially the top two in the upper tail but also the gene whose t-statistic is 20th from the top in Figure 5.1b lying exactly on the blue curve. Either we accept the blue line as reference and give up flagging this gene as DE, or we accept the red line and flag the gene together with hundreds of others. From a statistical perspective, too, there is no good justification for replacing the red line by the blue, but obviously the red line does not fit the true distribution at all. In summary, we do not have an off-the-shelf reference null distribution to carry out our DE tests.

To obtain meaningful p-values, we must resort to sample-label permutations (described in Section 5.2.3). At the gene level these calculations are quite costly. Let G be the number of genes and q be the researcher's tolerated FDR (typically in the 0.05–0.25 range). If we expect roughly g genes to be DE, we should perform more than G/qg permutations for rough preliminary detection. Current microarray chips have tens of thousands of genes, meaning that to generate valid gene-level p-values we may need to run 100 000 permutations, possibly more. Even with today's massive and cheap computing-power availability, this is quite a burden.

Moving one level up in the biological hierarchy from genes to GSs is a win-win solution for scientists and statisticians. Summary statistics based on groups of genes have the standard theoretical benefits promised by the laws of large numbers and the central limit theorem (CLT): simply put, they improve the signal-to-noise ratio. Summarizing across gene groups also means that we carry out only $K \ll G$ tests (with K being the number of GSs), thus greatly reducing the expected number of false positives and the number of required permutations. Scientifically, since these groups of genes are chosen according to biological criteria – for example, pathways, biological function, or chromosomal location – then the identification of a positive GS signal is often more meaningful than that of a single gene.

5.2.2
Some Notable GS Analysis Methods

The simplest type of GS analysis divides all genes into a single GS and all others, and tabulates this division in a contingency table versus membership in the individual-gene DE list. If the proportion of apparently-DE genes in the gene-set is unusually high, the GS as a whole will be flagged as DE. This is known as the "hypergeometric test," referring to the distribution of such a proportion under the null hypothesis that the GS is not really different [5]. While this test is extremely simple to perform, the information reduction is quite severe: we use only a binary outcome (DE or not) for each gene. This type of information may not be sufficient to detect small or medium-sized DE gene-sets. Moreover, an arbitrary individual-gene cutoff used to generate the DE list opens the door to distortions.

A more sophisticated approach is the one that introduced the term "gene-set enrichment analysis" (GSEA), which often serves as a synonym for any GS analysis [6, 7]. Here, too, the starting point is an individual-gene list. The list is ordered according to the strength of association with phenotype (e.g., via a *t*-test statistic as shown in Figure 5.1). For each GS, a meta-statistic based on the order of the GSs genes within the list is calculated and then compared with a permutation-generated reference distribution. While it provides better detection power than the hypergeometric test, the GSEA method is a tailor-made stand-alone product. As such, it derives little benefit from more general statistical methodology (an approach exhibiting similar advantages and limitations has been introduced more recently by Efron and Tibshirani [8].)

A more standard approach views the DE detection challenge (single-gene or GS) as a *regression* problem. Regression is the most widely used family of statistical tools to detect patterns in some response Y, as a function of explanatory variables (or covariates) X. The simplest and most accessible type of regression is the linear model [9]. The GS analysis field has made a decisive turn towards linear models in recent years [10–13]. The approach usually begins at the gene level (step 8), where a generic expression model can be written as:

$$y_{gi} = \beta_{g0} + \sum_{j=1}^{p} X_{ij}\beta_{gj} + \varepsilon_{gi} \tag{5.1}$$

where

$y_{gi}, g = 1, \ldots G, i = 1, \ldots n$ is the gene expression value of gene g in sample i;
p = the number of covariates (explanatory variables) in the model;
X_{ij} = the value of the j-th covariate for the i-th sample; for dichotomous covariates such as phenotype, one typically sets X to zero or one;
β_{gj} = the true magnitude of the effect of covariate j upon the expression of gene g (β_{g0} is the intercept, or baseline expression for gene g),
ε_{gi} = a random error ("noise"); this term encompasses all the randomness in the signal. It is assumed to be (at least approximately) Normal with mean zero. Its variance σ_g^2 may be equal or unequal across genes. Errors are assumed to be mutually independent.

The data and model are used to calculate $\hat{y}_{gi}$, a fitted value for each observation, an estimate for each effect's magnitude, denoted as $\hat{\beta}_{gj}$, and a *t*-statistic t_{gj} for each covariate quantifying the strength of evidence for its effect. Under model assumptions and the null hypothesis (H_0) of no true effect, the *t*-statistics follow the *t*-distribution with $n-p-1$ degrees of freedom (DF). The model form (5.1) is fitted to all genes independently and simultaneously. A simple gene-by-gene two-sample *t*-test is identical to a linear model with $p = 1$ and with the sole covariate taking on only two values: zero or one. However, the advantage of linear models is not their equivalence to a *t*-test but their ability to simultaneously correct DE estimates for the effect of other variables, such as age or sex, and the access to a wide variety of theoretical and practical tools.

The simplest linear-model based GS method was introduced under the acronym PAGE [10]. It looks at the mean of all *t*-statistics from the covariate of interest, averaged over genes in a given GS S_k. Under the null hypothesis that S_k is not DE, and assuming inter-gene independence, this mean is Normal with expectation zero and a variance inversely proportional to $|S_k|$, or the GS size. Jiang and Gentleman [12] suggest the rescaling:

$$\tau_k = \sum_{g \in S_k} t_g / \sqrt{|S_k|} \qquad (5.2)$$

which has the attractive feature of retaining a variance of 1 under the same assumptions, regardless of GS size (the covariate subscript *j* has been dropped for simplicity; it is assumed we focus on a single predetermined covariate of interest). Hummel and coworkers [13] introduced an expanded framework for (5.1) that integrates steps 8 and 9 together. This model, available via the *GlobalAncova* package, also allows for various forms of intra-sample correlations. It provides a statistical *F* test between an expanded model and a reduced model containing a subset of the expanded model's covariates. Rejection of H_0 provides evidence that the set of additional covariates, taken as a whole, has a true effect upon expression. This approach views membership in a specific GS as a zero–one covariate in the model, whose value is one for genes in the GS and zero otherwise. Identifying a GS as DE is equivalent to finding a significant *interaction* between that gene-set's covariate and the covariate of interest (e.g., phenotype). Tests can be performed either versus a reference distribution value or via permutations. When examining a large number of GSs, the authors recommend performing a multiple-test-correction procedure such as FDR to generate a shortlist of DE gene-sets.

Oron and coworkers [14] introduced the *GSEAlm* package with somewhat overlapping functionality. The model (5.1) is implemented with either equal or unequal variance across genes and no direct model for inter-gene correlation. Instead, inference is performed via a sample-label permutation test that indirectly accounts for correlations. The test examines the effect of the addition of a single covariate of interest to the model. This package also allows (via the *gsealmPerm* function) to test all GSs of interest simultaneously, using a $G \times K$ binary incidence matrix, which is simply a collection of gene-membership vectors as described above for *GlobalAncova*. In principle, the incidence-matrix framework allows to code genes known to be positively, negatively, or partially coordinated, within a single GS; this is true for both the Oron et al. and Hummel et al. approaches. However, in its simplest form the matrix has only 0s and 1s, and the author is not aware of any published study making use of a more sophisticated GS membership coding. Like with *GlobalAncova*, accounting for multiple testing via the FDR approach or otherwise is recommended for *GSEAlm*, although the correction is not automatically performed on the test output, and is left up to the user. The *GSEAlm* package also provides a suite of standard linear-model diagnostics, most prominently residuals, to examine model fit and identify outlying observations.

The *GlobalAncova* approach has the distinct advantage of offering a more comprehensive and coherent modeling framework, and the reader is warmly encouraged to explore it. The *GSEAlm* package's modeling options are more limited. However, it runs much faster, is simpler to use, and enables access to diagnostic tools that (as will be soon demonstrated) are immensely valuable. For these reasons, as well as the sheer coincidence of this chapter's author also being *GSEAlm*'s main author and maintainer, the walk-through example of Section 5.3 will rely upon that package.

5.2.3
Correlations and Permutation Tests

Regression-related GS analysis developers originally suggested comparing the GS statistic with a theoretical reference distribution – Normal, *t*, or *F*; some notable researchers still recommend it (Chapter 13 in Reference [15]). This assumes independence between genes within the same sample. However, in microarray experiments there are two extremely strong reasons to doubt such an assumption. The first is that all genes in a given sample come from the same organism, and thus we expect their expression levels to be correlated in multiple ways. In general, it is impossible for a regression model to perfectly capture all such correlations. Moreover, genes in the same sample are arrayed together – that is, they belong the same *experimental unit*. According to basic experimental-design principles, some intra-unit correlation should be expected. The correlations arising from both sources tend to be positive. Positive intra-sample correlations are observed (equivalently) as positive gene–gene correlations.

Even mildly positive gene–gene correlations can seriously distort inference and make it overly optimistic. For example, the rescaled τ_{kj} from (5.2) will have a variance that increases with increasing $|S_k|$ instead of remaining constant. But it is not always easy to detect such correlations; looking for them among the τ_{kj}'s is problematic, because it is not known how many GSs really obey H_0. To our aid come regression *residuals*. Rather than use the raw residuals $e_{gi} \equiv y_{gi} - \hat{y}_{gi}$, we normalize them to have unit variance [16]. Most preferable are (externally-)Studentized residuals, which under model assumptions are *t*-distributed with $n-p-2$ degrees of freedom. These can be used, analogously to (5.2), to produce rescaled GS-level residuals:

$$R_{ki} = \sum_{g \in S_k} r_{gi} / \sqrt{|S_k|} \tag{5.3}$$

where r_{gi} is the Studentized residual from sample i and gene g. There are n GS residuals per gene-set. Under inter-gene independence, $\text{Var}(R_{ki}) = 1$ regardless of GS size; in the presence of positive correlations the variance will increase with size. Therefore, plotting the per-GS sample variance of the R_{ki}'s versus the GS size $|S_k|$ provides a quick and reliable answer to the correlation question. Figure 5.2 shows such plots for the ALL dataset (which will be described below) using chromosome-locus GSs. The roughly linear increasing pattern indicates not only positive correlation, but also suggests the source: a linear pattern would result from differing baseline expression levels across samples (i.e., imperfect normalization). Figure 5.2a shows GS residuals from a phenotype-only *t*-test, while Figure 5.2b shows the same calculation after renormalization via removal of each sample's median expression level, and the addition of three covariates to the model. The trend is diminished, but has not disappeared; this can be explained technically (intra-sample correlations not stemming only from baseline offsets, model not yet complete, etc.) and biologically – as different chromosomal loci may be associated with different levels of expression intensity and variability [17]. In any case, intra-sample correlations seem to be an inherent feature of microarrays that needs to be acknowledged and addressed, rather than artificially eliminated.

As mentioned earlier, for inference we address correlations by calculating GS effect *p*-values via sample ("column") label permutations. In each permutation, sample labels are scrambled among groups of samples, in such a way that only the covariate of interest changes while the adjusting covariates remain constant [18]. Each time, the linear model (5.1) is calculated for all genes, and GS-level statistics [e.g., the GSEA statistic or (5.2)] calculated for all GSs. This is repeated a large number of times, to produce an *ensemble* of statistics for each GS. Permutation *p*-values are generated by calculating the ensemble proportion of permutation statistics that are at least as extreme as the observed one; each GS has its own reference ensemble. As mentioned, correction for multiple testing of many GSs simultaneously is still advised. The permutation-test null hypothesis is that GS-wide expression levels are indifferent to the covariate of interest, when the adjusting covariates are taken into

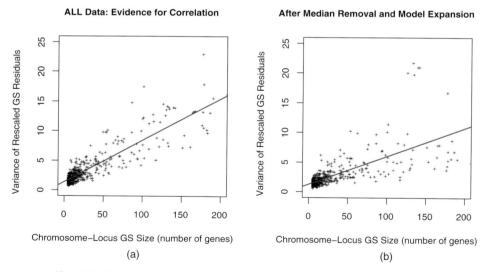

Figure 5.2 Demonstration of positive inter-gene correlations in the ALL dataset. (a) Variance of GS residuals (5.3) from a phenotype-only model as a function of GS size, for chromosome-locus GSs – the blue line indicates a least-squares linear fit; (b) the same as in (a) but after re-normalizing expression levels by sample, and adding age, sex, and hyperdiploidy covariates to the model.

account. Since permutations are performed on samples as single units, the correlation effect is neutralized. We are also relieved of the need to worry whether the data are close enough to Normality to justify the use of regression inference, because the ensemble simulates the true null distribution of the various statistics.

Correlations affect all GS methods outlined above, not only the regression-related ones. For example, the hypergeometric test's null hypothesis also assumes inter-gene independence. With positive correlations, the null-distribution tails are much heavier and therefore "unusually" high proportions of DE genes are in fact rather usual. Sample-label permutations are able to address these problems regardless of test method. Until something better comes along, they should be taken as the method of choice for GS-level and gene-level microarray inference (see also Reference [19]).

5.3
Demonstration with the "ALL" Dataset

5.3.1
The Dataset

The dataset comes from an adult and adolescent acute lymphoblastic leukemia (ALL) clinical trial [20] (hereafter: "the ALL dataset"). It contains 128 samples, each hybridized to an Affymetrix HG-U95Av2 chip containing 12 625 unique cDNA fragments (usually known as "features"). A log-transformed, normalized and annotated expression matrix with a wealth of phenotypical information is available on the Bioconductor repository as a dataset named ALL. A major research interest in this dataset is how the B-cell BCR/ABL mutation ("Philadelphia chromosome"), associated with poor prognosis for adult patients, affects gene expression. In this mutation, parts of chromosomes 9 and 22 exchange material, and a tyrosine kinase coded by a gene on chromosome 22 (the *ABL* gene) assumes a carcinogenic form. Incidentally, the *ABL* gene is the one at the very top right in Figure 5.1a and b.

The BCR/ABL phenotype group is compared with the mutation-free NEG phenotype of the disease; these two together account for 79 samples, 37 of them BCR/ABL. The nature of the mutation and the research question naturally lead us towards using chromosomal loci as GSs. This particular GS structure forms a hierarchical tree graph: the trunk is the organism, the first branches are complete chromosomes, and so forth – down to the lowest-resolution sub-bands, which are known in graph-theory as the tree's leaves. A lower GS-size cutoff was imposed: only loci with ≥ 5 genes post-filtering were included in the analysis.

5.3.2
The Gene-Filtering Dilemma

In a technology where no single standard exists for any step, gene filtering (step 7) is perhaps among the most questionable, yet it is seldom studied and easily overlooked. At this stage a huge chunk of the features on the array – quite often, the majority – are summarily discarded and never used again for subsequent analysis. This includes technical reference spots, unidentifiable features, and multiple features pointing towards the same gene. As to the latter group, simply averaging values from different features may introduce biases; instead, often all but one feature per gene are discarded. It is unclear which feature best represents a gene's expression. The MAQC studies suggested this depends upon the oligonucleotide's relative location on the gene, but unfortunately such detailed information is not always available. Instead, a simple common solution is to choose the feature exhibiting the highest variability across samples. This is the solution hard-coded into the standard R function *nsFilter* (package *genefilter*); one can choose whether or not to eliminate duplicate features, but not the elimination method. On the ALL dataset, out of 12 625 features 19 were identified as purely technical, 502 had no known associated gene, and 3088 were low-variability "duplicates," pointing to the same genes as some of the 9016 remaining features.

However, we are not done yet. It is known that in any given tissue only a fraction of genes are actually expressed. A commonly-quoted fraction is 40%; a recent study claims that only about 8–16% of genes are expressed in most human tissues, but the approach there has been decidedly conservative (see supplementary Figure 1E in Reference [21]). In any case, including all genes in the analysis tends to dilute the signal with too much noise; most unexpressed genes need to be filtered out prior to DE analysis.

Conceptually, in any given gene-microarray dataset there are three groups of genes: (1) genes not expressed at all in any sample, (2) genes expressed but roughly at the same level across samples, often called "housekeeping genes," and (3) genes whose expression level varies significantly across samples. Group 1 provides noise whose only use might be for estimating background levels. Group 2, which is often called "uninformative" by some researchers, can in fact serve rather useful purposes. Moreover, its exclusion might distort our inference. For example, take a GS S_k having 57 genes of which 50 are expressed equally across samples, and 7 are expressed differentially, for various reasons unrelated to S_k. If we see group 2 as "uninformative" and discard it we may reach the erroneous conclusion that S_k is a DE gene-set. Therefore, ideally both groups 2 and 3 should be included in DE analysis.

Unfortunately, it is not easy to distinguish group 2 from group 1. The current default implemented by *nsFilter* removes half of the genes with smallest expression inter-quartile range (IQR) across samples. This type of removal probably splits either group 1 or group 2 somewhere in the middle. Both the fraction of genes removed and the reference function can be changed, so if a function is developed that reliably leaves out only group 1 genes, the readers are urged to substitute it for the IQR. Alternatively, one can use manufacturer-provided "present/absent" calls if they are deemed reliable enough. In our particular case, we chose to use the standard deviation for reasons that will be apparent soon, and to remove half the genes, which is the default fraction; however, compared with the original number of features, we retain only 37%. Subsequently, a handful of remaining genes could not be mapped to any chromosomal locus (mapping was accomplished via the

5.3 Demonstration with the "ALL" Dataset | 99

HGU95-Av2 annotation database and other tools, all available on Bioconductor), leaving us with 4500 genes on 79 samples – hereafter, "the working dataset" – mapped to 526 chromosomal-loci GSs.

5.3.3
Basic Diagnostics: Testing Normalization and Model Fit

We next run the model (5.1) with phenotype as the sole covariate, and use the diagnostics in *GSEAlm* to see if anything suspicious turns up before proceeding. The simplest diagnostic plot (Figure 5.3) summarizes gene-level Studentized residuals by sample. It is a more thorough examination of normalization than that provided by standard microarray quality control packages, and it is also much closer in spirit to the DE signal-detection process since residuals are normalized for each gene separately, just like DE *t*-statistics. The ALL dataset now seems rather poorly normalized. Some

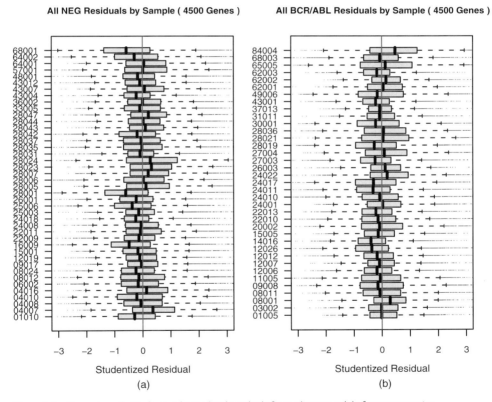

Figure 5.3 Raw externally-Studentized gene-level residuals from a linear model of gene expression on phenotype for the ALL dataset, grouped by sample, arranged by phenotype [(a) NEG, (b) BCR/ABL], and sorted by sample ID.

samples emerge as gross outliers, for example, 28 001,68 001 on the low side (28 001's residuals are about 70% negative) and 04 007,84 004 on the high side. How is this possible? The dataset is supposed to be post-normalization.

The answer is related to filtering. Dataset normalization is performed on all features. When Figure 5.3 is reproduced without filtering out genes, inter-sample offsets are much milder, samples 28 001 and 68 001 are not low outliers, and sample 84 004 morphs from highest-expressed in the dataset to lowest! In 80% of the features discarded as "redundant" or "uninformative," 84 004's residuals were negative; in 64% of the remaining features it has positive residuals. In short, the discarded genes have different normalization behavior from the retained ones. Potential explanations for this interesting phenomenon, which was observed in other datasets as well, are deferred to the summary. Right now, the lesson learned is that normalization needs to be revisited post-filtering; or perhaps filtering and normalization should occur simultaneously.

Before rushing to correct these between-sample offsets, we examined whether they result from true biological differences rather than technical normalization issues. One way to inspect this is to group residuals together by GSs as in (5.3). A heat map of the R_{ki}s with two-way clustering enabled (Figure 5.4) may be of help: if there are only vertical patterns, then the offsets have nothing to do with chromosomal loci. If a block pattern emerges, there are unaccounted-for associations between groups of samples and chromosomal loci, and the regression model needs to be expanded. To avoid overlaps, only the 264 leaves of the chromosome-loci tree are shown.

It turns out that both vertical and block patterns are visible. Sample 28 001, for example, shows as a narrow predominantly-blue vertical strip somewhat right of center. Unless we realign expression levels, sample 28 001 and the others mentioned above are likely to appear as outliers during more detailed analysis and possibly also distort inference. Thus, there is certainly a normalization problem. We resolve it by matching sample medians.

More conspicuous in Figure 5.4 is the apparent block or checkerboard pattern of the heat map. In particular, there is a relatively tight cluster of 20 samples (left-hand side of map), whose expression pattern is roughly the opposite of most other samples. Among the dataset's 21 descriptive variables, we identified hyperdiploidy – that is, the presence of extra chromosome copies in the sample's cells – to be most strongly associated with the pattern-induced grouping of samples. The association between hyperdiploidy and gene expression of chromosomal loci or complete chromosomes among pediatric ALL patients has been well-documented in research [22, 23], and we can plausibly assume it holds for adult patients as well. In the ALL dataset hyperdiploidy was determined via qualitative visual methods, with no further details about extra copies. In the colored band at the top of Figure 5.4, red indicates hyperdiploid samples, gray diploid samples, and white samples of unknown status. Even though only 19 of 79 samples are hyperdiploid, they form a clear majority in the 20-sample cluster described above, and are further differentiated from diploid samples within that cluster as well.

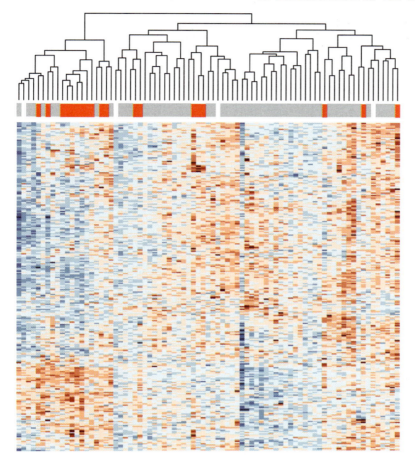

Figure 5.4 GS residuals from the linear model of gene expression on phenotype, for each lowest-level chromosome band (row) and sample (column). Residuals in each row were standardized to have mean zero and standard deviation of 1. Heat map colors change in increments of 0.8 (on the normalized scale), with reds positive and blues negative. The horizontal band at the top indicates the value of the "kinet" variable: red for hyperdiploid, gray for diploid, and white for unknown.

Hierarchical clustering is rather fickle and sensitive to minor changes; how certain are we that this is not an artifact, that if we change some clustering parameters or gene-filtering criteria, this apparent signal won't disappear? The predominantly-hyperdiploid cluster appears quite robust to the filtering threshold (it survives, in some form, when 30 to 70% of the genes are discarded). However, a change in filtering *method*, for example, changing the variability criterion from SD to IQR (which is the default), affects the clustering more strongly. This is because IQR completely ignores the top and bottom 25% of samples for each gene, and our cluster is composed of barely a quarter of the samples. If enough genes carrying the cluster-causing signal are replaced by others lacking that signal, it will be diluted. Additionally, Figure 5.4 includes another non-default choice: the clustering distance between samples' expression values was one minus their pairwise correlation, while the default of the heat-map function is simple Euclidean distance. Two samples with highly correlated patterns, but separated by a baseline offset, may be "Euclideally far" and yet very close in correlation-distance terms. If one uses the two default choices and reproduces Figure 5.4, both the block pattern and the hyperdiploid-related clustering become far less apparent, and might be overlooked (figure not shown).

5.3.4
Pinpointing Aneuploidies via Outlier Identification

We leave the original phenotype-related research question aside for the moment, and follow the unexpected lead suggested by Figure 5.4. Can we pinpoint, based upon expression patterns alone, which sample has what extra (or missing) chromosomes? Before undertaking this task, it is important to note the way microarray normalization works. Since we have realigned expression levels across samples, each sample's median gene expression is now pegged at zero on the $\log_2$ scale. There is nothing unusual here: this is what the original normalization had attempted to achieve. In other words, microarray expression measurements are only meaningful in the *relative* sense; hence the difficulty in information synergy across experiments and platforms [2].

On the plus side, we have at our disposal two comparison perspectives: between genes on the same sample, and between samples on the same gene (or GS). The latter perspective can reveal the baseline expression variation between chromosomes and sub-chromosomal loci [17], and is left for the reader to attempt (see, for example, Figure 5.4 in Reference [14]). Here we focus on between-sample comparisons: on the complete-chromosome level, aneuploidies (samples with extra or missing copies) are expected to emerge as gross outliers, since in general it is known that having extra copies of the same chromosome substantially increases that chromosome's expression levels [24], and we can logically assume the opposite also holds.

Hertzberg and coworkers [25] recently performed a similar identification task on a pediatric ALL dataset, with reasonable success. They used two *ad hoc* measures to flag suspect aneuploidies: one similar to outlier identification and the other setting an absolute threshold to the proportion by which a chromosome is over- or under-expressed on average. Here we also use this dual approach, but incorporate a more formal outlier identification procedure, via standard robust location and scale estimation of each chromosome's baseline level across samples [26]. Since the reference distribution is not theoretically known, we numerically generated an outlier-free reference distribution [27]. FDR thresholds of 0.05, 0.1, and 0.2 were applied to flag outliers, and the absolute-proportion threshold was set at $> 7/6$ or $< 6/7$ of the inter-sample baseline for each chromosome. Figure 5.5 shows the residual distributions for chromosomes 7 and X.

The overall suspected-aneuploidy map is shown in Figure 5.6. Most hyperdiploid samples, and about a dozen diploid samples, are flagged for at least one aneuploidy.

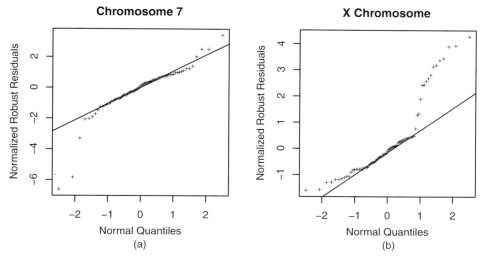

Figure 5.5 Demonstration of the outlier method for aneuploidy detection. Shown is each sample's mean chromosome-wide expression deviation from the bulk of all other samples, normalized by a robust location and scale estimate across samples, for chromosomes 7 (a) and X (b). For convenience the standard normal distribution is used on the horizontal axis; however, actual outlier testing was performed against a simulated null distribution that is somewhat more heavy-tailed. On chromosome 7, one sample was flagged for an extra copy and two for a missing copy. On the X chromosome, 12 samples were flagged for extra copies.

Observing Figure 5.6 from the perspective of chromosomes, chromosome X is by far the most prevalent, with 12 samples flagged as potential multisomies at the 0.2 FDR level. The next most prevalent multisomies are of chromosomes 21 and 14, respectively. This is in close agreement with current knowledge about childhood ALL aneuploidies [23, 25]. Since the truth is not known for this dataset, we examined the method against the pediatric ALL dataset used by the Hertzberg team to calibrate their own method, with reasonable success (see Reference [14] web supplement). From comparing Figures 5.5 and 5.6, we can see that in general the method is conservative. For example, on the X chromosome 12 samples were flagged for extra copies, but the visual distribution suggests as many as 15–16 gross positive outliers. Another important observation is that at least for ALL, there is a variety of hyperdiploidy patterns rather than a single one, and hence the group called "hyperdiploid" is really a collection of several sub-groups.

5.3.5
Signal-to-Noise Evaluation: The Sex Variable

We have just seen how the most evident diagnostic pattern, beside the need to renormalize the dataset, is driven by strong and clear physical differences between

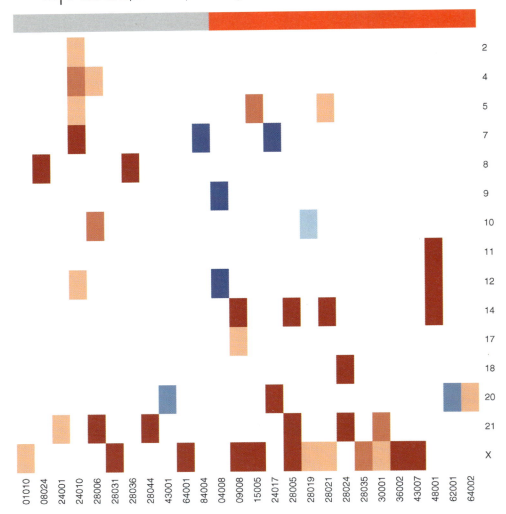

Figure 5.6 Map of suspected aneuploidies in the ALL dataset, by chromosome (rows) and sample (columns). Red-brown hues correspond to extra copies, and blue hues to missing copies. Dark, medium, and light shades correspond to FDR levels of 0.05, 0.1, and 0.2, respectively. The top bar indicates hyperdiploidy, as in Figure 5.4. Samples and chromosomes with no flags have been omitted.

samples, namely, different numbers of chromosomes. As suggested in the introduction, microarrays can usually be trusted to detect such gross differences, albeit noisily. We turn our attention to another clear chromosome-related signal: sex.

The working dataset has 50 males, 28 females and one sample with a missing sex entry. Females do not have the Y chromosome, but some Y-chromosome genes, known as autosomal, have functionally identical copies on the X chromosome, and are not expected to show drastic sex-related expression differences. The remaining Y genes are the equivalent of an a priori known subcellular pattern. Therefore, they can serve several functions at once: a benchmark for microarray technology, a test of GS analysis methodology, and a test for data-entry errors. The Y chromosome has relatively few genes, and only 18 in the working dataset. It is represented in Figure 5.4 by two rows, mixing autosomal and non-autosomal genes, and so its effect is virtually unnoticeable in that figure. Instead, we examine Y genes directly, and use the annotation database to find out whether each gene is autosomal. According to this database, out of 18 Y genes ten are Y-only, seven are autosomal and one has no precise mapping. Fortunately, that gene's name is available and betrays its identity (a testis-specific transcript). Moreover, one of the supposedly Y-only genes displays no noticeable expression differences between males and females, and therefore we reclassify it as autosomal (or unexpressed). Note that this type of data cleaning can only be performed when we are absolutely sure of the science! There is every reason to suspect that similar inaccuracies are present throughout annotation databases.

We treat the ten verified Y-only genes as a single GS, and compare mean expression levels between males and females (Figure 5.7a). The overall sex effect is evident, but several samples deviate towards the opposite sex so strongly as to suggest a possible sex mislabeling in the dataset. A more detailed analysis (see Reference [14] web supplement) led to the conclusion that two females had been mislabeled as males and

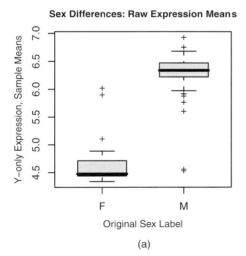
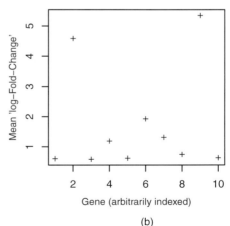

Figure 5.7 (a) Box plots of sample-specific expression means by sex (on the log-intensity scale), calculated on the set of Y-chromosome non-autosomal genes. Sex assignment is as originally given. (b) Gene-specific expression differences between males and females for the same genes (on the log-intensity scale). Expression data are post-renormalization. Sex assignment was changed for the three strongest outliers, and one missing-entry sample labeled as male based on expression.

one male mislabeled as female. These samples' sex labels where changed. Three additional females displayed intermediate expression patterns, and their labels were left unchanged. The sample with missing sex entry was easily identified as male by its Y-only expression patterns. Beyond the Y-chromosome and a few scattered X-chromosome genes, sex seems to play a very minor role in the expression of other chromosomal loci.

We now examine Y-only gene signal-to-noise. To begin on a positive note, sex differences on Y-only genes seem unrelated to the baseline unexpressed intensity, as estimated via the female samples (data not shown). On the other hand, Figure 5.7b shows estimated mean log fold-change for each gene, after correcting the mislabeled samples. The mean of all ten genes is 1.75 $\log_2$ fold-change, and the median is 0.97. Only two genes exhibit what we would like to see, namely a male–female intensity gap far in excess of the female baseline, resulting in fold-change estimates of magnitude $\gg 1$. Most Y-only genes show a sex effect that would be communicated, had it occurred on a different gene, as "this gene is expressed by males roughly twice as strongly as by females." Given that females *do not even have* these genes, the signal-to-noise ratio here is roughly 1 : 1, at best (probably worse, considering that for Y-only genes we do know the true signal's direction and were able to fix annotation errors). This, as well as the inability to determine the true sex of three samples, is a stark reminder of microarrays' quantitative limitations.

5.3.6
Confounding, and Back to Basics: The Age Variable

An unpleasant surprise awaits us when comparing ages between the two phenotype groups (Figure 5.8). The NEG group is considerably younger: nearly half its members

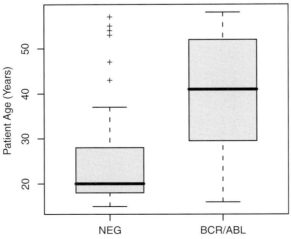

Figure 5.8 Box plots of patient age by phenotype group.

are teenagers 15–19 years old, compared with only two BCR/ABL patients. This imbalance leads to the classic data-analysis quagmire known as confounding, which occurs whenever two covariates (here, age and phenotype) and the modeled response (here, expression) are connected via three-way pairwise correlations. If there is no clear and unidirectional causal relationship between the two covariates, an imbalance as strong as shown here makes it very difficult to tell which of the two would better explain the response. Therefore, basic statistical principles dictate the inclusion of both in the model [28].

Besides this statistical perspective, the science further complicates matters: ALL is known to have rather different dynamics and prognoses among children and adults. These differences may translate into GS-level expression patterns. Biologically, perhaps all patients under ~ 20 years should be considered adolescents. Therefore, I have chosen here to omit the adolescent cohort altogether, adjust for age on the remaining patients, and thus focus the analysis on same-age phenotype differences for adult patients.

5.3.7
How it all Reflects on the Bottom Line: Inference

We implement the linear model (5.1) for phenotype, adjusting for hyperdiploidy and age categorized into the ranges 20–24, 25–49, and 50–58. We categorize age rather than use it as a continuous variable, to enable label-permutation tests. This model allows the incorporation of 55 out of 79 patients; beside patients under 20, we also lose three patients with missing age. Three more patients with missing hyperdiploidy status were classified as diploid, based on their clustering into diploid-dominant groups in Figure 5.4 and their non-appearance as aneuploidy suspects in Figure 5.6. Even though there are methods to adjust for multiple comparisons on hierarchically nested tests, we prefer to keep matters simple by choosing a subset of chromosomal loci that does not include any overlap. Here we chose chromosome sub-bands that seem to offer an optimum between resolution and efficiency: there are 208 sub-bands in the working dataset, containing 3580 of 4500 genes with practically no gene-level overlap. The vast majority of sub-bands have 5 to 25 genes, with the median at 11. Tables 5.1 and 5.2 present lists of sub-bands identified as DE between NEG and BCR/ABL by a phenotype-only model and by the expanded model, respectively, each controlled at 0.1 FDR; p-values were generated via 5000 sample-label permutations.

The phenotype-only list is strongly tilted towards overexpressed loci, while the expanded-model list is more balanced. Interestingly, the most significant GS in each direction under the phenotype-only model completely disappears from the list under the expanded model. However, many others remain. Among the changes between the two GS calculations – model, normalization, and sample removal – it seems that adjusting for age and removing teenage subjects had the strongest bottom-line impact. Overall, estimated phenotype effect sizes are rather mild: none exceed 0.3 on the $\log_2$ scale. In view of the Y-chromosome effect sizes depicted in Figure 5.7 and the implied noise level, the FDR-based "statistical guarantee" that the lists have only $\sim 10\%$ false signals seems rather optimistic.

Table 5.1 List of chromosome sub-bands flagged as DE (differentially expressed) by phenotype, at the two-tailed 0.1 FDR level using a phenotype-only model; p-values were calculated using 5000 phenotype-label permutations, and adding the true labels as the 5001-th. Overall, 208 sub-bands were tested.

	Loci up-expressed by BCR/ABL		
Sub-band	Number of genes	Permutation p-value	Effect size (log2 scale)
3q28	8	0.0002	0.21
8p22	7	0.0002	0.30
14q22	17	0.0006	0.20
7q31	9	0.0006	0.27
4p14	5	0.0006	0.27
5q23	8	0.0010	0.30
2q22	5	0.0016	0.14
6q27	5	0.0022	0.16
17q23	10	0.0024	0.22
9q31	8	0.0024	0.20
2q32	11	0.0030	0.16
13q32	10	0.0032	0.10
12q21	14	0.0040	0.16
3q25	14	0.0040	0.25
4q21	15	0.0040	0.23
15q11	6	0.0052	0.27
2q11	10	0.0058	0.17
1q25	13	0.0068	0.19
6q23	9	0.0074	0.27
6q14	5	0.0082	0.13
18p11	27	0.0102	0.14
	Loci down-expressed by BCR/ABL		
Sub-band	Number of genes	Permutation p-value	Effect size (log2 scale)
9p21	7	0.0036	−0.08

5.4
Summary and Future Directions

The data analysis example has been presented in lengthy detail. The intention is to show that each step in the tortuous microarray analysis route involves nontrivial decisions and inaccuracies. Specifically, the final GS-level step relies upon annotation information to correctly link microarray features and GSs. We have seen several examples for inaccurate or incomplete annotation (502 features having no known gene; two Y-chromosome genes with missing or questionable chromosome-coordinate mapping). In addition, we used a chip with one of the most complete annotations, and a GS type (chromosomal loci) that is the most physically clear-cut.

5.4 Summary and Future Directions

Table 5.2 List of chromosome sub-bands flagged as DE by phenotype, at the two-tailed 0.1 FDR level using a 3-covariate model (phenotype, age, hyperdiploidy), after re-normalizing expression values at the sample level and removing samples from patients younger than 20 years; *p*-values were calculated using 5000 phenotype-label permutations, and adding the true labels as the 5001-th. The "Rank in 'old' list" column refers to the sub-band's ranking (by *p*-value) in the list of over- (under-)expressed genes under the phenotype-only model (whose top GS list was shown above in Table 5.1).

		Loci up-expressed by BCR/ABL		
Sub-band	Number of genes	Permutation *p*-value	Effect size (log2 scale)	Rank in "old" list
4q21	15	0.0006	0.26	15
2q11	10	0.0006	0.17	17
14q22	17	0.0014	0.16	3
2q14	8	0.0016	0.15	24
4p14	5	0.0016	0.26	5
5q23	8	0.0020	0.30	6
2q32	11	0.0022	0.17	11
8p22	7	0.0024	0.25	2
6q25	9	0.0070	0.11	50
12q23	5	0.0088	0.22	41
17q23	10	0.0092	0.17	9
7q31	9	0.0092	0.26	4
		Loci down-expressed by BCR/ABL		
Sub-band	Number of genes	Permutation *p*-value	Effect size (log2 scale)	Rank in "old" list
1p34	22	0.0008	−0.13	34
7p13	7	0.0018	−0.28	6
20q13	41	0.0030	−0.13	2
1p35	11	0.0054	−0.12	38
7p22	14	0.0064	−0.13	4
3q21	17	0.0066	−0.06	94
7q22	22	0.0066	−0.13	9
4q12	8	0.0070	−0.20	15
19q12	5	0.0076	−0.15	50

When using stand-alone chips or more vaguely-defined GSs such as pathways, annotation quality drops sharply, placing the feasibility of GS analysis under serious doubt.

On a positive note, the linear-model toolset presented here is generic and platform-independent, and its use during the gene and GS-level steps is recommended. One can choose any test for the final GS-detection step (hypergeometric, GSEA, etc.), using as input the t-statistics from a gene-level regression model adjusting for all covariates deemed relevant. A key advantage of using regression tools is that the microarray analysis challenge is demystified and transferred to a more familiar terrain. It then turns out that such well-known concepts as outliers, a poorly-fitting model, and confounding are relevant and useful for microarrays, too.

Statistical tools, however, are not a replacement for thinking through the science. For example, without going into details it seems that many methods to summarize, transform, and normalize raw microarray data (steps 4–6 in Section 5.1) are not based on science as much as on the overriding goal of pounding the data into quasi-Normal behavior on the log scale. Log transformation implies that all effects are multiplicative; hence the "fold-change" terminology that has become dominant in the field. However, in truth both the signal (i.e., hybridization of expressed genes) and much of the baseline and background noise (both optical and biochemical) are *additive*. If not all noise is removed, then any "fold-change" estimate is inevitably biased towards zero [2]. The log-transformation of an additive signal + noise mix may also help explain why noise-only features display such different normalization behavior on the log scale from signal-containing genes, as discussed in Section 5.3.3. This has certainly happened here, since the ALL dataset's expression matrix was apparently calculated using only the chip's "perfect-match" probes, which means that the manufacturer's method for removing nonspecific-binding noise had been bypassed [20]. Unfortunately, recalculating and cleaning the expression matrix from the raw image files to include this adjustment and see whether it affects the bottom line is probably even more tedious than the entire data-analysis tour we have just completed.

In short, DE analysis in general and GS analysis in particular can be greatly affected by earlier-stage decisions. In many cases, the current stepwise approach is too lossy to retain anything but the strongest signals. Ideas for combining steps 7–9, or even 4–9, are being developed, and may hold a great promise for much clearer detection [B. Mecham, personal communication]. These approaches truly take advantage of the wealth of information stored in the image files.

Whether such a breakthrough will take place remains to be seen, since in this age the most common fix for an existing technology's problems is its replacement by a new one. This certainly appears to be the case for microarrays, with "next generations" already crossing over the horizon. I would not be surprised, however, if we find ourselves contending with the all-too-familiar themes of immense data reduction, excessive noise from various sources, signal attrition over multiple analysis steps, normalization and multiple testing issues, and other basic scientific and statistical constraints that are convenient (yet perilous) to ignore.

Acknowledgments

Thanks go to friends and colleagues Anna Freni-Sterrantino, Chen Yanover, and Golan Yona, who provided excellent feedback on this chapter. During the work leading to Reference [14] the author performed postdoctoral research in the Bioconductor core group at the Fred Hutchinson Cancer Research Center in Seattle, funded by NIH grants mentioned in that article. During the composition of this chapter, the author was supported in teaching roles at the Department of Statistics, University of Washington, Seattle.

References

1 Shi, L. et al. (2006) The microarray quality control (MAQC) project shows inter- and intraplatform reproducibility of gene expression measurements. *Nat. Biotechnol.*, **24**, 1141–1151.

2 Chen, J.J. et al. (2007) Reproducibility of microarray data: a further analysis of microarray quality control (MAQC) data. *BMC Bioinformatics*, **8**, 412.

3 Benjamini, Y. and Hochberg, Y. (1995) Controlling the false discovery rate - a practical and powerful approach to multiple testing. *J. R. Stat. Soc. B*, **57** (1), 289–300.

4 Benjamini, Y. and Yekutieli, D. (2001) The control of the false discovery rate in multiple testing under dependency. *Ann. Stat.*, **29** (4), 1165–1188.

5 Al-Shahrour, F., Diaz-Uriarte, R., and Dopazo, J. (2004) FatiGO: a web tool for finding significant associations of gene ontology terms with groups of genes. *Bioinformatics*, **20**, 578–580.

6 Mootha, V.K. et al. (2003) PGC-1α-responsive genes involved in oxidative phosphorylation are coordinately downregulated in human diabetes. *Nat. Genet.*, **34**, 267–273.

7 Subramanian, A. et al. (2005) Gene set enrichment analysis: A knowledge-based approach for interpreting genome-wide expression profiles. *Proc. Nat. Acad. Sci. USA*, **102** (43), 15545–15550.

8 Efron, B. and Tibshirani, R. (2007) On testing the significance of sets of genes. *Ann. Appl. Stat.*, **1** (1), 107–129.

9 Neter, J. et al. (1996) *Applied Linear Statistical Models*, McGraw-Hill Companies, Inc.

10 Kim, S.-Y. and Volsky, D.J. (2005) PAGE: Parametric analysis of gene set enrichment. *BMC Bioinformatics*, **6**, 144.

11 Kong, S.W. et al. (2006) A multivariate approach for integrating genome-wide expression data and biological knowledge. *Bioinformatics*, **22** (19), 2373–2380.

12 Jiang, Z. and Gentleman, R. (2007) Extensions to gene set enrichment analysis. *Bioinformatics*, **23**, 306–313.

13 Hummel, M., Meister, R., and Mansmann, U. (2008) GlobalANCOVA: exploration and assessment of gene group effects. *Bioinformatics*, **24** (1), 78–85.

14 Oron, A.P., Jiang, Z., and Gentleman, R. (2008) Gene set enrichment analysis using linear models and diagnostics. *Bioinformatics*, **24**, 2586–2591.

15 Hahne, F. et al. (2008) *Bioconductor Case Studies*, Use R, Springer.

16 Cook, R.D. and Weisberg, S. (1982) *Residuals and Influence in Regression*, Monographs on Statistics and Applied Probability, Chapman & Hall.

17 Caron, H. et al. (2001) The human transcriptome map: clustering of highly expressed genes in chromosomal domains. *Science*, **291** (5507), 1289–1292.

18 Ernst, M.D. (2004) Permutation methods: a basis for exact inference. *Stat. Sci.*, **19** (4), 686–696.

19 Goeman, J.J. and Bühlmann, P. (2007) Analyzing gene expression data in terms of gene sets: methodological issues. *Bioinformatics*, **23** (8), 980–987.

20 Chiaretti, S. et al. (2005) Gene expression profile of adult B-lineage adult acute lymphocytic leukemia reveal genetic patterns that identify lineage derivation and distinct mechanisms of transformation. *Clin. Cancer Res.*, **11** (20), 7209–7219.

21 Zilliox, M.J. and Irizzary, R.A. (2007) A gene expression bar code for microarray data. *Nat. Methods*, **4**, 911–913.

22 Ross, M.E. et al. (2003) Classification of pediatric acute lymphoblastic leukemia by gene expression profiling. *Blood*, **102**, 2951–2959.

23 Teixeira, M.R. and Heim, S. (2005) Multiple numerical chromosome aberrations in cancer: what are their causes and what are their consequences? *Sem. Cancer Biol.*, **15** (1), 3–12.

24 Pollack, J.R. et al. (2002) Microarray analysis reveals a major direct role of DNA copy number alteration in the transcriptional program of human breast tumors. *Proc. Nat. Acad. Sci. USA*, **99** (20), 12963–12968.

25 Hertzberg, L. *et al.* (2007) Prediction of chromosomal aneuploidy from gene expression data. *Genes Chromosome Cancer*, **46** (1), 75–86.

26 Huber, P.J. (1981) *Robust Statistics*, Wiley Series in Probability and Mathematical Statistics, John Wiley & Sons Inc., New York.

27 Wisnowski, J.W. *et al.* (2001) A comparative analysis of multiple outlier detection procedures in the linear regression model. *Comp. Stat. Data Anal.*, **36** (3), 351–382.

28 Friedman, D., Pisani, R., and Purves, R. (2007) *Statistics*, 4th edn, W. W. Norton and Company.

6
Multivariate Analysis of Microarray Data Using Hotelling's T^2 Test

Yan Lu, Peng-Yuan Liu, and Hong-Wen Deng

6.1
Introduction

Microarray technology is a powerful approach for genomic research, which allows the monitoring of expression profiles for tens of thousands of genes in parallel and is already producing huge amounts of data. Microarray data contain valuable information about gene functions, inter-gene dependencies, and underlying biological processes, and open a new avenue for discovering gene co-regulations, gene interactions, metabolic pathways and gene–environment interactions, and so on [1]. Microarray data are characterized with high dimensions and small sample sizes. Statistical inference from such high-dimensional data structures is challenging [2]. Several data-mining methodologies, such as clustering analysis and classification techniques, have been widely used to analyze gene expression data for identifying groups of genes sharing similar expression patterns [3–6].

While clustering and classification techniques have proven to be useful to search similar gene expression patterns, these techniques do not answer the most fundamental question in microarray experiments: which genes are responsible for biological differences between different cell types and/or states of a cell cycle? This question amounts to statistically testing the null hypothesis that there is no difference in expression under comparison. Various statistical methods have been proposed for identifying differentially expressed genes (DEGs), from using a simple fold change to using various linear models as well as Bayesian methods [7–12]. A common characteristic of these methods is that they are essentially of univariate nature.

Genes never act alone in a biological system – they work in a cascade of networks [13]. Expression profiles of multiple genes are often correlated and thus are more suitably modeled as mutually dependent variables in development of a statistical testing framework. However, most of the current statistical methods ignore the multidimensional structure of the expression data and fail to efficiently utilize the valuable information for gene interactions. Multivariate analyses take advantage of the correlation information and analyze the data from multiple genes jointly. As a result, multivariate statistical techniques are receiving increased attention in expression data analyses [14, 15]. However, applications of well-established multivariate statistical techniques for microarray data analyses are not straightforward because of the unusual features of the microarray data, such as high dimensions and small sample sizes.

In this chapter, we present a Hotelling's T^2 test that utilizes multiple gene expression information to identify DEGs in two test groups. The Hotelling's T^2 statistic is a natural multidimensional extension of the t-statistic that is currently a widespread approach for detecting DEGs in testing individual genes. The Hotelling's T^2 method has been applied to various aspects of life sciences, including genome association studies [16], microarray process control [17], and data control charts [18]. In this section, we briefly reviewed statistical methods for detecting differential gene expression in microarray experiments. A common characteristic of these statistical methods is the essentially univariate nature. In Section 6.2, we validated how the Hotelling's T^2 statistic is constructed for the identification of differential gene expression in microarray experiments. We implemented this method using a multiple forward search (MFS) algorithm that is designed for selecting a subset of feature vectors in high-dimensional microarray datasets. A resampling-based technique was also developed to smooth statistical fluctuation in T^2 statistic owing to large variability inherent in microarray data and to accommodate experiments with missing values for various spots on microarrays. In Section 6.3, we validated this new method by using a spike-in HGU95 dataset from Affymetrix. In Section 6.4, to illustrate its utility, we apply the Hotelling's T^2 statistic to the microarray data analyses of gene expression patterns in human liver cancers [19] and breast cancers [20]. Extensive bioinformatics analyses and cross-validation of DEGs identified in the application datasets showed the significant advantages of this new algorithm. Finally, extension of the Hotelling's T^2 statistic in microarray experiment is discussed in Section 6.5.

6.2
Methods

6.2.1
Wishart Distribution

The Wishart distribution plays an important role in the estimation of covariance matrices in multivariate statistics. Suppose X is an $n \times p$ matrix, each row of which is independently drawn from p-variate normal distribution with zero mean, $X \sim N_p(\mathbf{0}, V)$. Then, the probability distribution of the $p \times p$ random matrix $M(p \times p) = X^T X$ has the Wishart distribution $M(p \times p) \sim W_p(V, n)$ where n is the number of degree of freedom.

The Wishart distribution has the following useful properties:

1) It is a generalization to multiple dimensions of the χ^2 distribution, in particular, $W_1(V, n) = \sigma^2 \chi_n^2$.
2) The empirical covariance matrix S has a $\frac{1}{n} W_p(V, n-1)$ distribution.
3) In the normal case, $\bar{x}$ and S are independent.
4) For $M = W_p(V, n)$, $\frac{a^T M a}{a^T V a} \sim \chi_n^2$

6.2.2
Hotelling's T^2 Statistic

Hotelling's T^2 statistic is a generalization of Student's statistic that is used in multivariate hypothesis testing. Hotelling's T^2 statistic is defined as:

$$t^2 = n(X-\mu)^T W^{-1}(X-\mu) \tag{6.1}$$

where n is a number of data points, X is a column vector of p elements and W is a $p \times p$ sample covariance matrix.

If $X \sim N_p(\mu, V)$ is a random variable with a multivariate normal distribution and $W \sim W_p(m, V)$ has a Wishart distribution with the same non-singular variance matrix V and with $m = n - 1$, then the distribution of t^2 is $T^2(p,m)$, that is, Hotelling's T-square distribution with parameters p and m. It can be shown that:

$$\frac{m-p+1}{pm} T^2 \sim F_{p,m-p+1} \tag{6.2}$$

where F is the F-distribution.

6.2.3
Two-Sample T^2 Statistic

We consider a microarray experiment composed of n_D samples from a disease group and n_N samples from a normal group. Suppose that the expression levels of J genes are measured and used as variables to construct a T^2 statistic. Let X_{ij}^D be the expression level for gene j of sample i from the disease group and X_{kj}^N be the expression level for gene j of sample k from the normal group. The expression level vectors for samples i and k from the disease and normal groups can be expressed as $X_i^D = (X_{i1}^D, \cdots, X_{iJ}^D)^T$ and $X_k^N = (X_{k1}^N, \cdots, X_{kJ}^N)^T$, respectively. The mean expression levels of gene j in the disease and normal groups can be expressed as $\bar{X}^D = (\bar{X}_1^D, \cdots, \bar{X}_J^D)^T$ and $\bar{X}^N = (\bar{X}_1^N, \cdots, \bar{X}_J^N)^T$, respectively. The pooled variance–covariance matrix of expression levels of J genes for the disease and normal samples is then defined as:

$$S = \frac{(n_D-1)S^D + (n_N-1)S^N}{n_D + n_N - 2} = \frac{1}{n_D + n_N - 2}$$
$$\times \left[\sum_{i=1}^{n_D} (X_i^D - \bar{X}^D)(X_i^D - \bar{X}^D)^T + \sum_{k=1}^{n_N} (X_k^N - \bar{X}^N)(X_k^N - \bar{X}^N)^T \right]$$

where S^D and S^N are the variance–covariance matrix of expression levels for J genes in the disease and normal groups, respectively. The covariance terms in S^D and S^N account for the correlation and interdependence (interactions) of gene expression levels.

Hotelling's T^2 statistic for gene differential expression studies is then defined as:

$$T^2 = \frac{n_D n_N}{n_D + n_N} (\bar{X}^D - \bar{X}^N) S^{-1} (\bar{X}^D - \bar{X}^N)^T \tag{6.3}$$

This statistic combines information from the mean and dispersion of all the variables (genes being tested) in microarray experiments. When we compare two groups of samples, both of which have a large sample size, see under the null hypothesis that the distributions in both groups are the same, that is, there is no differential expression for any genes being tested in the disease and normal groups, the central limit theorem dictates that:

$$\frac{n_D + n_N - J - 1}{J(n_D + n_N - 2)} T^2 \tag{6.4}$$

is asymptotically F-distributed with J degrees of freedom for the numerator and $n_D + n_N - J - 1$ for the denominator.

Proofs

1) Given that $\bar{X}^D \sim N_J(\mu, \frac{1}{n_D} V)$ and $\bar{X}^N \sim N_J(\mu, \frac{1}{n_N} V)$, then $\bar{X}^D - \bar{X}^N \sim N_J(0, \frac{n_D + n_N}{n_D n_N} V)$,

   that is, $\sqrt{\frac{n_D + n_N}{n_D n_N}} (\bar{X}^D - \bar{X}^N) \sim N_J(0, V)$

2) For $(n_D - 1) S^D \sim W_J(n_D - 1, V)$ and $(n_N - 1) S^N \sim W_J(n_N - 1, V)$, $(n_D + n_N - 2) S = (n_D - 1) S^D + (n_N - 1) S^N \sim W_J(n_D + n_N - 2, V)$

6.2.4
Multiple Forward Search (MFS) Algorithm

There are usually a relatively small number of independent samples used in microarray experiments, while a relatively large number of genes under comparison may actually be differentially expressed. Hence, the pooled sample variance–covariance matrix S in T^2 statistic may be singular and not invertible. As a remedy for this problem, we propose a MFS algorithm that sequentially maximizes expression differences between groups of genes. This algorithm allows for iteratively and exhaustively finding a set of target DEGs. The basic structure of the MFS algorithm is outlined below:

- **Step 1**: Calculate T^2 statistics for each of all the genes that are measured in datasets, and find the gene j_1 that maximizes T^2, denoted as $T^2_{j_1}$.
- **Step 2**: If p-value$_{(T^2_{j_1})} < \alpha$ (a predefined significance level), calculate T^2 statistics for two genes, one is the gene j_1 and the other is one of the remaining genes excepting the gene j_1. Find the gene j_2 that maximizes T^2 combining with the gene j_1, denoted as $T^2_{j_1, j_2}$.

- **Step 3:** If p-value$_{(T^2_{j_1 j_2})}$ < p-value$_{(T^2_{j_1})}$, repeat step 2 by adding one more gene that maximizes T^2 combining with the genes j_1 and j_2.
- **Step 4:** Repeat step 3 until p-value$_{(T^2_{j_1,\ldots,j_{n_g-1},j_n})}$ > p-value$_{(T^2_{j_1,\ldots,j_{n-1}})}$ or the number of genes is larger than $n_1 + n_2 - 2$. Then the selected genes $j_1, j_2, \ldots, j_{n-1}$ are the first subset of identified DEGs.
- **Step 5:** Exclude gene $j_1, \ldots, j_{n-1}$, and repeat steps 1–4.
- **Step 6:** Repeat step 5 until the p-value of T^2 statistic of the starting gene is larger than α, that is, p-value$_{(T^2_{j_1})}$ > α, and stop searching.

The structure of the MFS algorithm that adds one gene to T^2 statistics in each of steps 1–4 allows for a fast updated computation of T^2 statistics by avoiding matrix inverse. For example, the pooled variance–covariance matrix for n genes can be partitioned into a block form:

$$S_n = \begin{bmatrix} S_{n-1} & a \\ a^T & b \end{bmatrix}$$

where S_{n-1} is the variance–covariance matrix for $n-1$ genes, a is the covariance vector for the first $n-1$ genes and the n-th gene, a^T is the transpose of a, and b is the variance for the n-th gene. The inverse of S_n is then calculated as:

$$S_n^{-1} = \begin{bmatrix} \left(S_{n-1} - \frac{1}{b}aa^T\right)^{-1} & -\frac{1}{k}S_{n-1}^{-1}a \\ -\frac{1}{k}a^T S_{n-1}^{-1} & \frac{1}{k} \end{bmatrix} = \begin{bmatrix} S_{n-1}^{-1} + \frac{1}{k}S_{n-1}^{-1}aa^T S_{n-1}^{-1} & -\frac{1}{k}S_{n-1}^{-1}a \\ -\frac{1}{k}a^T S_{n-1}^{-1} & \frac{1}{k} \end{bmatrix} \quad (6.5)$$

where $k = b - a^T S_{n-1}^{-1} a$. We only need to invert S_1 for the starting gene and recursively calculate the inverse of S_n by formula (6.5). Singular value decomposition can be used to obtain the general inverse of covariance matrix when the iterative method fails.

6.2.5
Resampling

In microarray experiments it is not unusual that some data points are missing due to poor quality. Large inherent "noise" in microarray data also renders estimation of the pooled sample variance–covariance matrix unrobust and variable. We propose the following procedure to handle such incomplete multivariate data that are used in constructing Hotelling's T^2 statistics used in the MFS algorithm:

- **Step 1.** Resample N replicates with replacement of subjects from the original data, denoting a replicate as R_r, $r = 1, \ldots, N$.
- **Step 2.** Calculate T^2 statistic for each R_r, denoting T^2_r, $r = 1, \ldots, N$.
- **Step 3.** Exclude 5% the lower and upper tails of T^2_r, and obtain the mean T^2 using the remaining T^2_r.

The number of replicates N could be as large as possible but, however, is limited by computational capability. This resampling strategy can alleviate statistical fluctuation and reduce sampling errors. It can help identify a consistent subset of DEGs.

6.3
Validation of Hotelling's T^2 Statistic

6.3.1
Human Genome U95 Spike-In Dataset

While developing and validating the Affymetrix Microarray Suite (MAS) 5.0 algorithm, Affymetrix produced and provided data (containing 12 640 genes) from a set of 59 arrays (HGU95) organized in a Latin-square design (http://www.affymetrix.com/support/technical/sample_data/datasets.affx). This dataset consists of 14 spike-in gene groups at known concentrations in 14 experimental groups, consisting of 12 groups of three replicates (A–L) and two groups of 12 replicates (group M–P and group Q–T). In our analyses, the latter two groups of 12 replicates were used to validate the proposed Hotelling's T^2 method for identifying DEGs. The correlations among 14 genes, measured by their concentrations, ranged from −0.965 to 0.924. Since a single RNA source was used, any probe-set not in the list of 14 genes should be negative for differential expression. Conversely, all of the probes in the list of 14 genes should be positive for differential expression.

6.3.2
Identification of DEGs

The probe levels were obtained by robust multi-array analysis (RMA) [21] and MAS 5.0. The significance level 0.001 was adopted in the analyses. The t-test resulted in four false negatives and seven false positives using the expression levels from RMA, and two false negatives and 33 false positives using the expression levels from MAS 5.0. The Hotelling's T^2 method resulted in one false negative and six false positives using the expression level from RMA, and two false negatives and 16 false positives using the expression levels from MAS 5.0 (Table 6.1).

6.4
Application Examples

6.4.1
Human Liver Cancers

6.4.1.1 Dataset
We applied the Hotelling's T^2 method to publicly available datasets from the study of Chen et al. [19], who examined gene expression patterns in human liver cancers by cDNA microarrays containing 23 075 clones representing ∼17 400 genes. In their

Table 6.1 DEGs identified by two methods in human genome U95 spike-in dataset.

t-Test		T²-Test	
RMA	MAS 5.0	RMA	MAS 5.0
1024_at[a]	1024_at[a]	37 342_s_at	684_at[a]	36 202_at[a]	1047_s_at
1091_at[a]	1091_at[a]	37 420_i_at	1091_at[a]	684_at[a]	37 777_at[a]
1552_i_at	1552_i_at	37 777_at[a]	36 085_at[a]	36 085_at[a]	1547_at
32 115_r_at	1708_at[a]	38 377_at	36 202_at[a]	1024_at[a]	39 981_at
32 283_at	1991_s_at	38 513_at	36 311_at[a]	407_at[a]	33 117_r_at
33 698_at	286_at	38 518_at	40 322_at[a]	40 322_at[a]	
36 085_at[a]	31 804_f_at	38 729_at	37 777_at[a]	32 660_at	
36 202_at[a]	32 660_at	38 734_at	1024_at[a]	38 729_at	
36 311_at[a]	32 682_at	38 997_at	38 254_at	35 270_at	
36 889_at[a]	33 117_r_at	39 058_at[a]	1552_i_at	39 733_at	
38 254_at	33 715_r_at	39 091_at	39 058_at[a]	36 311_at[a]	
38 502_at	34 540_at	39 311_at	36 889_at[a]	36 889_at[a]	
38 734_at[a]	35 270_at	39 733_at	33 698_at	1091_at[a]	
38 953_at	35 339_at	39 939_at	38 734_at[a]	38 513_at	
39 058_at[a]	35 986_at	40 322_at[a]	38 953_at	36 986_at	
40 322_at[a]	36 085_at[a]	407_at[a]	1526_i_at	1552_i_at	
684_at[a]	36 181_at	41 285_at	407_at[a]	38 997_at	
	36 200_at	41 386_i_at	38 502_at	35 862_at	
	36 202_at[a]	644_at	1708_at[a]	39 058_at[a]	
	36 311_at[a]	677_s_at		39 939_at	
	36 839_at	684_at[a]		38 734_at[a]	
	36 889_at[a]	707_s_at		34 026_at	
	36 986_at			41 036_at	

a) Spike-in genes.

study, they profiled genomic expressions in >200 samples including 102 primary hepatocellular carcinoma (HCC) from 82 patients and 74 non-tumor liver tissues from 72 patients. Two-sample Welch t-statistic was adopted to identify DEGs between two sets of samples. A permutation procedure was used to determine p-values. Genes with permutation p-values <0.001 were considered to be differentially expressed. Data are available online at the Stanford Microarray Database (SMD; http://genome-www5.stanford.edu/).

We chose genes for our analyses using the same standard as the original study [19]. Namely, all non-flagged array elements for which the fluorescent intensity in each channel was >1.5 times the local background were considered well measured. Genes for which fewer than 75% of measurements across all the samples met this standard were excluded from further analyses (http://genome-www.stanford.edu/hcc/Figures/Materials_and_Methods_v5.pdf). After primary data processing, we performed the following three comparisons using Hotelling's T^2 tests:

1) **HCC versus non-tumor liver tissues.** We compared gene expression in 82 HCC versus 74 non-tumor liver tissue samples; 11 386 genes with good

measured data for more than 62 HCC and more than 56 normal livers were used in our analyses.

2) **HCC with negative versus positive p53 staining.** To investigate the relationship between p53 mutations and gene expression programs in HCC, Chen et al. [19] examined 59 HCC specimens by immunohistochemical staining for p53 protein. They found 23 of these HCC analyzed have positive p53 staining, which has been noted to correlate with p53 mutation or inflammation in HCC [22]. 11 744 genes with good measured data for more than 27 HCC with negative p53 staining and more than 17 HCC with positive p53 staining were used in our analyses.

3) **HCC with versus without venous invasion.** To identify the role of vascular invasion in tumor spread and metastasis, 81 tumor samples were classified by histopathological evaluation as 43 negative and 38 positive for vascular invasion [19]; 11 161 genes with good measured data for more than 32 HCC without venous invasion and more than 29 HCC with venous invasion were used in our analyses.

6.4.1.2 Identification of DEGs

Table 6.2 summarizes the total numbers of DEGs identified in the above three subdatasets by the two-sample Welch t statistic in the original paper [19] and those by the Hotelling's T^2 statistic we proposed. The Hotelling's T^2 statistic found more DEGs than the t-test. In the comparison of the HCC versus non-tumor tissues, *more than 2000 DEGs* were identified by both of the two methods. In the comparison of the HCC with positive versus negative p53 staining, two-thirds of DEGs declared by the t-test were also identified by the Hotelling's T^2 statistic. However, a relatively smaller proportion of the DEGs is shared by the two methods in the comparison of the HCC with versus without venous invasion.

Eight bioinformatics resources were used to evaluate the relative performance of the two statistical methods on the basis of our knowledge about the gene function that has been obtained by various aspects of empirical studies, including biochemical, genetic, epidemiological, pharmacological, and physiological. These eight bioinformatics resources were KEGG (Kyoto Encyclopedia of Genes and Genomes, http://www.genome.ad.jp/kegg/kegg2.html), MedGENE database (http://medgene.med.harvard.edu/MEDGENE/), OMIM (Online Mendelian Inheritance in Man™, http://www.ncbi.nlm.nih.gov/Omim/), Atlas of Genetics and Cytogenetics in Oncology and Haematology (http://atlasgeneticsoncology.org//index_genes_gc.html), Cancer GeneWeb (http://www.cancerindex.org/geneweb//X070601.htm), MTB (Mouse Tumor Biology Database, http://tumor.informatics.jax.org/mtbwi/index.do),

Table 6.2 Comparison of the DEGs discovered by the two methods in human liver cancers.

Datasets (sample sizes)	t-Test	T^2-Test	Shared
HCC versus non-tumor (82/74)	3964	4508	2051
HCC with negative versus positive p53 staining (36/23)	121	146	83
HCC without versus with venous invasion (43/38)	91	151	34

Table 6.3 Number of DEGs discovered in various pathophysiological pathways by the two statistical methods in human liver cancers.

Pathways	Only t-test	Only T^2-test	Both methods[a]
p53 signaling pathway	8	16	15
Wnt signaling pathway	21	19	23
Cell cycle	16	22	29
Apoptosis profile	12	21	22
Angiogenesis	15	7	22
MAP kinase signaling pathway	24	39	57
Growth factors	7	4	10
Signal transduction in cancer	20	13	23
DNA damage signaling pathway	13	13	12
Stress and toxicity	17	12	21
Metastasis	16	13	22
DNA repair pathway	4	23	11
TGFb BMP signaling pathway	14	13	21
JAK/STAT signaling pathway	13	16	21
Total	200	231	309

a) "Both methods" indicates the number of DEGs discovered by both the Hotelling's T^2 and t-tests. "Only t-test" indicates the number of DEGs that were only found by the t-test but not by the Hotelling's T^2 test. While "Only Hotelling's T^2" indicates the number of DEGs that were only found by the Hotelling's T^2 test but not by the t-test.

GeneCards™ (http://www.genecards.org/), and GenePool (http://www.genscript.com/cgi-bin/products/genome.cgi). In the following, we detail our bioinformatics analyses for the DEGs identified by each of the two methods in the comparison of the HCC versus non-tumor tissues.

Table 6.3 summarizes the numbers of DEGs discovered in several main pathways implicated in high correlation with HCC. The Hotelling's T^2 statistic found significantly more DEGs than the t-test in the p53 signaling pathway, cell cycle, apoptosis profile, MAP kinase signaling pathway, and DNA repair pathway. For some other pathways related to HCC such as the Wnt signaling pathway, DNA damage signaling pathway, metastasis, TGFb BMP signaling pathway, and JAK/STAT signaling pathway, the numbers of DEGs identified by the two methods are very close to each other. In total, the Hotelling's T^2 test identified 31 more DEGs than the t-test in these pathways.

Table 6.4 shows grouping categories of the DEGs according to their relationships with HCC as cited in literature using the database MedGENE. We classified the DEGs identified by the two methods into several different categories [23]: (i) first-degree associations, that is, genes that have been directly linked to this disease by gene term search; (ii) first-degree associations by gene family term, that is, genes that have been directly linked to this disease by gene family term search; and (iii) second-degree associations, that is, genes that have never been co-cited with this disease but have been linked (in the same pathway) to at least one first-degree gene. Others are genes that have not been previously associated with this disease. The two-sample Welch

Table 6.4 Categories of the DEGs discovered by the two methods for the comparison of HCC versus non-tumor tissues.

Categories	Only t-test	Only T^2-test	Both methods[a]
First-degree associations	165	139	318
First-degree associations by gene family term	127	85	156
Second-degree associations	509	675	571
Total	801	899	1045

a) "Both methods" indicates the number of DEGs discovered by both the Hotelling's T^2 and t-tests. "Only t-test" indicates the number of DEGs that were only found by the t-test but not by the Hotelling's T^2 test. While "Only Hotelling's T^2" indicates the number of DEGs that were only found by the Hotelling's T^2 test but not by the t-test.

t-test identified 26 and 42 DEGs more than the Hotelling's T^2 test in the categories of first-degree associations and first-degree associations by gene family term, respectively. However, the Hotelling's T^2 test identified 166 more DEGs than the t-test in the category of second degree associations. These results indicate that the Hotelling's T^2 test is sensitive to finding genes whose differential expression is not detectable marginally, in addition to the genes found by the one-dimensional criteria.

In our analyses, several important cancer-associated genes that were differentially expressed between the HCC and normal tissues were identified by the Hotelling's T^2 test but not by the t-test. These genes included, for example, pleiomorphic adenoma gene-like 2 (PLAGL2), budding uninhibited by benzimidazoles 1 homolog beta (BUB1B) and budding uninhibited by benzimidazoles 3 homolog (BUB3), centromere protein F (CENPF), hepatoma-derived growth factor (HDGF), interleukin 1 beta (IL1B), and catenin (cadherin-associated protein) beta 1 (CTNNB1). PLAGL2 is a zinc-finger protein that recognizes DNA and/or RNA. It displays typical biomarkers of neoplastic transformation: (i) loses cell–cell contact inhibition, (ii) shows anchorage-independent growth, and (iii) induces tumors in nude mice [24]. BUB1B and BUB3 are the mitotic checkpoint genes, which were found overexpressed in gastric cancer and associated with tumor cell proliferation [25, 26]. CENPF was identified as antigen-inducing novel antibody responses during the transition to malignancy [27]. RT-PCR and Western blot analyses detected increased HDGF expression in malignant hepatoma cell lines [28]. Polymorphisms in the IL-1B-511 genetic locus are one of the possible determinants of progression of hepatitis C to HCC [29]. The expression of CTNNB1 is highly correlated with tumor progression and postoperative survival in HCC [30]. One study also reported a new non-canonical pathway through which Wnt-5a antagonizes the canonical Wnt pathway by promoting the degradation of β-catenin [31].

6.4.1.3 Classification of Human Liver Tissues

Each of the above three sub-datasets in human liver cancers was divided into ten subsets, and the cross validation was repeated ten times. Each time, one of the ten subsets was used as a validation set and the other nine subsets were put together to form a learning set. We applied the most significant genes identified in the learning sets by each of the two methods to classify samples in the validation sets using the following discriminant analyses. The average error rate across all ten trials was then computed.

The discriminant analyses were based on Mahalanobis distance that accounts for ranges of acceptability (variance) between variables and compensates for interactions (covariance) between variables [32]. The distance between two samples can be calculated as:

$$D^2(T, G_i) = (X-\mu_i)^T V_i^{-1}(X-\mu_i)$$

where

$i=1$ and 2 represent group 1 and 2, respectively;
D^2 is the generalized squared distance of the test sample T from the i-th group G_i;
V_i is the within-group covariance matrix of the i-th group;
μ_i is the vector of means of gene expression levels of the i-th group;
X is the vector of gene expression levels observed in the test sample T.

If $D^2(T,G_1) < D^2(T,G_2)$, the test sample is from group 1, otherwise from group 2.

Table 6.5 lists the average error rates for classification of samples for the two statistics. The average error rates from the Hotelling's T^2 test are always lower than those from the t-test in all of the three sub-datasets when the numbers of genes used for classification are the same. Furthermore, the average error rates of the Hotelling's T^2 test were much more stable than the t-test when different numbers of DEGs are used for classification. For example, for the HCC versus non-tumor tissues, the average error rates of the Hotelling's T^2 test varied from 0.05 to 0.07 when the numbers of genes used for classification varied from 29 to 63, while the average error rates of the t-test varied from 0.17 to 0.51. When using the T^2 test, the average error rates for the sub-datasets of the HCC with negative versus positive p53 staining and the HCC with versus without venous invasion were higher than that for the HCC versus non-tumor tissues. This is because the sample sizes of learning sets in the former two datasets are much smaller than the latter one.

Table 6.5 Error rates of discriminant analyses with DEGs discovered by the two methods in human liver tissues.

Datasets	Number of genes used	Error rates	
		t-test	T^2-test
HCC versus non-tumor (82/74)	63	0.51	0.07
	29	0.17	0.05
HCC with negative versus positive p53 staining (36/23)	42	0.55	0.16
	19	0.34	0.14
HCC without versus with venous invasion (43/38)	56	0.51	0.23
	22	0.43	0.18

6.4.2
Human Breast Cancers

6.4.2.1 Dataset

We applied the Hoteling's T^2 method to another dataset from the study of van't Veer et al. [20]. This dataset contains in total 78 primary breast cancers: 34 from patients who developed distant metastases within 5 years and 44 from patients who continued to be disease-free after a period of at least 5 years. These data were collected for the purpose of finding a prognostic signature of breast cancers in their gene expression profiles.

6.4.2.2 Cluster Analysis

van't Veer et al. [20] found 70 optimal marker genes as "prognosis classifier." This classifier predicted correctly the outcome of disease for 65 out of the 78 patients (83%), with five poor prognosis and eight good prognosis patients, respectively, assigned to the opposite category (see Figure 2b in the study of van't Veer et al. [20]). We used the Hotelling's T^2 test to find the signature genes and applied the top 70 and 52 genes to classify the respective samples. Hierarchical clustering was used for classifying these 78 primary breast cancers. We obtained 8 out of 78 incorrect classifications, with four poor prognosis and four good prognosis patients assigned to the opposite category, when using the 70-genes classifier (Figure 6.1a); we obtained 5 out of 78 incorrect classifications, with one poor prognosis and four good prognosis patients assigned to the opposite category, when using the 52-gene classifier (Figure 6.1b).

6.5
Discussion

The exponential growth of gene expression data is accompanied by an urgent need for theoretical and algorithmic advances in integrating, analyzing, and processing the large amount of valuable information. The Hotelling's T^2 statistic presented in this chapter is a novel tool for analyzing microarray data. The proposed T^2 statistic is a corollary to its original counterpart developed for multivariate analyses [33]. Our statistic for microarray data analysis possesses two prominent statistical properties. First, this new method takes into account multidimensional structure of microarray data. The utilization of the information for gene interactions allows for finding genes whose differential expressions are not marginally detectable in univariate testing methods. Second, the statistic has a close relationship to discriminant analyses for classification of gene expression patterns. The proposed search algorithm

Figure 6.1 Hierarchical clustering analyses of 78 primary human breast tumors using the 70-gene classifier (a) and the 52-gene classifier (b). Each row represents a single gene and each column represents a single tumor; <5 represents patients developing distant metastases within 5 years; >5 represents patients continuing to be disease-free after a period of at least 5 years. The samples marked with red dashes were incorrectly classified.

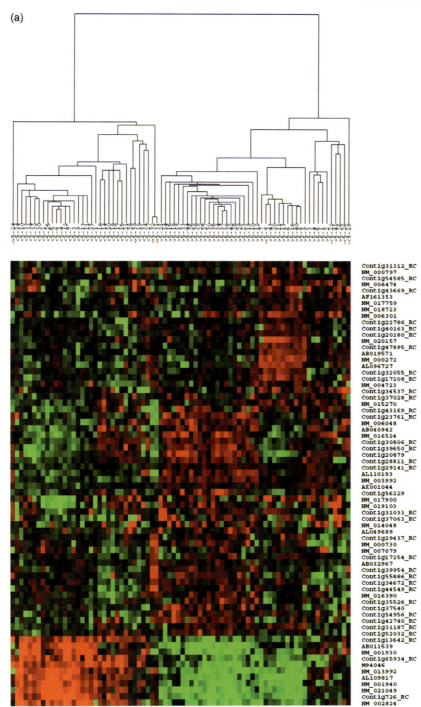

Figure 6.1 (Continued)

(b)

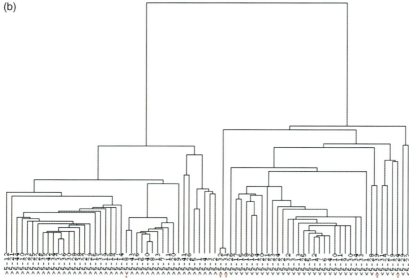

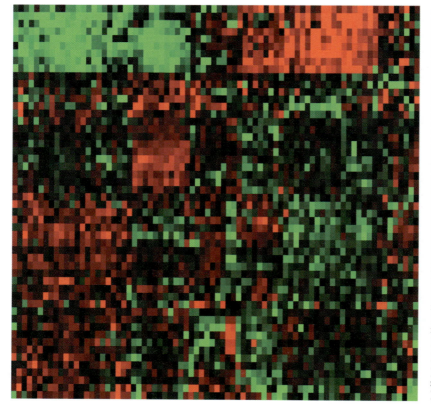

Figure 6.1 (Continued)

sequentially maximizes gene expression difference/distance between two comparison groups. Inclusion of such a set of DEGs into initial feature variables may increase the power of classification rules. In addition, The Hotelling's T^2 test gives one p-value for groups of genes rather than a p-value for each gene. Multiple testing problems are hence much less serious than univariate testing methods, unless too many groups of genes are tested.

We first validated the new T^2 method by using a spike-in HGU95 dataset from Affymetrix. This dataset consists of 14 spike-in genes at known concentrations. The Hotelling's T^2 method gave fewer false positives and negatives than t-test. For example, the new method produced one false negative and six false positives, while the t-test produced four false negatives and seven false positives, using the expression levels from RMA. We then applied the new T^2 method to the analyses of gene expression patterns in human liver cancers [19]. Extensive bioinformatics analyses and cross-validation of the DEGs identified in the study illustrated several significant advantages over the univariate t-test. First, our method discovered more DEGs in pathways related to HCC. Though p-values of the t-statistics for several genes do not exceed the threshold for significance level, these genes contribute significantly to the Hotelling's T^2 statistic in our study. These genes *per se* usually show marginal differential expressions but are correlated with other strong DEGs [14]. Second, our method identified significantly more DEGs in the category of second-degree associations with HCC. Interestingly, these genes have never been co-cited with HCC in the literature but have been linked to at least one gene that has been directly linked to this disease by gene term search, using the MedGene database [23]. Their roles in HCC tumors are worthy of further examination. This may also reflect a potential bias in the literature, where either HCC was investigated on an individual gene-by-gene study or multiple-gene expression profiles were analyzed univariately. In this sense, it is not surprising that the t-test found more DEGs in the categories of first-degree associations since current available databases seem to unduly favor the univariate approaches such as the t-test here. Third, we found several novel cancer-associated genes such as PLAGL2 and BUB1B that were also highly expressed in HCC tumors. They play important roles in the process of tumor formation and development as evidenced in a considerable body of literature [25–31]. Fourth, we reduced the misclassification to as low as 5% using <30 genes identified by the T^2 tests. This holds great promise in clinical diagnoses and classification of tumors. Large training samples, such as those we have examined here, are imperative to establish highly predictive classification functions. Finally, we applied our method to find signature genes in human breast cancers [19]. These signature genes used in hierarchical clustering resulted in higher accuracy of predicting disease outcome.

Several studies have proposed multivariate approaches for selecting subsets of DEGs [14, 15]. In their pioneering efforts, a measure of distance between vectors of gene expressions is defined for simultaneously comparing a set of genes. However, the final chosen DEGs are dependent on the choice of the predetermined cluster size, k: larger values of k typically lead to a larger list of DEGs found in a study [15]; in our method, a variable entering into T^2 statistic depends on its excess contribution to the maximization of two-group differences, thus circumventing some of the problems inherent in variable selection. This was implemented by a heuristic MFS algorithm that is designed for selecting a subset of feature vectors in high-dimensional microarray datasets. Another prominent feature of our method is that we developed a resampling-based approach to smoothen out statistical fluctuations of the T^2 statistic owing to large variability inherent in microarray data, which is very helpful for finding a consistent set of DEGs. The resampling technique can also be used for handling incomplete multivariate data, a common problem in microarray experiments.

More recently, Goeman et al. [34] have developed a score test for testing whether some pre-specified groups of genes are differentially expressed. The groups of genes could be those that are involved in a particular biochemical pathway or a genomic region of interest and should be specified before testing. This method is very valuable for testing some known pathways that affect clinical outcome in combination with groups of genes. However, the score statistic merely tests gene-expression differences in pre-specified groups of genes between two tissue types and is not intended for group wise search for DEGs. Intuitively, the Hotelling's T^2 statistic can also be used for testing pre-specified group differences and its relative performance requires further investigations in comparison with the score statistic.

One of the stopping rules associated with our search algorithm is when the number of genes entering into the T^2 statistic is smaller than $n_1 + n_2 - 2$, where n_1 and n_2 are sample sizes of two different tissue types under comparison. This restriction can be released by using principal component analysis (PCA) to reduce the dimensionality of variables entered in the Hotelling's T^2 statistic [35]. Within the framework of stabilized multivariate tests [36], the Hotelling's T^2 statistic can be performed on the basis of linear scores that are derived from the original variables using PCA. Incorporating the PCA technique into our method is valuable, especially for microarray experiments with small sample sizes. However, a small sample size may not warrant multivariate normal distribution of the data, in which permutation tests using the T^2 statistic may be necessary.

References

1 Slonim, D.K. (2002) From patterns to pathways: gene expression data analysis comes of age. *Nat. Genet.*, **32** (Suppl.), 502–508.

2 Mehta, T., Tanik, M., and Allison, D.B. (2004) Towards sound epistemological foundations of statistical methods for high-dimensional biology. *Nat. Genet.*, **36**, 943–947.

3 Alon, U., Barkai, N., Notterman, D.A., Gish, K., Ybarra, S., Mack, D., and Levine, A.J. (1999) Broad patterns of gene expression revealed by clustering analysis of tumor and normal colon tissues probed by oligonucleotide arrays. *Proc. Natl. Acad. Sci. USA*, **96**, 6745–6750.

4 Brazma, A. and Vilo, J. (2000) Gene expression data analysis. *FEBS Lett.*, **480**, 17–24.

5 Eisen, M.B., Spellman, P.T., Brown, P.O., and Botstein, D. (1998) Cluster analysis and display of genome-wide expression patterns. *Proc. Natl. Acad. Sci. USA*, **95**, 14863–14868.

6 Golub, T.R., Slonim, D.K., Tamayo, P., Huard, C., Gaasenbeek, M., Mesirov, J.P., Coller, H. et al. (1999) Molecular classification of cancer: class discovery

and class prediction by gene expression monitoring. *Science*, **286**, 531–537.

7 Baldi, P. and Long, A.D. (2001) A Bayesian framework for the analysis of microarray expression data: regularized t-test and statistical inferences of gene changes. *Bioinformatics*, **17**, 509–519.

8 Chen, Y., Dougherty, E.R., and Bittner, M.L. (1997) Ratio-based decisions and the quantitative analysis of cDNA microarray images. *J. Biomed. Opt.*, **2**, 364–374.

9 Kerr, M.K., Martin, M., and Churchill, G.A. (2000) Analysis of variance for gene expression microarray data. *J. Comput. Biol.*, **7**, 819–837.

10 Tusher, V.G., Tibshirani, R., and Chu, G. (2001) Significance analysis of microarrays applied to the ionizing radiation response. *Proc. Natl. Acad. Sci. USA*, **98**, 5116–5121.

11 Wang, S. and Ethier, S. (2004) A generalized likelihood ratio test to identify differentially expressed genes from microarray data. *Bioinformatics*, **20**, 100–104.

12 Wettenhall, J.M. and Smyth, G.K. (2004) limmaGUI: a graphical user interface for linear modeling of microarray data. *Bioinformatics*, **20**, 3705–3706.

13 Leung, Y.F. and Cavalieri, D. (2003) Fundamentals of cDNA microarray data analysis. *Trends Genet.*, **19**, 649–659.

14 Chilingaryan, A., Gevorgyan, N., Vardanyan, A., Jones, D., and Szabo, A. (2002) Multivariate approach for selecting sets of differentially expressed genes. *Math. Biosci.*, **176**, 59–69.

15 Szabo, A., Boucher, K., Carroll, W.L., Klebanov, L.B., Tsodikov, A.D., and Yakovlev, A.Y. (2002) Variable selection and pattern recognition with gene expression data generated by the microarray technology. *Math. Biosci.*, **176**, 71–98.

16 Xiong, M., Zhao, J., and Boerwinkle, E. (2002) Generalized T2 test for genome association studies. *Am. J. Hum. Genet.*, **70**, 1257–1268.

17 Model, F., Konig, T., Piepenbrock, C., and Adorjan, P. (2002) Statistical process control for large scale microarray experiments. *Bioinformatics*, **18** (Suppl 1), S155–S163.

18 Mason, R.L., Tracy, N.D., and Young, J.C. (1995) Decomposition of T2 for multivariate control chart interpretation. *J. Qual. Technol.*, **27**, 99–108.

19 Chen, X., Cheung, S.T., So, S., Fan, S.T., Barry, C., Higgins, J., Lai, K.M. et al. (2002) Gene expression patterns in human liver cancers. *Mol. Biol. Cell*, **13**, 1929–1939.

20 van't Veer, L.J., Dai, H., van de Vijver, M.J., He, Y.D., Hart, A.A., Mao, M., Peterse, H.L. et al. (2002) Gene expression profiling predicts clinical outcome of breast cancer. *Nature*, **415**, 530–536.

21 Irizarry, R.A., Bolstad, B.M., Collin, F., Cope, L.M., Hobbs, B., and Speed, T.P. (2003) Summaries of Affymetrix GeneChip probe level data. *Nucleic Acids Res.*, **31**, e15.

22 Hsu, H.C., Tseng, H.J., Lai, P.L., Lee, P.H., and Peng, S.Y. (1993) Expression of p53 gene in 184 unifocal hepatocellular carcinomas: association with tumor growth and invasiveness. *Cancer Res.*, **53**, 4691–4694.

23 Hu, Y., Hines, L.M., Weng, H., Zuo, D., Rivera, M., Richardson, A., and LaBaer, J. (2003) Analysis of genomic and proteomic data using advanced literature mining. *J. Proteome Res.*, **2**, 405–412.

24 Hensen, K., Van Valckenborgh, I.C., Kas, K., Van de Ven, W.J., and Voz, M.L. (2002) The tumorigenic diversity of the three PLAG family members is associated with different DNA binding capacities. *Cancer Res.*, **62**, 1510–1517.

25 Cahill, D.P., Lengauer, C., Yu, J., Riggins, G.J., Willson, J.K., Markowitz, S.D., Kinzler, K.W. et al. (1998) Mutations of mitotic checkpoint genes in human cancers. *Nature*, **392**, 300–303.

26 Grabsch, H., Takeno, S., Parsons, W.J., Pomjanski, N., Boecking, A., Gabbert, H.E., and Mueller, W. (2003) Overexpression of the mitotic checkpoint genes BUB1, BUBR1, and BUB3 in gastric cancer--association with tumour cell proliferation. *J. Pathol.*, **200**, 16–22.

27 Casiano, C.A., Landberg, G., Ochs, R.L., and Tan, E.M. (1993) Autoantibodies to a novel cell cycle-regulated protein that

accumulates in the nuclear matrix during S phase and is localized in the kinetochores and spindle midzone during mitosis. *J. Cell Sci.*, **106** (Pt 4), 1045–1056.

28 Hu, T.H., Huang, C.C., Liu, L.F., Lin, P.R., Liu, S.Y., Chang, H.W., Changchien, C.S. et al. (2003) Expression of hepatoma-derived growth factor in hepatocellular carcinoma. *Cancer*, **98**, 1444–1456.

29 Tanaka, Y., Furuta, T., Suzuki, S., Orito, E., Yeo, A.E., Hirashima, N., Sugauchi, F. et al. (2003) Impact of interleukin-1beta genetic polymorphisms on the development of hepatitis C virus-related hepatocellular carcinoma in Japan. *J. Infect. Dis.*, **187**, 1822–1825.

30 Inagawa, S., Itabashi, M., Adachi, S., Kawamoto, T., Hori, M., Shimazaki, J., Yoshimi, F. et al. (2002) Expression and prognostic roles of beta-catenin in hepatocellular carcinoma: correlation with tumor progression and postoperative survival. *Clin. Cancer Res.*, **8**, 450–456.

31 Topol, L., Jiang, X., Choi, H., Garrett-Beal, L., Carolan, P.J., and Yang, Y. (2003) Wnt-5a inhibits the canonical Wnt pathway by promoting GSK-3-independent beta-catenin degradation. *J. Cell Biol.*, **162**, 899–908.

32 Taguchi, G. and Jugulum, R. (eds) (2002) *The Mahalanobis-Taguchi Strategy*, John Wiley & Sons, Inc., New York.

33 Hotelling, H. (1947) Multivariate quality control, in *Techniques of Statistical Analysis* (eds C. Eisenhart, M.W. Hastay, and W.A. Wallis), McGraw-Hill, New York, pp. 111–184.

34 Goeman, J.J., van de Geer, S.A., de Kort, F., and van Houwelingen, H.C. (2004) A global test for groups of genes: testing association with a clinical outcome. *Bioinformatics*, **20**, 93–99.

35 Mardia, K.V., Kent, J.T., and Bibby, J.M. (eds) (1979) *Multivariate Analysis*, Academic Press, London.

36 Lauter, J., Glimm, E., and Kropf, S. (1996) New multivariate tests for data with an inherent structure. *Biomet. J.*, **38**, 5–23.

7
Interpreting Differential Coexpression of Gene Sets

Ju Han Kim, Sung Bum Cho, and Jihun Kim

7.1
Coexpression and Differential Expression Analyses

Microarray data analysis has been successfully applied to a wide variety of functional genomics. It enables identification of disease marker genes [1–3] and gene expression regulatory networks [4–6]. It can also be used to evaluate evolutionary conservation of gene coexpression [7].

Clustering algorithms that put similar things together and different things apart have been used in microarray data analysis, providing information about genetic regulatory relationships [8–10]. Clustering algorithms (and other unsupervised methods) applied to microarray data analysis can be considered as coexpression analysis, determining correlated groups of genes that are tightly coregulated [11].

Coexpression analysis typically generates lists of coexpressed genes (Figure 7.1c). The most challenging and rate-liming step is to determine what the resulting list(s) mean(s) biologically. Biological interpretation of coexpression clusters is based on the assumption that the genes showing similar expression profile may exhibit similar biological function. Coexpression analysis hence tends to be accompanied by the following biological knowledge-based annotation analysis. Neither statistical significance nor the biological knowledge alone is sufficient, but the two in combination are able to help better understanding of the results.

Although statistical significance analysis to determine differentially expressed genes (DEGs) between conditions is different from coexpression analysis, biological interpretation of the resulting lists of significantly down- or upregulated DEGs (Figure 7.1a) may also be benefited by the same ontology and pathway-based annotation analysis.

One naive approach is to retrieve all descriptive information concerning each gene for a particular list of genes (or a cluster) to comprehend the collective meaning of the descriptors under the biological systems context. Many statistical significance analysis methods have been developed to test whether certain gene ontology (GO)

Medical Biostatistics for Complex Diseases. Edited by Frank Emmert-Streib and Matthias Dehmer
Copyright © 2010 WILEY-VCH Verlag GmbH & Co. KGaA, Weinheim
ISBN: 978-3-527-32585-6

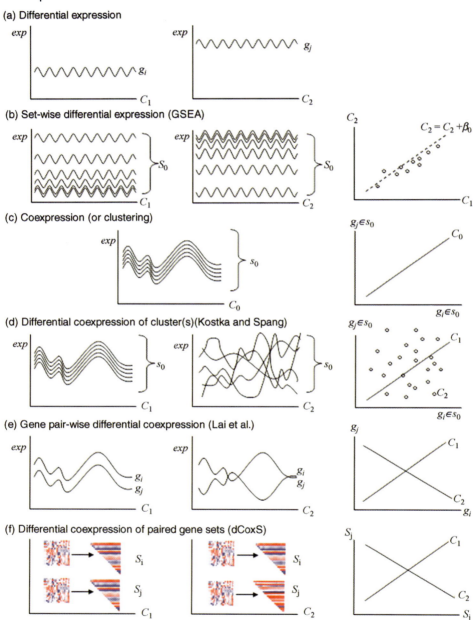

Figure 7.1 Illustration of different statistical strategies in DNA microarray data analysis. C: conditions, g: genes, s: gene clusters, S: a priori defined gene sets (e.g., pathways), exp: level of gene expression; (d) [26], (e) [24], (f) [28].

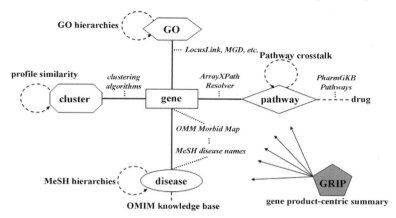

Figure 7.2 Collection of biological knowledge-based annotation resources for genes and gene clusters. (Courtesy of Nucleic Acid. Res.)

or biological pathway-based annotations are significantly enriched within a particular list of genes when compared to a reference list [12–14]. Many GO and biological pathway-based tools for gene expression analysis have been developed and proven to be useful [12, 15–21].

In principle, any attribute of genes can be applied for the "annotation analysis," including transcription factors [12], clinical phenotypes like disease associations, MeSH terms, micro-RNA binding sites, and so on, as well as GO terms and biological pathways. Moreover, these features may in turn have their own ontological structures (Figure 7.2). ArrayXPath provides one of the most comprehensive collections of these structured features for annotation analysis [18, 21].

7.2
Gene Set-Wise Differential Expression Analysis

Gene set enrichment analysis (GSEA) tests, for each a priori defined gene set, significant association with phenotypic classes in DNA microarray experiment [22]. While "annotation analysis" determines overrepresented GO terms or biological pathways after determining significant coexpression clusters or DEG lists, GSEA takes the "reverse-annotation" or "gene set-wise" approach. GSEA first creates a ranked list of genes according to their differential expression between experimental conditions and determines, for each a priori defined gene set, whether members of a gene set tend to occur toward the top (or bottom) of the ranked list, in which case the gene set is correlated with the phenotypic class distinction (Figure 7.1b).

This gene set-wise differential expression analysis method successfully identified modest but coordinated changes in gene expression that were missed by conventional "single gene-wise" differential expression analysis. Moreover, the gene set-wise approach provides straightforward biological interpretation because the gene sets are defined by biological knowledge.

7.3
Differential Coexpression Analysis

Coexpression analysis determines the degree of coexpression of a group (or cluster) of genes under a certain condition. In contrast, differential coexpression analysis determines the degree of coexpression difference of a gene pair or a gene cluster across different conditions, which may relate to key biological processes provoked by changes in environmental conditions [23–27]. Three types of differential coexpression analysis methods have been introduced to identify differentially coexpressed (i) gene cluster(s) (Figure 7.1d), (ii) gene pairs (Figure 7.1e), and (iii) paired (a priori defined) gene-sets (Figure 7.1f) between two (or more) conditions.

To identify differentially coexpressed gene cluster(s) between two conditions, Kostka and Spang used an additive model-based scoring system and determined whether a cluster shows significant conditional difference in the degree of coexpression [26]. After creating gene expression clusters, Watson used t-statistic for each cluster to evaluate the difference of the degree of coexpression between conditions [27]. These methods can be viewed as an attempt to find gene clusters that are tightly co-regulated (i.e., highly coexpressed) in one condition (i.e., normal) but not in another (i.e., cancer).

To identify differentially coexpressed gene pairs, Lai *et al.* calculated the expected conditional F-statistic (ECF), a modified F statistic [24], for all pair of genes between two conditions. Choi *et al.* detected gene pairs with significant differential coexpression between normal and cancer samples through a meta-analytic approach [25]. These methods can be viewed as an attempt to find gene pairs that are, in principle, positively correlated in one condition (i.e., normal) and negatively correlated in another (i.e., cancer).

Identification of differentially coexpressed gene clusters or gene pairs usually do not use a priori defined gene sets or pairs but try to find the best ones among all possible combinations without considering prior knowledge. Thus the biological interpretation of the clusters or pairs may also need the ontology and pathway-based annotation analysis.

Interestingly, to my best knowledge, no method has been presented for finding a gene cluster that shows positive correlation in one condition and negative correlation in another. It seems that there is very little chance for such a cluster to exist. Similarly, one can hardly find such a set among a priori defined gene sets (i.e., pathways). It is even hard to find a biological pathway for which all members are highly positively (or negatively) coexpressed in a condition because a biological pathway is a complex functional system with both interacting positive and negative feedback loops. Thus, members of a biological pathway may not be contained in a single coexpression cluster, especially when the cluster is not very big, but be split into different clusters.

7.4
Differential Coexpression Analysis of Paired Gene Sets

The dCoxS (differential coexpression of gene sets) algorithm (available at http://www.snubi.org/publication/dCoxS/) for differential coexpression analysis of paired (a priori defined) gene sets between conditions has the benefits of both differential coexpression and gene set-wise analyses [28]. For the purpose of illustration, we used biological pathways as predefined gene sets.

Figure 7.3 demonstrates how the dCoxS algorithm identifies differentially coexpressed biological pathway pairs. Expression matrices of two gene sets consist of the same samples (or columns) and different genes (or rows). Computing all sample pairwise distances for each condition for each gene set, given the same set of samples, returns the same number of sample-wise distances. Sample pair-wise similarities are

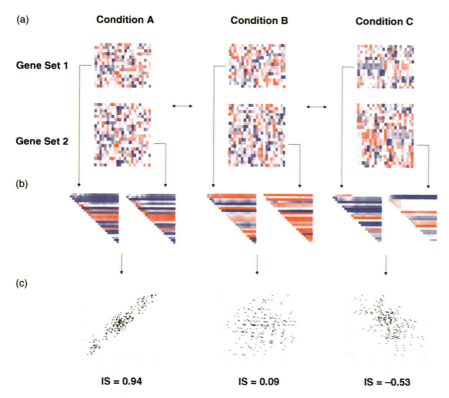

Figure 7.3 Overview of the dCoxS algorithm. Expression matrices of two gene sets (a) are transformed into Rényi relative entropy matrices by all sample pair-wise comparisons (b). The interaction score (IS), a kind of correlations coefficients, between a pair of entropy matrices is obtained for each condition. Upper diagonal heat maps (b) are transformed into scatter plots (c), where ISs are depicted as fitted lines. (Modified, courtesy of *BMC Bioinformatics*.)

computed in terms of the Rényi relative entropy, creating upper (or lower) diagonals of the entropy matrices.

To measure the expression similarity between paired gene-sets under the same condition, dCoxS defines the interaction score (IS) as the correlation coefficient between the sample-wise entropies (or diagonal elements). Although the numbers of the genes in different pathways are usually different, dCoxS can always compute the IS because it uses only sample-wise distances regardless whether the two pathways have the same genes or not. For example, when we compute the IS of a pair of pathway expression matrices with dimensions 25 by 20 and 15 by 20 (genes by samples) for a condition we calculate 190 [= (20 × 19)/2] sample pair-wise entropy distances for each pathway expression matrix. Then the IS is obtained by calculating the correlation coefficient between the two entropy vectors.

Finally, the statistical significance of the difference of the Fisher's Z-transformed ISs between two conditions is tested for each pathway pair. The validity of dCoxS is evaluated with simulation datasets and two public microarray datasets.

7.5
Measuring Coexpression of Gene Sets

To measure the degree of coexpression between two gene sets, dCoxS uses the variation of expression levels determined by the Rényi relative entropy, which is a generalized form of Shannon entropy [29]. It is given by Equation (7.1), where X is a stochastic variable with a probability density function fx:

$$H_R = \frac{1}{1-\alpha} \log \left(\int (fx)^\alpha dx \right) \alpha > 0, \alpha \neq 1 \tag{7.1}$$

dCoxS uses the quadratic Rényi relative entropy because of its convenience of estimation in a nonparametric manner [30]:

$$\left[D_2(P||Q) = \frac{1}{\alpha-1} \log \left(\int (p)^\alpha (q)^{1-\alpha} \right) = 2\log\left(\frac{p}{q}\right) \approx \log \frac{\hat{f}_h(S_i)}{\hat{f}_h(S_j)} \right] \tag{7.2}$$

where $\hat{f}_h(S_i)$ and $\hat{f}_h(S_j)$ denote the probabilistic density of the different samples i and j in an estimated multivariate distribution from a gene set expression matrix. Since $\alpha = 2$ and one sample is used, the log ratio of the density of the different samples approximates the quadratic Rényi relative entropy. Although $\log(p^\alpha) = \alpha \log(p)$, α is deleted because it has no effect on the calculation of the IS. The density is estimated using the Parzen window density estimation with the Gaussian kernel function. We used a multiplicative kernel for the density estimation, which can be expressed as:

$$\hat{f}(x)_h = \frac{1}{n} \sum_{i=1}^{n} \left\{ \prod_{j=1}^{d} h_j^{-1} K\left(\frac{x - X_{ij}}{h_j}\right) \right\} \tag{7.3}$$

where

d is the number of variables,
n is the sample size,
K denotes a univariate kernel function [31].

In this analysis, n and d are the numbers of samples in a condition and of genes in a gene set, respectively. In Equation (7.3), X_{ij} is the expression value from the i-th observation of the j-th gene in a gene set expression matrix and x is a vector containing the expression values of d genes in a sample. For bandwidth (h_j) selection of each dimension, we used Scott's rule in Equation (7.4), where $\hat{\sigma}_j$ is the estimated variance of the j-th variable [31]:

$$\hat{h}_j = n^{1/(d+4)} \hat{\sigma}_j \qquad (7.4)$$

For each condition for each gene set, one relative entropy matrix of all sample pairs can be obtained.

As a measure of the degree of coexpression between a pair of gene sets given a condition, we define the IS in Equation (7.5), which is the Pearson's correlation coefficient between the upper-diagonal elements of the relative entropy matrices of a paired gene sets:

$$IS = \frac{\sum_{i<j}(RE^{G_1} - \overline{RE^{G_2}})(RE^{G_1} - \overline{RE^{G_2}})}{\sqrt{\sum_{i<j}(RE^{G_1} - \overline{RE^{G_1}})^2}\sqrt{\sum_{i<j}(RE^{G_2} - \overline{RE^{G_2}})^2}} \qquad (7.5)$$

where RE^{G_1} and RE^{G_2} are the matrices of the Rényi relative entropy of gene sets G_1 and G_2, respectively. RE^G is computed using:

$$RE^G = \left\{ x : x_{ij} = \log\frac{\hat{f}_h(S_i)}{\hat{f}_h(S_j)}; \quad i,j = 1,2,3,\ldots,N \right\} \qquad (7.6)$$

7.6
Measuring Differential Coexpression of Gene Sets

dCoxS uses Fisher's Z-transformation of the IS in (7.7) to measure the degree of differential coexpression between paired gene sets under different conditions:

$$Zf = \frac{1}{2} \times \ln\left(\frac{1+IS}{1-IS}\right) \qquad (7.7)$$

The p-value of the difference in the Zf values is calculated using the standard normal distribution in Equation (7.8):

$$P\left(Z \geq \left|\frac{(Zf_1 - Zf_2)}{\sqrt{1/(N_1-3) + 1/(N_2-3)}}\right|\right) \qquad (7.8)$$

Zf_1 and Zf_2 are the Fisher's Z-transformed values of the IS under two different conditions and N_1 and N_2 are the numbers of upper-diagonal elements, which are calculated by $n(n-1)/2$ ($n=$ number of samples) for each condition.

dCoxS first obtains parametric p-values and selects significant ones according to the threshold determined from the p-value distribution. The selected pathway pairs are retested in a nonparametric fashion. The nonparametric p-value is determined by the number of cases where the difference of permuted ISs is larger than that of the original ISs. Hypothesis testing by gene-wise and sample-wise permutation is performed. Random resampling of the equal number of genes within each gene set is used for gene permutation. Shuffling sample class labels is used for sample permutations:

$$P = \frac{\sum_{i=1}^{N}\sum_{j=1}^{M} I[dZf(IS_{C1}, IS_{C2}) < dZf_{ij}(pIS', pIS'')]}{N \times M} \qquad (7.9)$$

In Equation (7.9), N and M represent the numbers of gene and sample permutations, respectively; $dZf(IS_{C1}, IS_{C2})$ is the absolute value of the difference of Z-transformed ISs (ZISs) computed from conditions C1 and C2; dZf_{ij} indicates the absolute value of the difference between pIS' and pIS'', which are ISs calculated from the i-th gene and j-th sample permutations, respectively. Gene- and sample-wise permutations generate a pair of random gene set expression matrices for each condition. After transforming expression matrices to the relative entropy matrices, the entropy matrices are permuted. Permuted ISs (pIS' and pIS'') are then computed with the permuted entropy matrices following the nonparametric test method of the Mantel test [32]. $I(\cdot)$ is an indicator function, which equals one when the absolute value of the dZf of the permuted entropy matrices is larger than that of the original dZf or otherwise is zero. More permutation is recommended for genes than for samples because there are more probes than samples.

Pathway pairs often share common genes, requiring a different strategy. For pathway pairs with shared genes, dCoxS applies three methods to calculate dZISs: (i) non-assigning method by applying the standard method disregarding the shared ones and (ii) assigning method by assigning the shared ones to one of the pathways and (iii) then the other. The most significant dZIS among the three is selected.

7.7
Gene Pair-Wise Differential Coexpression

For comparison, a gene pair-wise differential coexpression analysis similar to Figure 7.1f is tested. All gene pair-wise Zf values are calculated for each condition and the conditional difference of the Fisher's Z-transformed correlation coefficients is tested for each gene pair as follows:

$$Zf = \frac{1}{2} \times \ln\left(\frac{1+CC}{1-CC}\right) \qquad (7.10)$$

$$p\left(Z \geq \left|\frac{(Zf_1 - Zf_2)}{\sqrt{1/(N_1-3) + 1/(N_2-3)}}\right|\right) \qquad (7.11)$$

where

CC indicates the correlation coefficient of a gene pair,
Zf_i is the Fisher's Z-transformed correlation coefficient,
N_i the number of samples in conditions i.

The p-value for differential coexpression is obtained according to the difference between the Z values from the normal distribution. For each gene pair, three p-values are obtained, one from each condition and another from the difference between the conditions. Bonferroni correction is applied and the gene pairs whose three p-values are all lower than the Bonferroni adjusted p-value are selected (adjusted p-value 6.274×10^{-10} for 79 689 000 gene pairs).

7.8
Datasets and Gene Sets

7.8.1
Datasets

One simulation dataset and two microarray datasets, lung cancer (http://www.broad.mit.edu/) [33] and Duchenne's muscular dystrophy (DMD) (GSE1004, http://www.ncbi.nlm.nih.gov/geo/) [34], are tested. The lung cancer dataset consists of 17 normal lung and 21 squamous cell carcinoma samples and the DMD dataset of 11 normal and 12 DMD patient muscle samples, both using the Affymetrix HU-95 Av2 platform. The Robust Multichip Averaging (RMA) [35] package is used for data normalization.

7.8.2
Gene Sets

Biological pathway information is used to define gene sets. We use human biological pathways in the ArrayXPath knowledge base available at http://www.snubi.org/software/ArrayXPath/ [18, 21] and map the microarray probes onto pathway nodes. We arbitrarily set the minimum size (i.e., the number of member nodes) of a valid gene set as 10, resulting in 350 pathways for the Affymetrix HU 95 Av2 platform.

7.9
Simulation Study

To validate whether the IS represents the similarity between two gene expression matrices, simulated expression matrices are generated from reference expression

Table 7.1 Evaluation of distance measures by simulation study.

Distance metric	SD[a]					
	0.05	0.1	0.2	0.3	0.4	0.5
IS[b]	0.9982	0.8633	0.6133	0.4232	0.3000	0.2367
Gower	0.9989	0.9177	0.7715	0.6178	0.5016	0.4128
Canberra	0.9994	0.9477	0.8314	0.6846	0.5567	0.4571
Bray	0.9995	0.9571	0.8575	0.7248	0.6056	0.5085
Manhattan	0.9995	0.9574	0.8587	0.7276	0.6102	0.5137
Euclidean	0.9998	0.9748	0.9031	0.7950	0.6819	0.5851

a) SD: standard deviation.
b) IS: interaction score.

matrix by adding random values, where SX_{ij} and X_{ij} indicate the j-th gene expression values of the i-th sample in the simulated and reference matrices, respectively.

Random values are generated from the normal distribution with six different standard deviations ($\mu = 0$, $\sigma = SD$, $SD = 0.05$, 0.1, 0.2, 0.3, 0.4, and 0.5). Matrix similarity hence decreases as SD increases. Two real datasets are used to generated 700 [=350 (pathways × 2 (datasets)] simulated expression profiles. ISs are calculated between the reference and simulated matrices.

For validation, the IS is compared to the Mantel statistics computed by five different metrics (Bray, Canberra, Euclidean, Gower, and Manhattan). Average similarity between the reference and simulation data decreases as SDs increases for all six computations (Table 7.1). The mean ISs has the lowest similarity scores at all SD levels and the difference of the mean ISs across different SD groups is statistically significant (paired t-test, $p < 0.001$). The IS shows statistically significant differences to all others at all SD levels ($p < 0.001$).

7.10
Lung Cancer Data Analysis Results

We tested 61 075 pairs from the 350 pathways to determine differentially coexpressed pathway pairs in the lung cancer dataset. We used a very strict threshold (p-value $= 2.2 \times 10^{-16}$) since 53% of p-values from parametric tests were lower than the Bonferroni adjusted p-value, 8.187×10^{-7} ($\alpha = 0.05$, $n = 61\,075$ gene set pairs). We chose the strict threshold to focus only on more significant results, representing one percentile of the p-values obtained from dCoxS analysis of all pathway pairs. We obtained three p-values, one from the normal, a second from lung cancer, and the third from the difference between them. We selected significant pairs only when all three p-values were lower than the threshold.

Sixty-five (0.11%) among the 61 075 pathway pairs were significant within the criteria. All pairs were also statistically significant in the permutation test

7.10 Lung Cancer Data Analysis Results

Table 7.2 The ten pathway pairs showing significant differences in dZIS in lung cancer dataset[a].

Pathway pair	Number of OGs	IS NL	IS SCC	dZIS
Cytokine network (37) / TNF/stress-related signaling (54)[b]	7	0.97	0.56	13.8
Estrogen-responsive protein Efp controls cell cycle and breast tumor growth (24) / Propanoate_metabolism (26)	0	0.97	0.55	13.6
Activation of Src by protein-tyrosine phosphatase α (22) / Nuclear_receptors (51)	0	0.96	0.59	12.2
Double-stranded RNA-induced gene expression (15) / Neuroregulin receptor degradation protein-1 controls ErbB3 receptor recycling (13)	0	0.96	0.56	11.8
Acute myocardial infarction (23) / Angiotensin-converting enzyme 2 regulates heart function (18)[b]	11	0.96	0.60	11.5
ALK in cardiac myocytes (52) / Inositol_phosphate_metabolism (146)	0	0.96	0.61	11.4
p38 MAPK signaling pathway (69) / Apoptosis (73)[b]	10	0.95	0.54	11.3
fMLP-induced chemokine gene expression in HMC-1 cells (62)[b] / PTEN-dependent cell cycle arrest and apoptosis (25)	2	0.95	0.56	11.2
BRCA1-dependent Ub-ligase activity (18) / Aminosugars_metabolism (13)	0	0.96	0.61	11.2
Endocytotic role of NDK, phosphins, and dynamin (21) / Pyruvate_metabolism (40)	0	0.96	0.65	11.0

a) Number of OGs: number of overlapping genes in two gene sets, NL: normal lung, SCC: squamous cell carcinoma, dZIS: difference of Z-transformed IS, (): number of genes in a gene set, nonparametric p-value $< 8.0 \times 10^{-7}$.
b) Shared genes are assigned to this pathway.

(p-value $< 8.0 \times 10^{-7}$). Among the 65 pairs, 38 did not have and 27 had shared members. All of the 27 were determined to be significant by using an assigning method after being non-significant by the non-assigning method.

Table 7.2 shows the top ten pathway pairs sorted by the dZIS values. The cytokine network and TNF/stress-related pathway pair yielded the highest dZIS. The estrogen-responsive protein Efp-related and propanoate-metabolism pathway pair was the second highest. Many important carcinogenesis-associated pathways such as cell cycle, apoptosis, and telomerase pathways were found in the 65 pairs.

For gene pair-wise differential coexpression tests, the correlation coefficients of each gene pair were obtained, and the conditional difference of the correlation coefficients was tested using Bonferroni's multiple testing correction. In contrast to the dCoxS analysis, we found no significant gene pair.

Figure 7.4 shows the expression profiles and the ISs of the cell cycle: G1/S check point (a) and inhibition of cellular proliferation by Gleevec (b) pathways. The expression profiles of the pathways seem by human eyes less similar in lung cancer than in normal lung. This difference, however, is more evident in the IS scatter plots (Figure 7.4c).

One can simply expand the differential coexpression dyads into a network of interacting pathways, representing close collaborators. Table 7.3 shows the pathways showing significant differential coexpression with more than two pathways. The thrombin signaling and protease-activated receptors pathway showed differential coexpression with five other pathways, which was the highest number of interacting pathways.

7.11
Duchenne's Muscular Dystrophy Data Analysis Results

In the DMD data analysis, we used ten percentile of the p-values ($=1.18 \times 10^{-8}$) obtained from the parametric test as a cutoff threshold because only three pairs of gene sets were significant within one percentile threshold. It was still much lower than the Bonferroni adjusted p-value ($=8.187 \times 10^{-7}$). Thirty pathway pairs were significant and the permutation test were all significant, too ($p < 8.0 \times 10^{-7}$). Among the 65 pairs, 38 did not have and 27 had shared members. All of the 27 were determined to be significant by using the assigning method after being non-significant by the non-assigning method. Among the 30 pairs, 25 did not have and five had shared members. All of the five were determined to be significant by using the assigning method after being non significant by the non-assigning method. Like the lung cancer data, gene pair-wise differential coexpression analysis resulted in no significant pairs.

Table 7.4 shows the pathways showing more than one differentially coexpressed pathways in the DMD dataset. The D4-GDI signaling pathway has the biggest number of interacting pathways ($n = 10$). The Monoamine_GPCRs and Trka receptor signaling pathway are connected to three others. Figure 7.5 depicts the differential coexpression (or pathway interaction) network of DMD dataset.

Table 7.5 shows the pathway pairs that have the top ten dZISs. The pathway pair β-arrestins in GPCR desensitization and D4-GDI signaling had the highest dZIS value. The D4-GDI signaling and "role of arrestins in the activation and targeting of MAP kinases" pathway pair had the second highest dZIS. Figure 7.5 shows IS scatter plots for the six selected pathway pairs, which may be related to the pathophysiology of DMD.

7.11 Duchenne's Muscular Dystrophy Data Analysis Results

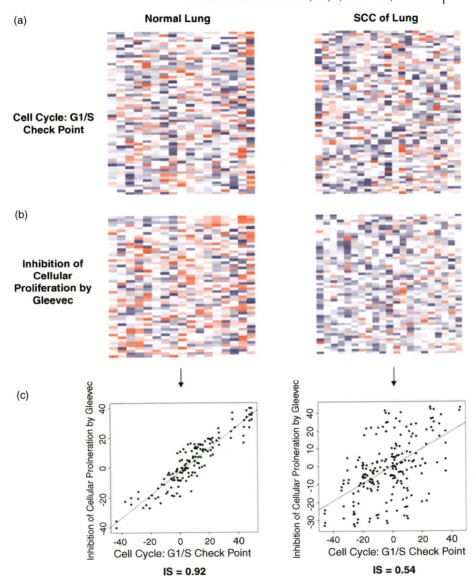

Figure 7.4 Lung cancer dataset. The similarity between the pathways – cell cycle: G1/S check points (a) and inhibition of cellular proliferation by Gleevec (b) – exhibiting conditional changes represented by the IS plots (c). Unlike the heatmap representations, IS plots clearly represent the quantitative difference of coexpression of a pathway pair between normal and cancer tissues. (Courtesy of BMC Bioinformatics)

Table 7.3 Pathways showing differential coexpression with more than one pathway in the lung cancer dataset[a].

Pathway	K	Sum (ZIS)
Thrombin signaling and protease-activated receptors (30)	5	43.9
Cell cycle: G1/S check point (42)	4	39.0
Activation of Src by protein-tyrosine phosphatase α (13)	3	31.6
TNF/stress related signaling (29)	3	31.5
Pyruvate_metabolism (18)	3	30.3
fMLP induced chemokine gene expression in HMC-1 cells (22)	3	30.1
ALK in cardiac myocytes (23)	3	30.0
Nuclear_receptors (28)	3	29.9
Sphingoglycolipid_metabolism (22)	3	29.6
Role of MEF2D in T-cell apoptosis (20)	3	28.3
T cell receptor signaling pathway (28)	3	27.3
Cell cycle: G2/M checkpoint (50)	3	27.3
Insulin signaling pathway (15)	3	27.3
Bioactive peptide induced signaling pathway (32)	3	27.2
Translation_factors (52)	3	26.9
Nicotinate_and_nicotinamide_metabolism (18)	3	25.8
B lymphocyte cell surface molecules (65)	2	21.3
Apoptotic DNA fragmentation and tissue homeostasis (19)	2	19.9
Keratinocyte differentiation (11)	2	19.3
CDK regulation of DNA replication (12)	2	18.8
IL-2 receptor β chain in T cell activation (43)	2	18.2
Nuclear_receptors (35)	2	18.0
Glycine_serine_and_threonine_metabolism (47)	2	17.8
Control of skeletal myogenesis by HDAC & calcium/calmodulin-dependent kinase (CaMK) (22)	2	17.6

a) K: no. of pathways showing differential coexpression, Sum(ZIS): total sum of Z-transformed IS, (): number of genes in a gene set.

Table 7.4 Pathways showing more than one differentially coexpressed pathways in DMD dataset[a].

Pathway name	K	Sum (ZIS)
D4-GDI signaling pathway (30)	10	111.5
Monoamine_GPCRs (42)	3	30.6
Trka receptor signaling pathway (13)	3	29.2
Aspirin blocks signaling pathway involved in platelet activation (29)	2	23.1
Msp/Ron receptor signaling pathway (18)	2	21.4
TGF β signaling pathway (22)	2	20.7
AKT signaling pathway (23)	2	18.3

a) K: number of pathways showing differential coexpression, Sum(ZIS): total sum of Z-transformed IS, (): number of genes in a gene set.

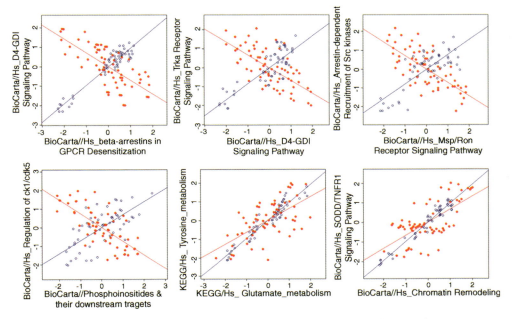

Figure 7.5 Differentially coexpressed pathway pairs in the DMD dataset. Blue and red indicate the normal and DMD samples, respectively. (Courtesy of *BMC Bioinformatics*.)

7.12 Discussion

The idea of measuring matrix similarity is rooted in the Mantel statistic, which measures the similarity of two matrices using correlation coefficient of sample-wise distances [32]. Instead of using well-known distance metrics, however, dCoxS applies the quadratic Rényi relative entropy with multivariate kernel density estimation. The Rényi relative entropy is calculated by subtracting each sample's Rényi entropy, which has a metric property [30]. Therefore, it is equivalent to the distance between samples. Gene sets are defined by biological knowledge such that the member genes are likely to have internal correlation structure. The Rényi relative entropy may be a plausible distance metric to model this correlation structure because the entropy was estimated according to the multivariate density.

As shown in the simulation study, the IS represents the similarity between two pathway expression matrices. Average IS decreases as the SD increases and the differences of the mean ISs are significant (Table 7.1). Therefore, the Rényi relative entropy and the IS may be a valid similarity measure for gene expression matrices.

All five distance metrics for the Mantel statistic (see below) take the form of the summation of squared or absolute values of the differences for the i-th dimension, $x_{ij} - x_{ik}$, and hence have more chance to have equal or similar distances than the IS

Table 7.5 Top ten pairs showing significant dZIS in DMD dataset[a].

Pathway pair	Number of OGs	IS NM	IS DMD	dZIS
β-Arrestins in GPCR desensitization (15) / D4-GDI signaling pathway (22)	0	0.95	−0.71	14.7
D4-GDI signaling pathway (22) / Role of arrestins in the activation and targeting of MAP kinases (22)	0	0.94	−0.65	13.2
Eicosanoid metabolism (25) / Lysine_degradation (28)	0	0.94	−0.66	13.2
Regulation of hematopoiesis by cytokines (28) / Monoamine_GPCRs (34)	0	0.92	−0.66	12.6
Aspirin blocks signaling pathway involved in platelet activation (35) / D4-GDI signaling pathway (22)	0	0.90	−0.68	12.3
D4-GDI signaling pathway (22) / RB tumor suppressor/checkpoint signaling in response to DNA damage (23)	0	0.79	−0.80	11.5
T helper cell surface molecules (16) / TGF β signaling pathway (34)	0	0.88	−0.64	11.4
D4-GDI signaling pathway (22) / Trka receptor signaling pathway (22)	0	0.84	−0.68	11.0
Aspirin blocks signaling pathway involved in platelet activation (35) / Msp/Ron receptor signaling pathway (14)	0	0.81	−0.72	10.8
Msp/Ron receptor signaling pathway (14) / Roles of arrestin-dependent recruitment of Src kinases in GPCR signaling (28)	0	0.79	−0.72	10.5

a) Number of OGs: number of overlapping genes in two gene sets, NM: normal muscle, DMD: Duchenne's muscular dystrophy, dZIS: difference of Z-transformed IS, (): number of genes in a gene set, nonparametric p-value $< 8.0 \times 10^{-7}$.

using Rényi relative entropy that uses multivariate kernel density estimation. For example, two distances, $d(v_R, v_1)$ and $d(v_R, v_2)$ from three vectors, v_R, v_1, and v_2, become similar when the i-th dimension of the two vector pairs have similar $|x_{ij} - x_{ik}|$ values. In contrast, the Rényi relative entropy distinguishes these differences. This may explain why all Mantel statistics are higher than the IS (Table 7.1). In a biological sense, distances from a (sample) vector to two different ones should be different. Therefore, the strength of IS as a representative distance measure for gene expression profiles is supported:

Euclidian $d_{jk} = \sqrt{\sum_i (x_{ij} - x_{ik})^2}$

Manhattan $d_{jk} = \sum_i |x_{ij} - x_{ik}|$

$$\text{Gower } d_{jk} = \frac{1}{M} \sum_i \frac{|x_{ij} - x_{ik}|}{\max x_i - \min x_i} \quad \text{where } M \text{ is the number of columns}$$
(excluding missing values)

$$\text{Canberra } d_{jk} = \frac{1}{N_Z} \sum_i \frac{|x_{ij} - x_{ik}|}{x_{ij} + x_{jk}} \quad \text{where } N_Z \text{ is the number of non-zero entries}$$

$$\text{Bray } d_{jk} = \frac{\sum_i |x_{ij} - x_{ik}|}{\sum_i (x_{ij} + x_{ik})}$$

Pathways often share common genes and one can use both the assigning and non-assigning methods. When the shared members are assigned to one of the pathways, the other pathway has to have a subset excluding the shared ones. Therefore, biological interpretation of the pathway pairs should be careful, especially when the shared genes occupy a large portion of the original pathway. This property can be used to find a novel subset (or module) of a pathway that is differentially coexpressed with another pathway (or module).

Although dCoxS results provide the ease of biological interpretation by using gene sets that are defined by a priori biological knowledge, exploratory analysis like clustering still has advantages in discovering novel clusters or modules of interacting genes. The differential coexpression network constructed in Figure 7.6 is an attempt to organize the significant biological knowledge structure extracted by dCoxS for further insight into the underlying biological processes. One can apply the dCoxS algorithm for the clusters created not by prior knowledge but by exploratory algorithms to find and organize novel differentially-coexpressed clusters or modules. Then, the following step of "annotation analysis" becomes essential again.

The next step is to organize the annotated results. BioLattice is a mathematical framework for such integration based on concept lattice analysis available at http://www.snubi.org/software/biolattice/ [36]. By considering explored gene clusters as objects and associated annotations as attributes and by applying set inclusion theory, BioLattice orders them into a lattice of biological "concepts" defined by the sets of objects that share common knowledge attributes and the attributes that are annotated to the objects. The concepts are arranged in a hierarchical order to provide an "executive summary" of the experimental context, representing the correlation structure implied in the results (Figure 7.7) [36].

dCoxS detected many pathways related to the pathophysiology of lung cancer. The pathway pair cytokine network and TNF/stress related signaling, for example, showed the highest dZIS (Table 7.2). Many of the member genes of these pathways are known to be associated with squamous cell cancer of the lung [37, 38]. The "thrombin signaling and protease-activated receptors pathway" showing the highest number of interacting pathways and sum of corresponding dZISs (Table 7.3) is known to be involved in the angiogenesis of lung cancer [39]. Notably, the cell cycle, pathway pair G1/S check point and inhibition of cellular proliferation by Gleevec, is shown up (Figure 7.4). Although the Gleevec was developed for the treatment of chronic myelogenous leukemia, it has already been used for treating many kinds of solid tumors, including lung cancer [40]. Lung cancer samples show a strong tendency to

148 | *7 Interpreting Differential Coexpression of Gene Sets*

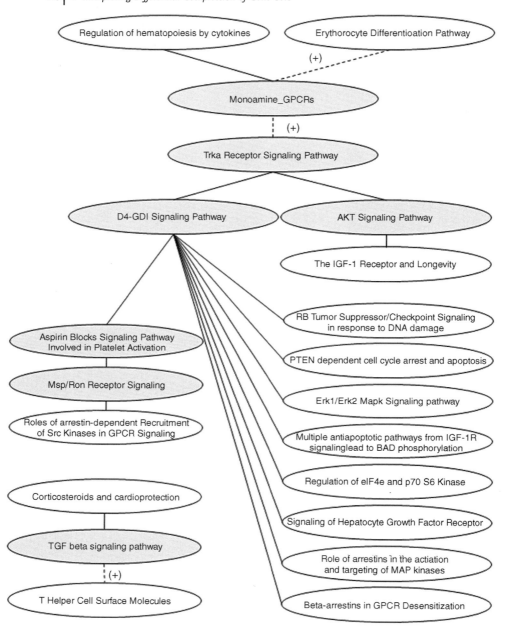

Figure 7.6 Part of differential coexpression networks from the DMD dataset. Two-member networks are omitted. "Hub" pathways involved in more than one differential coexpression pairs are in gray. ISs of many pairs show the opposite signs between DMD and normal muscle, that is, positive in one and negative in another or vice versa. Three pairs with no sign change between conditions are linked by broken lines labeled with "(+)" symbols.

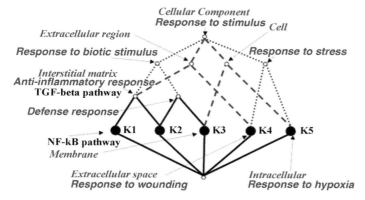

Figure 7.7 BioLattice as an "executive summary" for the biological interpretation of the combined results from coexpression analysis and the following annotation analysis of microarray experiment. (Courtesy of *Journal of Biomedical Informatics*.)

have lower ISs in most of the pathway pairs than normal samples (Table 7.2). This may suggest perturbed normal molecular regulatory mechanisms in cancer.

In DMD samples, the D4-GDI signaling pathway with the biggest number of interacting pathways (Table 7.4 and Figure 7.6) shows the highest dZIS with the β-arrestins in GPCR desensitization pathway (Table 7.5). D4-GDI has been known to be associated with cytoskeletal changes in apoptotic cells [41]. The significant changes in the ISs in interaction with others imply that the D4-GDI signaling pathway may play an important role in propagating the abnormal genetic features of DMD.

A differential coexpression network of DMD is constructed by linking the significant dyads. Only the two networks with more than two members are shown in Figure 7.6, omitting 11 isolated dyads. Sixteen and three among the 19 edges in the two networks show the opposite and the same signs of ISs between conditions, respectively, that is, positive IS in one and negative IS in another condition or vice versa. Seven and four among the omitted eleven dyads show the opposite and the same signs, respectively. Overall, 23 among the significant 30 pairs show the opposite signs of ISs between conditions. The abundance of opposite signs of ISs in DMD dataset is in strong contrast to the lung cancer dataset, whose 65 significant pathway pairs show all positive ISs in both normal lung and lung cancer samples. This suggests that lung cancer and DMD may impact a different degree of perturbation in a gene expression regulation network.

The lung cancer dataset shows much more significant pathway pairs than the DMD dataset. Massive genetic alterations in cancer, including mutation, insertion, deletion, and translocation, may result in severe perturbations of gene and pathway regulations, as shown in previous studies [37, 42]. DMD, conversely, has one mutated gene (dystrophin) only and the pathology is largely confined to muscle tissue. The small number of significant results in the DMD dataset compared to the lung cancer dataset may be explained by the limited change of gene expression within dystrophin-related genes. Previous studies support this assumption [43, 44].

Acknowledgments

This work is supported by a grant from the Ministry of Education Science and Technology, Korea (M10729070001-07N2907-00110).

References

1 Golub, T.R. (1999) *Science*, **286**, 531–537.
2 Lossos, I.S. (2004) *New Engl. J. Med.*, **350**, 1828–1837.
3 van de Vijver, M.J. (2002) *New Engl. J. Med.*, **347**, 1999–2009.
4 Livesey, F.J. (2000) *Curr. Biol.*, **10**, 301–310.
5 Segal, E. (2003) *Nat. Genet.*, **34**, 166–176.
6 Wang, Y. (2006) *Bioinformatics*, **22**, 2413–2420.
7 Stuart, J.M. (2003) *Science*, **302**, 249–255.
8 Ge, H. (2001) *Nat. Genet.*, **29**, 482–486.
9 Jansen, R., Greenbaum, D., and Gerstein, M. (2002) *Genome Res.*, **12**, 37–46.
10 Lee, H.K. (2004) *Genome Res.*, **14**, 1085–1094.
11 Eisen, M.B. (1998) *Proc. Natl. Acad. Sci. USA*, **95**, 14863–14868.
12 Tavazoie, S. (1999) *Nat. Genet.*, **22**, 281–285.
13 Kanehisa, M. and Goto, S. (2000) *Nucleic Acid. Res.*, **28**, 27–30.
14 Dennis, G.Jr., (2003) *Genome Biol.*, **4**, P3.
15 Dahlquist, K.D. (2002) *Nat. Genet.*, **31**, 19–20.
16 Al-Shahrour, F., Diaz-Uriarte, R., and Dopazo, J. (2004) *Bioinformatics*, **20**, 578–580.
17 Boyle, E.I. (2004) *Bioinformatics*, **20**, 3710–3715.
18 Chung, H.J. (2004) *Nucleic Acid. Res.*, **32**, W460–W464
19 Zhang, B. (2004) *BMC Bioinformatics*, **5**, 16.
20 Zhong, S. (2004) *Appl. Bioinformatics*, **3**, 261–264.
21 Chung, H.J. (2005) *Nucleic Acid. Res.*, **33**, W621–W626
22 Mootha, V.K. (2003) *Nat. Genet.*, **34**, 267–273.
23 Li, K.C. (2002) *Proc. Natl. Acad. Sci. USA*, **99**, 16875–16880.
24 Lai, Y. (2004) *Bioinformatics*, **20**, 3146–3155.
25 Choi, J.K. (2005) *Bioinformatics*, **21**, 4348–4355.
26 Kostka, D. and Spang, R. (2004) *Bioinformatics*, **20** (Suppl 1), i194–i199
27 Watson, M. (2006) *BMC Bioinformatics*, **7**, 509.
28 Cho, S.B. (2009) *BMC Bioinformatics*, **10**, 109.
29 Rényi, A. (1960) On measures of entropy and information, in *Proceedings of the Fourth Berkeley Symposium on Mathematical Statistics and Probability, Volume 1: Contributions to the Theory of Statistics* (ed. J. Neyman), University of California Press, Berkeley, pp. 547–561.
30 Jenssen, R. (2003) *Proceedings of the International Joint Conference on Neural Networks*, vol. **1**, International Neural Network Society, pp. 523–528.
31 Scott, D.W. (1992) *Multivariate Density Estimation: Theory, Practice, and Visualization*, John Wiley & Sons, Inc., New York.
32 Shannon, W.D. (2002) *Genet. Epidemiol.*, **23**, 87–96.
33 Bhattacharjee, A. (2001) *Proc. Natl. Acad. Sci. USA*, **98**, 13790–13795.
34 Haslett, J.N. (2002) *Proc. Natl. Acad. Sci. USA*, **99**, 15000–15005.
35 Bolstad, B.M. (2003) *Bioinformatics*, **19**, 185–193.
36 Kim, J. (2008) *J. Biomed. Inform.*, **41**, 232–241.
37 Chen, Y., Okunieff, P., and Ahrendt, S.A. (2003) *Semin. Surg. Oncol.*, **21**, 205–219.
38 Villaflor, V. and Bonomi, P. (2005) *Semin. Oncol.*, **32**, S30–S36
39 Roselli, M. (2004) *Clin. Cancer. Res.*, **10**, 610–614.
40 Vlahovic, G. (2007) *Br. J. Cancer*, **97**, 735–740.
41 Essmann, F. (2000) *Biochem. J.*, **346**, 777–783.
43 Sato, M. (2007) *J. Thorac. Oncol.*, **2**, 327–343.
42 Deconinck, N. and Dan, B. (2007) *Pediatr. Neurol.*, **36**, 1–7.
44 Nowak, K.J. and Davies, K.E. (2004) *EMBO Rep.*, **5**, 872–876.

8
Multivariate Analysis of Microarray Data: Application of MANOVA
Taeyoung Hwang and Taesung Park

8.1
Introduction

Microarray technology enables the simultaneous monitoring of expression profiles on a genome scale and has become an important tool for biology [1]. Much of the initial research with expression data has focused on evaluating the significance of individual genes in a comparison between two groups of samples [2]. Comparing a healthy group with a diseased one is an example for such an analysis. A statistical significance is assigned to each gene through statistical tests such as two sample t-test, ANOVA, and so on [3–9]. After genes are ranked according to their statistical significance, a list of differentially expressed genes (DEGs) is determined from a cutoff threshold value. The list is then investigated with sets of genes derived from the Gene Ontology database or some pathway databases to determine whether any set in the list is overrepresented compared with the whole list. The Fisher's exact test is typically used to assess the significance for overrepresentation [10]. Finally, further experimental analysis or biological interpretations can be conducted based on significant ontology terms or pathways. This type of analysis is typically called individual gene analysis (IGA) [11].

Several studies have shown that DEGs could be utilized for disease markers to help in diagnosis and prognosis of diseases [12–14]. However, it is still daunting to develop robust gene markers in that several studies have only a few genes in common [15]. Such a disparity might be explained by the following hypothesis: Changes in expression of the relatively few genes governing disease mechanism may be subtle compared to those of the downstream effectors, which may vary considerably from patient to patient [16]. In IGA, researchers often use the conservative cutoff threshold values. This could not detect moderate but essential expression changes.

The difficulty in detecting moderate expression changes has been partially compromised by extending the level of analysis from a single gene to multiple genes. This analysis first constructs sets of individual genes (hereafter referred to as "gene sets") from prior biological data, and then scores these predefined gene sets.

Medical Biostatistics for Complex Diseases. Edited by Frank Emmert-Streib and Matthias Dehmer
Copyright © 2010 WILEY-VCH Verlag GmbH & Co. KGaA, Weinheim
ISBN: 978-3-527-32585-6

Gene sets with high scores or significant ones are investigated for biological interpretations. This method is usually called gene set analysis (GSA) [11]. There are various ways by which gene sets can be defined. For example, gene sets can be defined according to the information provided by several databases, such as Gene Ontology, KEGG, BioCarta, and Pfam [17]. In addition to the construction of gene sets, GSA requires an adequate scoring method to deal with multiple genes in a gene set. In general, a gene-specific statistic, known as a "local" statistic is first computed for each gene. A "global" statistic for a gene set is then built as a function of the local statistic for each gene within the gene set [18–29]. The significance of a global statistic is usually assessed by a permutation test. Importantly, GSA could achieve a high power for detecting differentially expressed gene sets by integrating expression changes of genes in the same gene set, even when the expression changes of individual genes are modest. In addition, because the gene sets have already been annotated by their common functions in the databases, the biological interpretation for a given list of significant gene sets is clear [17]. Furthermore, GSA is reasonable from a biological perspective because biological phenomena occur through the interactions of multiple genes, via signaling pathways, networks, or other functional relationships [10].

The main difference between IGA and GSA is that GSA directly assesses the expression patterns of gene sets that are defined by shared biological themes, while IGA assesses the significance of individual genes first and searches for the enriched biological themes later [11]. We now look at the difference between two methods from a statistical perspective. No matter what analysis is selected between IGA and GSA, a gene is regarded as a dependent variable in a statistical analysis. While the individual gene analysis corresponds to a univariate statistical analysis, the gene set analysis is regarded as a multivariate analysis (Figure 8.1). There are plenty of statistical theories for multivariate data analysis [30]. It could be effective to apply multivariate statistical analysis to GSA instead of using a global statistic mentioned above. When multivariate analysis is performed, one important matter is to take the correlation structures among genes (dependent variables) into consideration. In reality, expression profiles of multiple genes are often correlated. However, the complex structure of gene interactions within a gene set could not be fully captured using a function of univariate statistics. In this chapter we present specifically why correlation among genes should be considered in the study of multiple gene approach and introduce multivariate analysis of variance (MANOVA) as one of the useful statistical tools to tackle this problem. Some examples are provided to illustrate how MANVOA can be applied to real datasets.

8.2
Importance of Correlation in Multiple Gene Approach

It is well known that genes never act alone in a biological system – they work in a cascade of networks. Genes in a gene set are functionally related and expression profiles in the same pathway or complex tend to be correlated. Therefore, they are

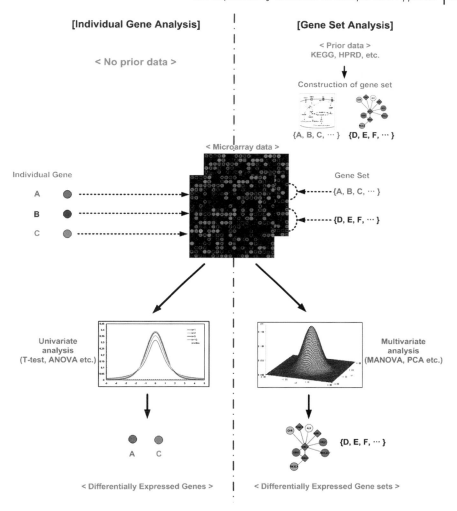

Figure 8.1 Schematic overview of individual gene analysis and gene set analysis. In the individual gene analysis, no prior data is used to identify phenotype-significant genes. After identifying the differentially expressed genes, biological interpretation is carried through GO (Gene Ontology) analysis or additional experiments. However, in the gene set analysis, biological information is utilized as a prior data to construct gene sets. Therefore the results from gene set analysis are more easily interpreted biologically without further tasks.

more suitably modeled as mutually dependent variables in development of a statistical testing framework. However, most of the current statistical methods ignore the multivariate structure of the expression data and fail to utilize efficiently the information valuable for gene interactions [31]. In this section, we discuss why multivariate analysis is important with a specific example. The importance of correlation will also be accounted for.

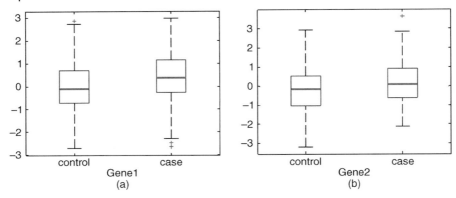

Figure 8.2 Box plots of (a) gene 1 and (b) gene 2.

8.2.1
Small Effects Coordinate to Make a Big Difference

By extending the level of analysis from an individual gene to multiple genes, we can identify genes with small changes that are not identified by the single gene level analysis [2]. For example, assume that there are expression profiles consisting of two groups (control, case) and two genes (gene 1, gene 2). Each group has 100 observations. Figure 8.2 shows the box plots of these data.

As shown in Figure 8.2, the mean difference between the case group and the control group for each gene is very small but the variance of each gene is quite large. In fact, their p-values from two sample t-test are larger than 0.05, indicating that there is no significant mean difference between two groups in both cases of gene 1 and gene 2. However, if we consider gene 1 and gene 2 simultaneously, these small differences can make significant changes. As indicated in Table 8.1, applying MANOVA to the gene set consisting of gene 1 and gene 2 can produce p-values smaller than 0.05. Note that the results depend on the correlation between gene 1 and gene 2. We see how this happens in the following discussion.

Table 8.1 The p-values obtained from univariate and multivariate analyses; r denotes a correlation coefficient between gene 1 and gene 2.

	Gene 1	Gene 2
Univariate:		
Two sample t-test	0.074	0.078
Multivariate:		
MANOVA ($r = -0.954$)	0	
MANOVA ($r = 0.017$)	0.045	
MANOVA ($r = 0.982$)	0.205	

8.2.2
Significance of the Correlation

In the multivariate analysis, correlation among dependent variables plays an important role in assessing the significance of null hypothesis. If the correlation structure among genes in a gene set is ignored, the probability of type I error may increase. For example, take the case of two dependent variables from the two populations. Suppose that a researcher considers the two-dimensional analysis ignoring the correlation between two dependent variables. Note that the significance of difference between two mean vectors increases as the statistical distance between two mean vectors increases. The distance between two mean vectors can be measured as follows:

$$d^2 = (\bar{X}_{11} - \bar{X}_{21} \quad \bar{X}_{12} - \bar{X}_{22}) D^{-1} \begin{pmatrix} \bar{X}_{11} - \bar{X}_{21} \\ \bar{X}_{12} - \bar{X}_{22} \end{pmatrix}, D = \begin{pmatrix} s_1^2 & 0 \\ 0 & s_2^2 \end{pmatrix}$$

where $\bar{X}_{ij}$ is the sample mean of jth dependent variable in the i th group and s_j is the sample variance of j th dependent variable. We call this measure "standardized Euclidean distance." However, if we consider the correlation between two dependent variables, it is modified like the following:

$$d^2 = (\bar{X}_{11} - \bar{X}_{21} \quad \bar{X}_{12} - \bar{X}_{22}) S^{-1} \begin{pmatrix} \bar{X}_{11} - \bar{X}_{21} \\ \bar{X}_{12} - \bar{X}_{22} \end{pmatrix}, S = \begin{pmatrix} s_1^2 & rs_1 s_2 \\ rs_1 s_2 & s_2^2 \end{pmatrix}$$

where $\bar{X}_{ij}$, s_j are the same as the above and r is the sample correlation coefficient. This is called as "Mahalanobis distance" and it is the statistic of Hotelling's T^2 test which is essentially the same as MANOVA when there are two populations. When r is non-zero, which means there exists the correlation between the dependent variables, the Mahalanobis distance can differ from the standardized Euclidean distance because the off-diagonal terms in S contribute to the calculation of S^{-1}. This is why the MANOVA statistic in Table 8.1 varies according to the correlation coefficient. Two extreme cases in Table 8.1 are plotted in Figure 8.3. Although the mean difference between control and case group is same in each case, the distinction between control and case group is more evident in Figure 8.3b than Figure 8.3a. This shows how different correlation values can produce difference results and how ignoring the correlation in multivariate analysis can lead to wrong results. In particular, when the distance between two mean vectors is measured larger than a true one due to ignoring the correlation, the type I error could be increased.

8.3
Multivariate ANalysis of VAriance (MANOVA)

MANOVA is an extension of analysis of variance (ANOVA) that covers cases where there is more than one dependent variable. While ANOVA compares the mean differences in expression among the phenotypes for an individual gene, MANOVA

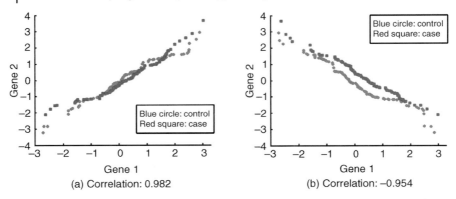

Figure 8.3 Scatter plots of two cases in Table 8.1: scatter plots for (a) a highly positive correlation value (0.982) and (b) a highly negative correlation value (−0.954). In each plot, blue circles denote control group and red squares describe case group.

compares the mean differences for a set of genes simultaneously taking the correlation structure into consideration. Therefore, ANOVA is used to identify differentially expressed genes, while MANOVA is used to identify differentially expressed gene sets in an expression profile analysis. In this section, we present a statistical review of MANOVA. We use the same notation as Johnson et al. [30].

8.3.1
ANOVA

A review of the univariate analysis of variance (ANOVA) will facilitate our discussion of MANOVA. Assume there are G population and n_g samples for g populations ($g = 1, 2, \ldots, G$). Let $X_{g1}, X_{g2}, \ldots, X_{gj}, \ldots, X_{gn_g}$ be an independent random sample from $N(\mu_g, \sigma^2)$ population. Suppose we want to test the null hypothesis of equality of means, which is formulated as:

$$H_0 : \mu_1 = \mu_2 = \cdots = \mu_G$$

Since $\mu_g = \mu + \tau_g$ where μ is an overall mean, the above null hypothesis can be restated as:

$$H_0 : \tau_1 = \tau_2 = \cdots = \tau_G = 0$$

The response X_{gj}, distributed as $N(\mu + \tau_g, \sigma^2)$, can be expressed in the suggestive form:

$$X_{gj} = \mu(\text{overall mean}) + \tau_g(\text{treatment effect}) + e_{gj}(\text{random error}),$$

where e_{gj} are independent random variables from $N(\mu_g, \sigma^2)$.

Analysis of variance is based on an analogous decomposition of the observations:

$$x_{gj} = \bar{x} + (\bar{x}_g - \bar{x}) + (x_{gj} - \bar{x}_g)$$

8.3 Multivariate ANalysis of VAriance (MANOVA)

Table 8.2 ANOVA table.

Source of variation	Sum of squares	Degree of freedom (d.f.)
Treatments	$\sum_{g=1}^{G} n_g(\bar{x}_g - \bar{x})^2$	$G-1$
Residual (error)	$\sum_{g=1}^{G} \sum_{j=1}^{n_g} (x_{gj} - \bar{x}_g)^2$	$\sum_{g=1}^{G} n_g (=N) - G$
Total	$\sum_{g=1}^{G} \sum_{j=1}^{n_g} (x_{gj} - \bar{x})^2$	$\sum_{g=1}^{G} n_g (=N) - 1$

$$(\text{observation}) = (\text{overall sample mean}) + (\text{estimated treatment effect}) + (\text{residual})$$

Subtracting $\bar{x}$ from both sides and squaring gives:

$$(x_{gj} - \bar{x})^2 = (\bar{x}_g - \bar{x})^2 + (x_{gj} - \bar{x}_g)^2 + 2(\bar{x}_g - \bar{x})(x_{gj} - \bar{x}_g)$$

We can sum both sides over j, note that $\sum_{j=1}^{n_g} (x_{gj} - \bar{x}_g) = 0$, and obtain:

$$\sum_{j=1}^{n_g} (x_{gj} - \bar{x})^2 = n_g (\bar{x}_g - \bar{x})^2 + \sum_{j=1}^{n_g} (x_{gj} - \bar{x}_g)^2$$

Next, summing both sides over g we obtain:

$$\sum_{g=1}^{G} \sum_{j=1}^{n_g} (x_{gj} - \bar{x})^2 = \sum_{g=1}^{G} n_g (\bar{x}_g - \bar{x})^2 + \sum_{g=1}^{G} \sum_{j=1}^{n_g} (x_{gj} - \bar{x}_g)^2$$

Total SS (SS_{total}) = between SS (SS_{tr}) + within SS (SS_{res})

Analysis of variance proceeds by comparing the relative sizes of SS_{tr} and SS_{res}. If H_0 is true, variances computed from SS_{tr} and SS_{res} should be approximately equal. To make inference for population, the degree of freedom should be provided. Table 8.2 summarizes the basic information to test the null hypothesis.

Since:

$$\frac{SS_{\text{tr}}/(G-1)}{SS_{\text{res}}/(N-G)}$$

follows $F_{G-1, N-G}$ under H_0, the p-value can be calculated using F distribution. H_0 is rejected when the p-value is smaller than a given significance level (usually, 0.05 or 0.01).

8.3.2
MANOVA

Usually, the data include simultaneous measurements on many variables, which means there are more than one dependent variable. For the statistical analysis of such data, multivariate analysis, considering dependent variables simultaneously, is needed. MANOVA is well-known multivariate statistical analysis to test the equity of mean vectors among several populations. We review MANOVA by analogy to ANOVA. There are four MANOVA test statistics: Wilks' λ, Pillai's trace, Lawley–

Hotelling trace, and Roy's largest root. For large samples, all of these statistics are essentially equivalent. Here, we limit the discussion to Wilks' λ for the purpose of a brief introduction.

In the MANOVA model, $\boldsymbol{X}_{gj}$ denotes a random sample of $p \times 1$ vector:

$$\boldsymbol{X}_{gj} = \begin{pmatrix} X_{gj1} \\ X_{gj2} \\ \vdots \\ X_{gjp} \end{pmatrix}$$

when there are p dependent variables.

In the same way, $\boldsymbol{x}_{gj}$ describes an observation of $p \times 1$ vector. Then we can decompose multivariate sum of squares on the analogy of univariate case using matrix notation:

$$\sum_{g=1}^{G}\sum_{j=1}^{n_g}(\boldsymbol{x}_{gj}-\bar{\boldsymbol{x}})(\boldsymbol{x}_{gj}-\bar{\boldsymbol{x}})' = \sum_{g=1}^{G} n_g(\bar{\boldsymbol{x}}_g-\bar{\boldsymbol{x}})(\bar{\boldsymbol{x}}_g-\bar{\boldsymbol{x}})' + \sum_{g=1}^{G}\sum_{j=1}^{n_g}(\boldsymbol{x}_{gj}-\bar{\boldsymbol{x}}_g)(\boldsymbol{x}_{gj}-\bar{\boldsymbol{x}}_g)'$$

We call each term in the above formula "total sum of squares and cross products," "treatment (between) sum of squares and cross product," and "residual (within) sum of squares and cross product." The null hypothesis of equity of mean vectors in the MANOVA is formulated as the following:

$$H_0 : \tau_1 = \tau_2 = \cdots = \tau_G = \boldsymbol{0}, \quad \text{where} \quad \tau_g = \begin{pmatrix} \tau_{g1} \\ \tau_{g2} \\ \vdots \\ \tau_{gp} \end{pmatrix}$$

Analogous to the univariate result, the hypothesis of no treatment effects is tested by considering the relative sizes of the treatment and residual sums of squares and cross products. Table 8.3 summarizes the formulas for the calculations of the test statistic.

Wilks proposed that the null hypothesis is rejected when the quantity $\Lambda = |\boldsymbol{W}|/|\boldsymbol{B}+\boldsymbol{W}|$ is significantly small [32]. It is known that when the sample size (N) is large:

$$-\left(N-1-\frac{p+G}{2}\right) \times \ln \Lambda \sim \chi^2_{p(G-1)}$$

Table 8.3 MANOVA table.

Source of variation	Sum of squares	Degree of freedom (d.f.)
Treatments	$\boldsymbol{B} = \sum_{g=1}^{G} n_g (\bar{\boldsymbol{x}}_g - \bar{\boldsymbol{x}})(\bar{\boldsymbol{x}}_g - \bar{\boldsymbol{x}})'$	$G-1$
Residual (error)	$\boldsymbol{W} = \sum_{g=1}^{G}\sum_{j=1}^{n_g}(\boldsymbol{x}_{gj}-\bar{\boldsymbol{x}}_g)(\boldsymbol{x}_{gj}-\bar{\boldsymbol{x}}_g)'$	$\sum_{g=1}^{G} n_g (= N) - G$
Total	$\boldsymbol{B} + \boldsymbol{W} = \sum_{g=1}^{G}\sum_{j=1}^{n_g}(\boldsymbol{x}_{gj}-\bar{\boldsymbol{x}})(\boldsymbol{x}_{gj}-\bar{\boldsymbol{x}})'$	$\sum_{g=1}^{G} n_g (= N) - 1$

The significance of test can be determined using this result. More precise test procedures about MANOVA are easily found in References [30, 33].

8.4 Applying MANOVA to Microarray Data Analysis

In this section we discuss MANOVA from the perspective of microarray data analysis. Since each gene in the microarray data is regarded as a dependent variable, MANOVA can be properly applied to gene set analysis that deals with multiple genes simultaneously. Suppose there are G phenotype groups and p genes. For the i-th gene in group g, let μ_{gi} ($g = 1, \ldots, G$; $i = 1, \ldots, p$) be the expected value of its expression value. Then the following hypotheses are of interest in MANOVA test:

$$H_0 : \begin{pmatrix} \mu_{11} \\ \vdots \\ \mu_{1i} \\ \vdots \\ \mu_{1p} \end{pmatrix} = \begin{pmatrix} \mu_{21} \\ \vdots \\ \mu_{2i} \\ \vdots \\ \mu_{2p} \end{pmatrix} = \cdots = \begin{pmatrix} \mu_{G1} \\ \vdots \\ \mu_{Gi} \\ \vdots \\ \mu_{Gp} \end{pmatrix}$$

The alternative is that at least one gene is expressed differently in at least two conditions. That is, the null hypothesis is rejected if one or more of the mean differences among the genes in the gene set differ significantly from zero.

There are several advantages when MANOVA is used to analyze the microarray data. First of all, MANOVA could identify genes whose differential expressions are not marginally detectable in univariate testing methods, taking into account multidimensional structure of microarray data [31]. Second, it considers the correlation structure of multiple genes when it is used to compare the mean vectors of multiple genes, resulting in high power of test. Third, MANOVA can deal with the data of any number of groups. Many microarray experiments involve multiple experimental conditions. The different experimental conditions can be dose levels, time points, or treatment combinations [10].

However, there are some critical issues to be considered when applying MANOVA to microarray data: distributional assumptions under the MANOVA model and the singularity problem:

1) **Distributional assumptions under the MANOVA model**
   MANOVA assumes that the structure of the data follows three conditions:
   (i) the samples from different populations are independent;
   (ii) each population is multivariate normal;
   (iii) all populations have a common covariance matrix $\sum$, that is, the variances and covariances of the dependent variables should be homogenous across the phenotype groups.

2) **Singularity problem**
   The calculation of MANOVA involves the matrix inversion of the pooled within-groups sample variance-covariance matrix. If the number of variables is greater

than the number of samples, the sample covariance matrix is singular or not invertible. Therefore, MANOVA requires the number of samples be larger than the number of genes to avoid a singularity problem.

To successfully apply MANOVA to microarray data, the above two issues are managed properly. In the case of distributional assumptions, the second and third conditions are not often satisfied in microarray data. However, the second condition can be relaxed by appealing to the central limit theorem when the sample size n_g is large [30]. In addition, most of proposed algorithm involved in MANOVA uses the permutation method to generate the null distribution and calculate the p-values. A permutation test does not require the normality assumption on the underlying distribution of the microarray data, which means that the assumptions for MANOVA could be relaxed. With respect to the homogeneous variance-covariance assumption, several tests can be applied to check the validity of this condition. When the homogenous assumption is not satisfied, the transformation of the dependent variables is recommended [2].

The second issue, the singularity problem, can be solved mainly by two methods: The first is by developing the search algorithm to find best gene sets with the limited number of genes. For example, a sequential and iterative algorithm to search for a gene set that maximizes expression differences between groups of genes has been developed [31]. In addition, a greedy search algorithm over the protein–protein interaction data was utilized to identify phenotype-specific subnetworks [2]. The second method utilizes the data reduction method. Kong et al. [1] transformed the data onto an orthonormal subspace using principal components to calculate the score even for the subspaces whose dimension is larger than that of the samples.

In the next section we review several studies in which MANOVA is applied through the novel algorithm to microarray data analysis.

8.5
Application of MANOVA: Case Studies

MANOVA has been applied to various applications of life sciences. In the analysis of microarray experiment, MANOVA is a useful framework when a multiple gene approach is needed. In particular, this method has become a valuable tool in cancer research, disease diagnostics, and prediction. The following three studies apply MANOVA successfully to disease-relevant microarray data. They identify disease specific genes, pathways, and PPI subnetworks respectively. Note that first two examples utilize Hotelling's T^2 test, which is equivalent to MANOVA when the number of phenotype is two.

8.5.1
Identifying Disease Specific Genes

Lu et al. [31] used Hotelling's T^2 test to identify subsets of differentially expressed genes (DEGs) in two test groups. They proposed the multiple forward search (MFS) algorithm for applying Hotelling's T^2 to analyze microarray data, which is designed to select a set of genes and avoid singularity problem. First, the MFS algorithm calculates T^2 statistics for each of all the genes and selects the best one as a first gene in the gene set. Then another gene is searched by adding one more gene that maximizes T^2 when combined with the previous genes in the gene set. These steps continue iteratively until the stopping rules to avoid the singularity problem are satisfied. The detailed structure of the MFS algorithm is outlined below (Chapter 6, Section 6.2.4) [31]:

- **Step 1**: Calculate T^2 statistics for each of all the genes that are measured in datasets, and find gene j_1 that maximizes T^2, denoted as $T^2_{j_1}$.
- **Step 2**: If p-value $(T^2_{j_1}) < \alpha$ (a predefined significance level), calculate T^2 statistics for two genes, one is the gene j_1 and the other is one of the remaining genes excepting the gene j_1. Find gene j_2 that maximizes T^2 combining with gene j_1, denoted as $T^2_{j_1,j_2}$.
- **Step 3**: If p-value $(T^2_{j_1,j_2}) < p$-value $(T^2_{j_1})$, repeat step 2 by adding one more gene that maximizes T^2 combining with genes j_1, j_2.
- **Step 4**: Repeat step 3 until p-value $(T^2_{j_1,\ldots,j_{n-1},j_n}) > p$-value $(T^2_{j_1,\ldots,j_{n-1}})$ or the number of genes is larger than $n_1 + n_2 - 2$ (where n_1 and n_2 are sample sizes of two different tissue types under comparison). Then the selected genes $j_1, j_2, \ldots, j_{n-1}$ are the first subset of identified DEGs.
- **Step 5**: Exclude genes $j_1, j_2, \ldots, j_{n-1}$ and repeat steps 1–4.
- **Step 6**: Repeat step 5 until the p-value of T^2 statistic of the starting gene is larger than α, that is, p-value $(T^2_{j_1}) > \alpha$, and stop searching.

It was reported that Hotelling's T^2 gave fewer false positives and false negatives than the univariate t-test when a spike-in HGU95 dataset from Affymetrix was analyzed. In addition, the utility of this algorithm was demonstrated by the analyses of gene expression patterns in human liver cancers and breast cancers (Chapter 6, Section 6.4).

8.5.2
Identifying Significant Pathways from Public Pathway Databases

Kong et al. [1] have combined analysis of differential gene expression with biological knowledge databases. They utilized the functional pathways defined by Reactome, KEGG (Kyoto Encyclopedia of Genes and Genomes), BioCarta, and Gene Ontology databases as gene set information. They assessed the significance of gene set expression through Hotelling's T^2 test. When the number of genes in a given gene set is larger than the number of samples, the within-group covariance matrix is not convertible, resulting in a singularity problem. To address this, they used principal component analysis (PCA) which transforms a number of possibly correlated variables into a smaller number of uncorrelated variables called principal components [30]. They diagonalize the within-group covariance matrix by projecting the data onto an orthonormal subspace spanned by principal components of the covariance matrix [1].

This allows them to reduce the dimension of space of genes and prevent the singularity problem in the Hotelling's T^2 test. They applied their method to a heart failure dataset, resulting in the identification of relevant pathways that are not apparent by single-gene analysis.

8.5.3
Identification of Subnetworks from Protein–Protein Interaction Data

As protein–protein interaction (PPI) data become available, there has been a growing interest in combining PPI data with genome-wide expression data. In the integration of PPI and expression data, expression values of each gene are usually matched to its corresponding protein in the PPI network. Researchers then searched for significant subnetworks or connected sub-graphs. Subnetworks could be regarded as gene sets that consist of connected genes on PPI. For a given subnetworks or gene sets, the multivariate statistical tests can be applied to find the subnetworks with the maximum scores. However, the search algorithm for subnetworks or gene sets with the maximum scores is also needed since there are no predefined subnetworks. This approach is different from the original gene-set analysis that uses biological database information as predefined information. The combined analysis of expression data and PPI data allows us to detect the unknown gene sets that are not predefined in public database. Therefore, novel hypotheses about pathways or complexes could be generated. Hwang et al. [2] have proposed a MANOVA-based scoring method with a greedy search for identifying differentially expressed PPI subnetworks. They proposed using Wilks' λ statistic as a MANOVA-based score for a given subnetwork. Given the scoring method, a greedy search was performed to identify subnetworks within the PPI network (Figure 8.4). Initially, each candidate subnetwork had a single seed protein. To expand the subnetwork from a seed protein, they first constructed every possible subnetwork consisting of the seed and each of its neighboring proteins. After completing the score calculation for all of the possible subnetworks, they chose the neighboring proteins in the subnetworks with the maximum scores and included them as members of expanded subnetworks. This process was iterated until the termination conditions were met.

Three termination criteria were used:

1) The search stops when no addition of neighbor proteins increases the score over a specified relative improvement rate r, which is defined as the difference between the previous and current scores divided by the previous score.
2) The distance from the seed is adopted as another criterion. That is, only proteins within a specified distance d from the seed are added to an expanded subnetwork.
3) The maximum possible number of proteins in a subnetwork is also used as a termination criterion to avoid the singular matrix conversion in the process of calculating Wilks' λ statistic from MANOVA. The maximum number of nodes (genes) in a subnetwork is set to one less than the number of samples in the smallest group.

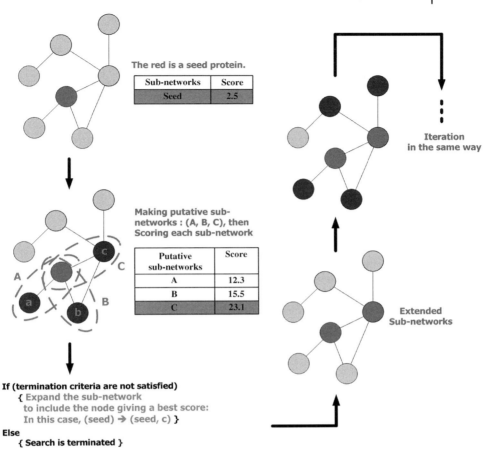

Figure 8.4 Greedy search: a greedy search is an iterative process. Starting from the seed protein, the subnetwork expands by including one of the neighbor nodes iteratively to improve the test statistic most efficiently until the termination criteria are satisfied.

When one of the three criteria is satisfied, the iteration stops. The significance of the subnetworks is determined by a permutation test.

8.6 Conclusions

High-throughput technology expands explosively data ranging from DNA sequence variations to mRNA expression and protein abundance. At present, data analysis, not data generation, is becoming the main bottleneck. In particular, the proper integration of various types of genome-wide data could fill gaps in the separate data, resulting in an exceptional opportunity to understand biological phenomenon at the system level. Multidimensional analysis provides the main framework for such integration. In this chapter we introduced MANOVA, which deals with multiple variables considering correlation structure among them. MANOVA could identify multiple genes whose differential expressions are not marginally detectable in univariate testing methods, by taking into account multidimensional structure among them. It also avoids the inflation of type I error by taking the correlation into account. The empirical results from case studies in the Section 8.5 show these advantages well. Lu et al. [31] have reported that Hotelling's T^2 statistic found more DEGs than the t-statistic and performed better at the discriminant analysis for classification of gene expression patterns. Hwang et al. [2] have argued that MANOVA-based scoring methods tended to construct significant subnetworks with a larger number of highly correlated proteins compared with other scoring methods such as t-statistic- and mutual information-based scoring methods.

However, when the statistical model is used to integrate or analyze the biological data, it is necessary to consider the characteristics of data for an effective application of the statistical models. In the application of MANOVA to microarray analysis, the main difficulty is that it requires the number of samples to be larger than the number of genes in the gene set to avoid singularity in the inversion of sample covariance matrix. An intuitive approach to account for the singularity is to use the generalized inverse matrix to compute the test statistic. However, this approach does not perform well [10]. Several methods have been suggested to avoid the singularity problem efficiently. As shown in the Section 8.5, Kong et al. [1] used Hotelling's T^2-statistic with PCA, a dimensional reduction method. They address the singularity problem by transforming the data onto an orthonormal subspace using principal components first. This allows them to calculate the score even for the subspaces whose dimension is larger than that of the samples [1]. In other ways, iterative search process can be applied until the number of genes is larger than the number of samples. The multiple forward search algorithm developed by Lu et al. [31] is a good example. In particular, Hwang et al. [2] have performed the greedy search iteratively on protein–protein interaction data to reduce the search space.

It is essential that when the statistical model is applied to real data the distributional assumptions underlying its model should be carefully checked. In the case of MANOVA, a permutation test can be performed to relax normality assumption as discussed in Section 8.4. In addition, large inherent "noise" in microarray data renders estimation of the pooled sample variance-covariance matrix unrobust and variable, thereby violating another assumption of MANOVA, namely, homogenous variance and covariance. Lu et al. [31] have proposed the resampling-based approach to construct Hotelling's T^2 statistics, alleviating statistical fluctuation and reducing sampling errors. Alternatively, Tsai et al. [10] have applied the shrinkage covariance matrix estimator to compute the MANOVA test statistic to tackle this problem.

Aside from MANOVA, there are many statistical models available for the integration and combined analysis of biological data. Increasing efforts and interest are encouraged to develop the proper algorithm for utilizing them.

Acknowledgments

This work was supported by the National Research Laboratory Program of the Korea Science and Engineering Foundation (M10500000126) and a fellowship for a Seoul citizen in Science.

References

1. Kong, S.W., Pu, W.T., and Park, P.J. (2006) *Bioinformatics*, **22**, 2373–2380.
2. Hwang, T. and Park, T. (2009) *BMC Bioinformatics*, **10**, 128.
3. Lonnstedt, I. and Speed, T.P. (2002) *Stat. Sinica*, **12**, 31–46.
4. Tusher, V., Tibshirani, R., and Chu, G. (2001) *Proc. Natl. Acad. Sci. USA*, **98**, 5116–5124.
5. Efron, B., Tibshirani, R., Storey, J.D., and Tusher, V. (2001) *J. Am. Stat. Assoc.*, **96**, 1151–1160.
6. Broberg, P. (2003) *Genome Biol.*, **4**, R41.
7. Baldi, P. and Long, A.D. (2001) *Bioinformatics*, **17**, 509–519.
8. Thomas, J.G., Olson, J.M., Tapscott, S.J., and Zhao, L.P. (2001) *Genome Res.*, **11**, 1227–1236.
9. Yan, X., Deng, M., Fung, W.K., and Qian, M. (2005) *J. Theor. Biol.*, **234**, 395–402.
10. Tsai, C.A. and Chen, J.J. (2009) *Bioinformatics*, **25**, 897–903.
11. Nam, D. and Kim, S.Y. (2008) *Brief. Bioinform.*, **9**, 189–197.
12. Ramaswamy, S., Ross, K.N., Lander, E.S., and Golub, T.R. (2003) *Nat. Genet.*, **33**, 49–54.
13. Golub, T.R., Slonim, D.K., Tamayo, P., Huard, C., Gaasenbeek, M., Mesirov, J.P., Coller, H., Loh, M.L., Downing, J.R., Caligiuri, M.A. *et al.* (1999) *Science*, **286**, 531–537.
14. Alizadeh, A.A., Eisen, M.B., Davis, R.E., Ma, C., Lossos, I.S., Rosenwald, A., Boldrick, J.C., Sabet, H., Tran, T., Yu, X. *et al.* (2000) *Nature*, **403**, 503–511.
15. Ein-Dor, L., Kela, I., Getz, G., Givol, D., and Domany, E. (2005) *Bioinformatics*, **21**, 171–178.
16. Chuang, H.Y., Lee, E., Liu, Y.T., Lee, D., and Ideker, T. (2007) *Mol. Syst. Biol.*, **3**, 140.
17. Yan, X. and Sun, F. (2008) *BMC Bioinformatics*, **9**, 362.
18. Mootha, V.K., Lindgren, C.M., Eriksson, K.F., Subramanian, A., Sihag, S., Lehar, J., Puigserver, P., Carlsson, E., Ridderstrale, M., Laurila, E. *et al.* (2003) *Nat. Genet.*, **34**, 267–273.
19. Subramanian, A., Tamayo, P., Mootha, V.K., Mukherjee, S., Ebert, B.L., Gillette, M.A., Paulovich, A., Pomeroy, S.L., Golub, T.R., Lander, E.S., and Mesirov, J.P. (2005) *Proc. Natl. Acad. Sci. USA*, **102**, 15545–15550.
20. Tian, L., Greenberg, S.A., Kong, S.W., Altschuler, J., Kohane, I.S., and Park, P.J. (2005) *Proc. Natl. Acad. Sci. USA*, **102**, 13544–13549.
21. Goeman, J.J. and Buhlmann, P. (2007) *Bioinformatics*, **23**, 980–987.
22. Efron, B. and Tibshirani, R. (2007) *Ann. Appl. Stat.*, **1**, 107–129.
23. Pavlidis, P., Qin, J., Arango, V., Mann, J.J., and Sibille, E. (2004) *Neurochem. Res.*, **29**, 1213–1222.
24. Jiang, Z. and Gentleman, R. (2007) *Bioinformatics*, **23**, 306–313.
25. Newton, M.A., Quintana, F.A., den Boon, J.A., Sengupta, S., and Ahlquist, P. (2007) *Ann. Appl. Stat.*, **1**, 85–106.
26. Barry, W.T., Nobel, A.B., and Wright, F.A. (2005) *Bioinformatics*, **21**, 1943–1949.
27. Adewale, A.J., Dinu, J., Potter, J.D., Liu, Q., and Yasui, Y. (2008) *J. Comput. Biol.*, **15**, 269–277.
28. Chen, J.J., Lee, T., Delongchamp, R.R., Chen, T., and Tsai, C. (2007) *Bioinformatics*, **23**, 2104–2112.

29 Dinu, I., Potter, J.D., Mueller, T., Liu, Q., Adewale, A.J., Jhangri, G.S., Einecke, G., Famulski, K.S., Halloran, P., and Yasui, Y. (2007) *BMC Bioinformatics*, **8**, 242.

30 Johnson, R.A. and Wichern, D.W. (2002) *Applied Multivariate Statistical Analysis*, 5th edn, Prentice Hall.

31 Lu, Y., Liu, P.Y., Xiao, P., and Deng, H.W. (2005) *Bioinformatics*, **21**, 3105–3113.

32 Wilks, S.S. (1932) *Biometrika*, **24** (3–4), 471–494.

33 Bartlett, M.S. (1938) *Proc. Cambridge Philos. Soc.*, **34**.

9
Testing Significance of a Class of Genes[1]
James J. Chen and Chen-An Tsai

9.1
Introduction

A common task in microarray gene expression studies is to identify a list of genes that express differently under different experimental (phenotypes) conditions. The objective is to establish a relationship between genes or gene classes and biological samples for identifying biological functions, clustering experimental samples (different tumor subtypes or bacteria species), classifying experimental conditions (exposed or un-exposed), or predicting biological outcomes (good or poor prognosis). This chapter focuses on the objective of analysis of differentially expressed gene sets (gene classes) under different experimental conditions (phenotypes). A gene class refers to a group of genes with related functions or a set of genes grouped together based on biologically relevant information, such as a metabolic pathway, protein complex, or GO (gene ontology) category. A multivariate statistical test to determine whether some functionally predefined classes of genes express differently (enrichment and/or deletion) in different phenotypes is referred to as gene class testing (GCT). In other words, GCT is an analysis of the association of a priori defined gene classes with the phenotypes; GCT is also called the gene set analysis (GSA).

The commonly used approach to GSA is first to identify a list of genes that express differently among two phenotypes using statistical significance testing (e.g., [1, 2]). Identification of differentially expressed genes can be separated into two steps. The first step is to calculate a discriminatory score based on the *p*-value of a test statistic that will rank the genes in order of evidence of differential expressions. The test statistic typically is a ratio (signal-to-noise ratio) of the mean difference between the two groups over an estimate of its standard deviation (in log scale), $T = M/s$ (e.g., [3]). The second step is to assign a significance level from the *p*-values to select the differentially expressed genes. Because multiple genes are tested, assigning a significance level should be done in terms of an overall false positive error for determining the set of significance genes. The FDR (false discovery rate) criterion [4]

---

[1] The views presented in this chapter are those of the authors and do not necessarily represent those of the US Food and Drug Administration.

Medical Biostatistics for Complex Diseases. Edited by Frank Emmert-Streib and Matthias Dehmer
Copyright © 2010 WILEY-VCH Verlag GmbH & Co. KGaA, Weinheim
ISBN: 978-3-527-32585-6

is commonly used for determining a significance cutoff in gene expression data analysis. The FDR error measure considers the expected proportion of the number of false positives among the selected genes. Essentially, FDR is the probability of the number of false selections over the number of genes declared as significant. The FDR approach allows the investigator to select the potential differentially expressed genes while accepting a small fraction of false findings, as compared with the family-wise error rate approach such as the Bonferroni adjustment (e.g., Chen, 2007). Much of initial research on methods for microarray data analysis has focused on the development of techniques to rank each individual gene for evidence of differential expressions and to determine a significance cutoff to divide the genes into the differential expression and non-differential expression. After selection of a list of differentially expressed genes, the list is then examined with biologically predefined gene sets to determine whether any sets are over-represented in the list compared with the whole list [5–7]. The analysis of comparing the number of genes in the differential expression list with the number in a predefined gene set is known as the over-representation analysis (ORA). Fisher's exact test is typically used to assess the significance for an over-representation [5]. The approach of performing individual gene analysis to identify a list of differential expression genes is referred to as IGA [8]. We refer to the use of the IGA in conjunction with the ORA for the gene set analysis as the IGA-ORA approach. An IGA-ORA approach is illustrated below.

Recently, Mootha et al. [9] and Subramanian et al. [10] proposed gene set enrichment analysis (GSEA), which used the Kolmogorov–Smirnov statistic to assess the significance of predefined gene-sets. The GSEA method considered the distributions of entire genes in the gene set rather than a subset from the differential expression list. The GSEA method is able to identify a significant gene set between the diabetic samples and normal muscles for which no single gene was found to be differentially expressed by the IGA. The key principle is that the individual genes in a gene set are closely related and often have similar expression patterns. By borrowing strength across the gene set, IGA will increase statistical power. The GSA approach essentially shifts the level of analysis of the microarray experiment from single genes to the sets of related genes. In other words, GSA provides a direct approach to the analysis of gene sets of interest. This approach should be more powerful and easier to interpret than IGA-ORA. Furthermore, as microarray experiments inherit various sources of biological and technical variability, the results from a gene set analysis is expected to more reproducible than from an individual gene analysis.

The work of Mootha et al. [9] has inspired the development of various GSA methods for alternatives to the IGA-ORA approach. Tian et al. [11] have proposed an approach based on two-sample t-statistics. The test statistic for a gene set is an aggregate of each individual gene test statistics. Chen et al. [12] have proposed two global statistics for one-sided test and two statistics for two-sided test. Dinu et al. [13] have proposed a test based on the SAM statistic [1]. Adewale et al. [14] have generalized the SAM-GS statistic from the framework of regression model. Efron and Tibshirani [15] have proposed a MaxMean statistic for summarizing gene sets, and a re-standardization for more accurate inferences. These tests are an aggregate of individual gene test statistics within the gene set. Kong et al. [16] have proposed using the Hotelling's T^2 statistic by projection of the original data to an ortho-normal substance, when the number of genes in the gene set is larger than the number of samples. Tomfohr et al. [17] have also used t-statistic after reducing the gene set to its first principal component. Tsai and Chen [18] have recently proposed a multivariate analysis of variance (MANOVA) test without dimensional reduction. The MANOVA test can be used for data collected from studies with two or more conditions. When there are two conditions, the MANOVA test becomes the Hotelling's T^2 test. The test has been applied to identify differentially expressed genes [19–21].

Alternatively, Goeman et al. [22] have proposed a global score test by modeling gene expressions as random effects in a logistic regression model. Mansmann and Meister [23] and Hummel et al. [24] have proposed an ANCOVA (analysis of covariance) test, which is similar to the Goeman et al. [22] model except that the roles of condition and gene are exchanged in the regression models. These two tests are equivalent in the case of independence among genes in the gene set. A third approach is a meta-analysis based on the individual p-values from the univariate test (e.g., [25, 26]). Goeman and Mansmann [27] have proposed a focus-level method for GSA analysis of GO terms. This method made use of the hierarchical structure of GO graphs. They proposed using the closed testing procedure [28] to account for multiple testing in GSA.

9.2
Competitive versus Self-Contained Tests

Tian et al. [11] have described two fundamental hypotheses, Q1 and Q2, for GCT:

- Q1: the genes in a gene set show the same pattern of associations with the phenotype compared with the rest of the genes.
- Q2: all the genes in the gene set are not associated with the phenotypes.

The hypothesis Q1 tests whether the association of a gene set with the phenotype is equal to those of the other gene sets. Q1 tests the relative strengths of the associations of the genes in a gene class with the phenotypes as compared to the genes outside the gene class. This hypothesis does not test whether the expression in the gene class is different in the phenotypes. Rather, it tests whether the observed difference between the phenotypes in the gene class is more or less than the average differences in the study. The hypothesis Q2 tests if the expression of a gene class differs by the phenotype. The null hypothesis is that the gene set does not contain any genes whose expression levels are associated with the phenotype. In other words, Q1 considers the relative association of differential expressions among the gene classes, while Q2 considers the association of each gene set with the phenotype, irrespective of the strength of the association of the other gene sets. Goeman and Bühlmann [29] denoted the tests for Q1 and Q2 as "competitive test" and "self-contained test" respectively.

A typical GCT approach can be summarized as follows: (i) grouping all genes based on the same annotation term together into gene classes; (ii) for each gene class, a GCT statistic is calculated as a summary measure of the class; (iii) re-sampling methods are used to generate the null distribution of the class score for each gene class; and (iv) statistical significance is assessed by comparing the observed functional score to the percentile of the null distribution of the gene class. Conceptually, the *p*-values of a GCT statistic can be calculated either by permuting genes or by permuting samples. Many authors have discussed the differences between gene and sample randomization in inferring the statistical significance of gene set test statistics under either the Q1 or the Q2 hypothesis (e.g., [11, 29]). The null distributions of statistic under Q1 are generated by permuting genes (gene sampling), and null distributions under Q2 are generated by permuting samples (subject-sampling). Various GSA methods have been proposed for testing either the Q1 or Q2 hypothesis or both. However, some methods hypothesized as the competitive test, but the *p*-values were calculated from the null distribution generated by subject-sampling. For example, GSEA formulated the Q1 hypothesis but generated the null distribution by subject-samplings. The competitive test and gene sampling methods are more popular [29]. Nam and Kim [8] provided a list of GSA methods with their hypotheses and sampling methods, and the references.

Nam and Kim [8] conducted a simulation study to examine the two hypotheses. They generated expression profiles of 2000 genes with two sample groups, each having 20 samples. The genes were divided into 100 gene sets, each of which contained 20 genes. The data were generated under Q1 (the competitive hypothesis) such that 30% of all genes were truly differentially expressed and each gene set was built such that 30% of genes in each gene set are differentially expressed. Under Q1 no gene set should be called differentially expressed since all gene sets have the same level of association with the phenotype. In contrast, under Q2 (the self-contained hypothesis), because 30% of genes in each gene set are differentially expressed, all genes sets should be called differentially expressed. Recently, Dinue et al. [30] have simulated the data under Q2 such that no gene was differentially expressed between the two groups for 100 gene sets. Under Q2 the *p*-values of the 100 gene sets were distributed uniformly. However, under Q1 it detected 27 of the 100 sets as differentially expressed with a *p*-value cutoff of 0.05. These results illustrated the key difference between the Q1 and Q2.

In principle, under the permutation test the sampling units (subjects or genes) are assumed to be independent and identically distributed. There are concerns with permutations of genes under the Q1 hypothesis [12]. Its empirical null distribution will not represent the distribution of genes that are not differentially expressed. The null distribution is essentially generated from the empirical distribution of the observed *p*-values, instead of the uniform distribution under the null hypothesis that there is no difference in gene expressions between two phenotypes. Permuting the genes only reassigns individual genes to different gene classes. Q1 is a conditional test, conditional on the association strength between phenotypes in expressions in the observed data. In Q1, a differently expressed gene set has a different interpretation from a differentially expressed gene identified from IGA. On the other hand, permutation of samples under Q2 is based on the random (independent) samples. The null distributions of different gene classes under Q2 are identically distributed, and their *p*-values are comparable. The Q2 hypothesis is consistent with the current use of permutation tests [1, 31] to select a list of differentially expressed genes in IGA; that is, GSA is a generalization of IGA. We consider only Q2-self-contained hypothesis and *p*-values are computed by sample permutations.

9.3
One-Sided and Two-Sided Hypotheses

The original GSEA statistic was a one-sided test to identify gene sets containing down-regulated genes in type 2 diabetes mellitus subjects [9]. The basic idea in this analysis is that the gene sets are closely related and, hence, will have similar expression patterns, either up or down. In GSA a one-sided test means that the changes of gene expressions in the gene set are in one direction: either up- or down-regulation. The two-sided test means that changes in the gene class can be both up- and down-regulation [12]. The Tian et al. [11] and Efron and Tibshirani [15] statistics were one-sided tests using the maximum in absolute values. Chen et al. [12] recommend the ordinary least squares (OLSs) statistic [32] and the standardized weighted sum statistic [33] for a one-sided test. These two global statistics were shown to perform well for GSA analysis. Most GSA statistics are for two-sided tests (e.g., [13, 18, 21–24]). The meta-analysis approaches based on the *p*-values of IGA are also two-sided tests (e.g., [25, 26]). When the goal is to detect coordinated changes in one direction, the one-sided hypothesis is appropriate. However, in an exploratory context, it is not possible to pre-specify how individual genes in a gene set will respond in different phenotypes.

9.4
Over-Representation Analysis (ORA)

In ORA, the statistical significance of a gene class is assessed by counting the number of statistically significant genes in the class from the list of significant genes from IGA. The null hypothesis that this count is a random sample of the significant genes on the array is tested versus an alternative hypothesis that count is enriched [5, 7]. The test is Fisher's exact test (e.g., [5]); the *p*-value of a gene set is calculated as:

$$P(x) = \sum_{l=x}^{k} \frac{\binom{N}{l}\binom{M-N}{K-l}}{\binom{M}{K}}$$

where

M is the total number of genes in the array,
N is the number of genes in the class,
K is the number of genes in the significant list,
x is the number of gene in the list from the class.

The p-values are computed using a hypergeometric distribution or one of its many approximations such as the chi-squared test, which approximates the hypergeometric distribution with a binomial distribution (e.g., [34]). The ORA approach has been proposed with minor variations by many different authors [5, 35–37]. IAG-ORA is the most commonly used method for gene set enrichment in the analysis of significant pathways or GO categories in the gene set annotation analysis. Khatri and Draghici [6] have provided an overview of ORA for the ontological analysis of gene expression.

There are several shortcomings with the IAG-ORA approach (e.g., [10, 11, 25]), which can be summarized as follow. First, the division of genes into differential and non-differential expression groups is arbitrary, and many genes with moderate but meaningful expression changes can be discarded by a strict cutoff value. Second, only the number of genes in the list is used in the ORA, those genes not in the list are treated as irrelevant although some insignificant genes may be on the borderline. Third, the order of genes on the significant gene list is not taken into consideration. The difference between those very significant genes and the less significant genes can be substantial if the list is long. Fourth, Fisher's exact test assumes independence among genes – the correlation structure of genes is not taken into consideration. Fifth, ORA may miss important effects on pathways where the genes having modest effects in concert may not be in the differential expression list. An increase of 20% in all genes in a metabolic pathway may dramatically alter the flux through the pathway and may be more important than a 20-fold increase in a single gene [10]. An ORA analysis of a gene set from the diabetes dataset presented by Mootha et al. [9] and Subramanian et al. [10] is illustrated below.

The diabetes dataset consisted of 318 gene classes from 15 056 genes measured on 17 subjects with normal glucose tolerance and 17 subjects with type 2 diabetes mellitus. Table 9.1 lists the unpaired t-statistics and p-values of the top 50 genes. Using the Benjamini and Hochberg [4] method, the smallest FDR value is 0.688. The number of significance genes is 0 even at the 0.25 level of significance. Of the 318 gene classes analyzed the gene set MAP00 252_Alanine_and_aspartate_metabolism is one of the most significant gene sets identified by two-sided tests (shown in Section 9.6). This gene set was used to illustrate and highlight a shortcoming of the ORA analysis. Table 9.2 shows the p-values from the Fisher's exact test according with the significant cutoff probability for the gene set MAP00 252. It can be seen that the p-values fluctuate as the cutoff changes. For example, using a p-value cutoff of 0.005 the Fisher's exact test has the p-value of 0.0701 (>0.05), but using a cutoff of 0.075 the corresponding p-value for the gene set is 0.0471 (<0.05).

9.5
GCT Statistics

Consider a microarray study of m genes with c phenotypes of sample sizes $n_1, \ldots, n_c$. Without loss of generality, consider a gene set consisting of m genes. Let

Table 9.1 The 50 smallest p-values from the analysis of diabetes dataset; the diabetes dataset consisted of 15 056 genes measured on 17 subjects with normal glucose tolerance and 17 subjects with type 2 diabetes mellitus.

Gene	1	2	3	4	5	6	7	8	9	10
t-Value	−4.713	−4.344	−4.249	−4.300	4.292	−4.110	−4.047	3.871	−3.846	−3.736
p-Value	00001	0.0001	0.0002	0.0002	0.0002	0.0004	0.0005	0.0005	0.0006	0.0008
Gene	11	12	13	14	15	16	17	18	19	20
t-Value	3.711	−3.604	3.694	3.516	−3.563	3.542	−3.527	−3.464	3.436	3.382
p-Value	0.0010	0.0011	0.0013	0.0014	0.0014	0.0015	0.0015	0.0016	0.0018	0.0019
Gene	21	22	23	24	25	26	27	28	29	30
t-Value	−3.489	−3.357	−3.457	−3.471	−3.318	3.342	3.270	3.326	3.341	−3.387
p-Value	0.0019	0.0021	0.0022	0.0022	0.0023	0.0024	0.0026	0.0028	0.0029	0.0031
Gene	31	32	33	34	35	36	37	38	39	40
t-Value	−3.200	−3.189	−3.238	3.192	−3.243	−3.209	3.216	3.189	−3.118	−3.117
p-Value	0.0031	0.0032	0.0032	0.0032	0.0033	0.0035	0.0038	0.0038	0.0038	0.0039
Gene	41	42	43	44	45	46	47	48	49	50
t-Value	−3.097	−3.084	−3.155	−3.074	−3.088	3.188	3.063	3.046	3.072	3.038
p-Value	0.0041	0.0042	0.0042	0.0043	0.0044	0.0045	0.0046	0.0047	0.0047	0.0047

Table 9.2 Over-representation analysis of the diabetes data from the Fisher's exact test. The diabetes dataset consisted of 318 gene classes from 15 056 genes. The gene set MAP00252_Alanine_and_aspartate_metabolism is one of the most significance gene sets identified with 21 genes in the gene set. For a given cutoff, K is the number of genes in the significant list and X is the number of gene in the list from the class.

	MAP00252_Alanine_and_aspartate_metabolism (N = 21)		
Cutoff	K	X	p-Value
0.001	11	1	0.0152
0.003	29	1	0.0397 ←
0.005	52	1	0.0701 ←
0.010	105	1	0.1367 ←
0.020	226	2	0.0391 ↓
0.050	642	2	0.2249 ←
0.060	790	2	0.3026 ←
0.070	929	3	0.1365 ↓
0.075	1002	4	0.0471 ↓
0.080	1081	4	0.0594 ←
0.090	1233	4	0.0875 ←

$y_{ij} = (y_{ij1}, \ldots y_{ijm})$ be the m-vector of intensities for simple j ($j = 1, \ldots, n_i$) in i-th phenotype ($i = 1, \ldots, c$). Two one-sided tests and three two-sided tests are considered described below.

9.5.1
One-Sided Test

9.5.1.1 OLS Global Test

Denote the standardized variable $y_{ijk}^* = (y_{ijk} - \bar{y}_k)/s_k$, where $\bar{y}_k$ is the overall sample mean for the k-th gene and s_k is the pooled standard deviation. Let $z_{ik} = \sum_j y_{ijk}^*/n_i$ be the mean of the standardized variable for the k-th in the i-th phenotype. Denote the $z_i = (z_{i1}, \ldots z_{im})$ as the m-vector of the standardized mean variable z_{ij}s for the i-th phenotype (i = 1, 2). Let d_i be a m-dimensional vector for the mean difference between two phenotypes $d_i = (z_1 - z_2)$. The O'Brien's OLS statistic [32] is:

$$T_{ols} = \frac{1' d_i}{(1' V_i 1)^{1/2}}$$

where 1 is a $m_i \times 1$ vector of 1s and V_i is the pooled sample covariance matrix of d_i. If d_i is a multivariate normal, then the OLS statistic T_{ols} has an approximately t-distribution with $n_1 + n_2 - 2$ degrees of freedom. An equivalent way to compute the test statistic is to add up the y_{ijg}^* over the m genes and then perform the two-sample t-test with this variable.

When sample size is small, T_{ols} does not keep the prescribed level of significance [33]. Läuter [33] have proposed an exact test by standardizing the variables by the overall mean and standard deviation, The permutation p-values for the OLS and the Laüter test are very close [12]. Therefore, only the OLS test is presented in this chapter.

9.5.1.2 GSEA Test

Gene set enrichment analysis (GSEA) [10] consists of the following steps. The first step is to rank the N genes based on some ranking metric, r_k, which reflects the degree of the correlation between the expression and the class phenotypes. The second step is to calculate an enrichment score (ES) for the gene set G of N_G genes in the ranked list $L = \{g_1, g_2, \ldots, g_N\}$. The score is composed of evaluating the fraction of genes in G ("hits") weighted by their correlation and the fraction of genes not in G ("misses") present up to a given position i in L. Defining the two quantities:

$$P_{hit}(G, i) = \sum_{\substack{g_i \in G \\ j \leq i}} \frac{|r_j|^p}{N_R}, \quad \text{where } N_R = \sum_{g_i \in G} |r_j|^p$$

$$P_{miss}(G, i) = \sum_{\substack{g_i \in G \\ j \leq i}} \frac{1}{(N - N_G)}.$$

The ES is the maximum deviation from zero of $(P_{hit} - P_{miss})$. When $p = 0$, $ES(G)$ reduces to the standard Kolmogorov–Smirnov statistic; when $p = 1$, the genes in G are weighted by their enrichment scores normalized by the total enrichment scores over all of the genes in G. The p-values are computed by the sample permutation.

9.5.2 Two-Sided Test

9.5.2.1 MANOVA Test

The MANOVA model [18] can be expressed as $y_{ij} = \mu_i + e_{ij}$, where e_{ij} is m-vector of residuals with $\text{Var}(e_{ij}) = \Sigma$, and μ_i is the m-vector of means for the i-th condition. The null hypothesis of no difference in gene expressions among the c phenotypes is given as: $\mu_1 = \ldots = \mu_c$; an alternative is at least one gene in the gene set express differently in at least two phenotypes. There are four MANOVA tests: Wilks' Λ, Pillai's trace, Hotelling's T^2, and Roy's largest root. The four tests are equivalent to Hotelling's T^2 when there are only two conditions. Tsai and Chen [18] considered the Wilks' Λ test:

$$\text{Wilks' } \Lambda = \Pi\, 1/(1 + \lambda_k)$$

where λ_ks are the eigenvalues of the matrix $S\ (= E^{-1}H)$, and E is within sum of squares matrix (sample covariance matrix) and H is between sum of squares matrix. The number of eigenvalues k is equal to the minimum of the number of genes (m) and the number of conditions minus 1 ($c - 1$). When the number of genes in the gene set is greater than the number of samples, the matrix E is singular and ill-conditioned. The shrinkage covariance matrix estimator (S_{ij}^*) proposed by Schäfer and Strimmer [38] is used to make the matrix well-condition given as:

$$S_{ij} = \begin{cases} S_{ii} & \text{if } i=j \\ r_{ij}\sqrt{S_{ii}S_{jj}} & \text{if } i \neq j \end{cases}$$

and $r_{ij}^* = r_{ij}\min\{1, \max(0, 1-\hat{\lambda})\}$, where s_{ii} and r_{ij} respectively denote the empirical sample variance and sample correlation, and the optimal shrinkage intensity $\hat{\lambda}$ is estimated by:

$$\hat{\lambda} = \frac{\sum \hat{Var}(r_{ij})}{\sum r_{ij}^2}$$

The distribution of Wilks' Λ (or Hotelling's T^2) under the null hypothesis of no difference in responses between the conditions was estimated by the permutation method. The null hypothesis is rejected if one or more of the mean differences or some combination of mean differences among the genes in gene set differs from zero.

The Wilks' Λ test is equivalent to Hotelling's T^2 when there are only two conditions:

$$T^2 = \frac{n_1 n_2}{n_1 + n_2}(\bar{x}_1 - \bar{x}_2)^t S_p^{-1}(\bar{x}_1 - \bar{x}_2)$$

where $\bar{x}_i$ and S_i denote the sample mean vector and sample covariance matrix of the i-th group ($i = 1, 2$), respectively, and $S_p = [(n_1-1)S_1 + (n_2-1)S_2]/(n_1+n_2-2)$ denotes the pooled covariance matrix.

9.5.2.2 SAM-GS Test

The SAM-GS test [13] extended the univariate SAM [1] single-gene analysis to gene-set analysis. The SAM-GS statistic is based on the sum of independence univariate t-type SAM statistics. For each gene k, the SAM statistic d_k is calculated as:

$$d_k = \frac{\bar{y}_{1,k} - \bar{y}_{2,k}}{s_k + s_0}$$

where

$\bar{y}_{i,k}$ is the sample mean of the k-th gene in the i-th phenotype,
s_k is a pooled standard deviation for the k-th gene,
s_0 is a small positive constant to adjust for the small variability [1].

SAM-GS is computed by summing the SAM statistics for all genes in the gene set:

$$\text{SAM-GS} = \sum_{k=1}^{m} d_k^2$$

The p-value of the SAM-GS test is computed by permutations. The permutation approach does not take the weighted Dempster's adjustment [39] for correlations into consideration; that is, like the ANVOVA test, SAM-GS assumes independence among genes in the gene set. In addition, like the t-test SAM-GS is for comparison of two phenotypes.

9.5.2.3 ANCOVA Test

The ANCOVA test [23] uses the analysis of variance (ANOVA) to account for covariate effects. The ANCOVA model uses a univariate gene-by-gene analysis; it does not account for the correlation structure among gene set. Let y_{ijk} denote the intensity for gene k ($k = 1, \ldots, m$) in the simple j ($j = 1, \ldots, n_i$) and condition i ($i = 1, \ldots c$). The model for the ANCOVA test is of the form: $y_{ijk} = \mu + \alpha_i + \beta_j + \gamma_{ij} + e_{ijk}$, with phenotype effects α, gene effects β, the gene–phenotype interaction γ, and e is the error term. The null hypothesis of no difference in a GSA is $H_0: \alpha_i = \gamma_{ij} = 0$. The test statistic is the F-statistic. The p-values of the ANCOVA F-statistic can be calculated either from the F-distributions or by the permutation method. The permutation approach has been shown to perform better than the distribution approach [40].

9.6 Applications

9.6.1 Diabetes Dataset

We first applied the GCT tests to the diabetes dataset. Table 9.3 lists the p-values of the top ten gene sets from the one-sided OLS (T_{ols}) and GSEA tests. The number of gene sets with p-values less than 0.05 are 8 and 9 (the last row) for OLS and GSEA tests, respectively. The two tests are very similar with some minor discrepancy for the mitochondria pathway. Table 9.4 lists the p-values of top eight gene sets from the two-sided MNOVA (T^2), SAM-GS, and ANCOVA tests. The numbers of f gene sets with

Table 9.3 GSA analysis of the diabetes data from the OLS and GSEA tests. The lists are the p-values of ten top ranked gene sets (ranks are in parentheses) of each test. The p-values are computed based on 1000 permutations.

ID	Size	T_{ols}	GSEA
P53_Down	18	0.004 (1)	0.000 (1)
ST_T_Cell signal transduction	42	0.008 (2)	0.010 (4)
VOXPHOS	83	0.015 (3)	0.006 (2)
Electron transport chain	85	0.015 (3)	0.008 (3)
MAP00500_Starch_and_sucrose_metabolism	21	0.027 (5)	0.050 (9)
MAP00120_Bile_acid_biosynthesis	22	0.034 (6)	0.016 (5)
MAP00561_Glycerolipid_metabolism	46	0.035 (7)	0.025 (6)
ST_MONOCYTE_AD_PATHWAY	27	0.036 (8)	0.028 (7)
Mitochondria pathway	21	0.053 (9)	0.260 (55)
GNF_female_Genes	85	0.057 (10)	0.053(10)
SA_B_CELL RECEPTOR COMPLEXES	24	0.061(11)	0.038 (8)
Number with $p < 0.05$		8	9

Table 9.4 GSA analysis of the diabetes data from the T^2, SAM-GS, and ANCOVA tests. The lists are the p-values of the eight top-ranked gene sets (ranks are in parentheses) of each test. The p-values are computed based on 1000 permutations.

ID	Size	T^2	SAM-GS	ANCOVA
GNF_Female_Genes	85	0.011 (1)	0.059 (4)	0.269 (72)
MAP00252_Alanine_and_aspartate_metabolism	21	0.013 (2)	0.038 (1)	0.014 (1)
achPathway	15	0.016 (3)	0.045 (2)	0.752 (217)
Matrix_Metalloproteinases	26	0.022 (4)	0.066 (6)	0.306 (80)
MAP00251_Glutamate_metabolism	20	0.025 (5)	0.128 (10)	0.312 (82)
INSULIN_2F_UP	196	0.034 (6)	0.164 (18)	0.628 (179)
MAP03020_RNA_polymerase	17	0.039 (7)	0.181 (21)	0.076 (26)
GLUCO	31	0.041 (8)	0.093 (7)	0.262 (70)
Electron_Transport_Chain	85	0.283 (87)	0.058 (3)	0.033 (11)
VOXPHOS	83	0.193 (57)	0.063 (5)	0.035 (13)
P53_DOWN	18	0.109 (26)	0.103 (8)	0.063 (19)
MAP00190_Oxidative_phosphorylation	43	0.122 (38)	0.142 (11)	0.018 (2)
MAP00193_ATP_synthesis	18	0.117 (34)	0.146 (12)	0.021 (3)
igf1mtorPathway	20	0.773 (248)	0.823 (248)	0.022 (4)
ptdinsPathway	20	0.626 (197)	0.730 (202)	0.025 (5)
mtorPathway	23	0.561 (176)	0.623 (165)	0.025 (5)
MAP00195_Photosynthesis	19	0.172 (53)	0.155 (14)	0.026 (7)
GO_0005739	161	0.112 (28)	0.304 (53)	0.029 (8)
Number with $p < 0.05$		8	2	10

p-values less than 0.05 are given in the last row. There are discrepancies among the three two-sided tests. The T^2 and SAM-GS tests are relatively similar in terms of the ranking of gene sets. T^2 appears to be more powerful in identifying significant gene sets than SAM-SG. The ANVOVA test shows considerably results different from the T^2 and SAM-GS tests. The ANCOVA test is more powerful.

The p-values from the one-sided OLS and GSEA tests are very different from the p-values from the two-sided T^2, SAM-GS, and ANCOVA tests; as are the gene set rankings. The gene set p53_Down is highly significant ($p < 0.01$) by OLS and GSEA but it is not significant by the three two-sided tests. Figure 9.1 is a "GCT" plot (a modified SAFE plot of [41]) of relative extent and direction of differential expression observed for the 18 genes in the p53_Down pathway. Nine of the 18 genes are underexpressed with p-values less than 0.05 in the diabetes samples compared to the normal samples. On the other hand, the gene set MAP00 252_Alanine_and_aspartate metabolism is highly significance in all three two-sided tests, but the one-sided test is not significant (Figure 9.2). Of the 21 genes in MAP00252, one gene showed up as significantly underexpressed and one as significantly overexpressed. Figure 9.3 is a plot for gene set GNF_Female_Genes; the p-values are 0.057 and 0.053 from the one-sided T_{ols} and GSEA, respectively, and 0.011, 0.059, and 0.269 for the two-sided T^2, SAM-GS, and ANCOVA tests, respectively.

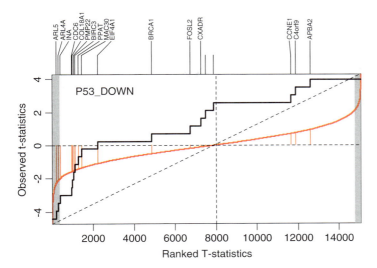

Figure 9.1 GCT-plots for the gene set P53_Down in the diabetes dataset. The solid line is the empirical cumulative distribution function of the ranked *t*-statistics for 15 056 in genes in the array. The two tailed shaded regions represent the *t*-statistics that had *p*-values below the 5%. The dashed line is expected *p*-values under the null hypothesis of no difference between groups. There are 18 tick marks above each plot that display the location of the *p*-value of the genes from the gene set. The gene set shows underexpression.

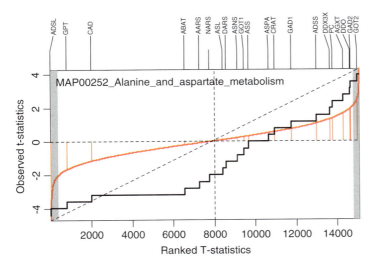

Figure 9.2 GCT-plots for the gene set MAP00252_Alanine_and_aspartate_ metabolism in the diabetes dataset. The solid line is the empirical cumulative distribution function of the ranked *t*-statistics for 15 056 in genes in the array. The two tailed shaded regions represent the *t*-statistics that had the *p*-values below the 5%. The dashed line is expected *p*-values under the null hypothesis of no difference between groups. There are 21 tick marks above each plot that display the location of the *p*-value of the genes from the gene set. The gene set shows both under- and overexpression.

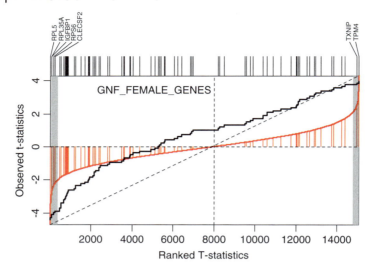

Figure 9.3 GCT-plots for the gene set GNF_Female_Genes in the diabetes dataset. The solid line is the empirical cumulative distribution function of the ranked *t*-statistics for 15 056 in genes in the array. The two tailed shaded regions represent the *t*-statistics that had the *p*-values below the 5%. The dashed line is expected *p*-values under the null hypothesis of no difference between groups. There are 167 tick marks above each plot that display the location of the *p*-value of the genes from the gene set. The gene set shows both under- and overexpression.

9.6.2
p53 Dataset

We next applied the GCT tests to a p53 study. The p53 dataset is a study to identify targets of the transcription factor p53 from 10 100 gene expression profiles in the NCI-60 collection of cancer cell lines. There are 308 gene sets in the p53 study. The mutation status of the p53 gene has been reported for 50 of the NCI-60 cell lines with 17 normal and 33 mutation samples. The dataset is publicly available at the GSEA website (http://www.broad.mit.edu/gsea). Dinu *et al.* [13] have analyzed this dataset for comparisons between SAM-GS and GSEA. Tsai and Chen [18] have analyzed this dataset with several GCT tests, including GSEA, T^2, SAM-GS, and ANCOVA, but without OLS.

Table 9.5 shows the number of gene sets with *p*-values less than 0.01 and 0.05 for the five GSA methods. For the one-sided tests, OLS and GSEA appear to be very similar. For the two-sided tests, unlike the diabetes dataset, Hotelling's T^2 and SAM-GS identify many more gene sets than ANCOVA. In addition, T^2 identifies slightly more gene sets than SAM-GS. Dinu *et al.* [13] have discussed that SAM-GS identified more gene sets than GSEA, and many of those additional gene sets identified by SAM-SG were associated with p53 genes or p53 signaling.

Table 9.5 Number of gene sets with p-values less than 0.01 and 0.05 by the global (T_{ols}), GSEA, Hotelling's T^2, SAM-GS, and ANCOVA for the p53 study; the number of gene sets is 308.

p-Value ≤	Method				
	T_{ols}	GSEA	T^2	SAM-GS	ANCOVA
0.01	10	10	39	32	7
0.05	29	27	77	60	16

9.7 Discussion

Biological phenomena often occur through the interactions of multiple genes, via signaling pathways, networks, or other functional relationships. Genes in a gene set are functionally related and are not independent; the complex structure of gene interactions within a gene set are not fully captured using univariate approaches. Some gene sets that may not seem to be different by univariate methods may show a difference by a simultaneous analysis of entire gene set. With rapid developments of genomic databases and availability of more comprehensive annotations, GCT can provide a powerful and more easily interpretable analysis.

The two one-sided tests OLS and GSEA are considered in the analysis. A one-sided test is used to detect coordinated changes in one direction. The OLS statistic is the most widely used global test for the analysis of multiple clinical endpoints [32]. This test is very powerful when the changes in the gene expression are in the same direction. There were concerns that the null distributions of the one-sided GSEA statistic were affected by the class sizes [11, 42]. The OLS statistics account for gene set size and correlation structure [12]. Both OLS and GSEA tests can identify either up- or down-regulated gene sets. In an OLS analysis, the direction of changes of significant gene sets can be checked from the OLS statistic (Table 9.1 and Figure 9.1). The GSEA test performs up- and down-regulation analyses separately to identify the direction of changes. Both one-sided tests are powerful when the changes are in the same direction [18].

Three two-sided tests, T^2, SAM-GS, and ANCOVA, are considered in this chapter. When the changes are a mixture of up- and down-regulations, the two-sided tests are more powerful in identifying the significant gene sets. Each significant gene set from a two-sided test may be checked for the direction of changes. Liu et al. [40] have compared statistical performance of the global test [22], ANCOVA test [23], and SAM-GS [13]. In the simulation experiment, they found that a proper standardization across genes is necessary for the global and ANOCOVA tests in order to obtain more accurate inference. Similarly, Tsai and Chen [18] have compared two one-sided tests, GSEA [10] and MaxMean [15], and five two-sided tests: MANOVA T^2 [18], principal component analysis (PCA) [16], SAM-GS [13], Global [22], and ANCOVA [23], using simulation. Under the models considered in the simulation, they showed that T^2 and ANCOVA were reasonably close to or below the 0.05 nominal level. PCA and SAM-GS showed anti-conservatism in few cases, while Global showed conservatism. The T^2 performed the best in terms of power. SAM-GS and PCA appeared to be comparable. The Global test had the lowest power. ANCOVA can be more powerful than T^2 and SAM-GS if the variances are equal across all genes in the gene set. MaxMean was shown to have an overly inflated size.

The MANOVA test described in this chapter is developed to identify differentially expressed gene sets for the data collected from studies with two or more experimental conditions. The MANOVA is a multivariate generalization of the univariate analysis of variance (ANOVA) as the Hotelling's T^2 test is the generalization of the univariate t-test. Like the ANOVA and t-test, the MANOVA and Hotelling's T^2 are the most commonly used multivariate data analysis methods; the tests are robust and most powerful under normality assumption, have been well studied, and perform well in many areas of applications. The shrinkage covariance matrix estimator is used in the standard MANOVA Wilks' statistic to incorporate the correlations structure among the genes in the test statistic and to account for the singularity and ill-condition of the sample covariance matrix. The T^2 test was shown to perform well for the two-sided test in terms of controlling the type I error and power in simulation and data analysis. This chapter considers the GCT for two experimental conditions. An analysis of dataset collected from three conditions using the MANOVA and ANCOVA tests was given in Tsai and Chen [18].

A GCT analysis assigns an overall statistical significance of differences in gene expression for a gene set. It does not identify which genes in the gene class actually contribute to the difference. After identifying gene classes that show a difference, the standard univariate test can be used to identify which genes in the gene class are significant. Dinue et al. [30] have proposed a significance analysis of microarray for gene set reduction (SAMGSR). This approach provides a tool to reduce a gene set that has previously been found differentially expressed to a core set. In testing individual genes in a gene set, the total number of the tests is the number of genes in the gene set, not the total number of genes in the array. In the follow-up analysis, the interest is in identifying which genes are significant in the given significant gene set. A gene may be significant in one gene set, but insignificant in another.

References

1 Tusher, V.G. et al. (2001) Significance analysis of microarrays applied to the ionizing radiation response. *Proc. Natl. Acad. Sci. USA*, **98**, 5116–5121.

2 Chen, J.J. (2007) Key aspects of analyzing microarray gene expression data. *Pharmacogenomics*, **5**, 473–482.

3 Chen, J.J., Wang, S.J., Tsai, C.A., and Lin, C.J. (2007) Selection of differentially expressed genes in microarray data analysis. *Pharmacogenom. J.*, **7**, 212–220.

4 Benjamini, Y. and Hochberg, Y. (1995) Controlling the false discovery rate: a practical and powerful approach to multiple testing. *J. R. Stat. Soc. B*, **57**, 289–300.

5 Draghici, S. et al. (2003) Global functional profiling of gene expression. *Genomics*, **81**, 98–104.

6 Khatri, P. and Draghici, S. (2005) Ontological analysis of gene expression data: current tools, limitations, and open problems. *Bioinformatics*, **21**, 3587–3595.

7 Rivals, I. et al. (2007) Enrichment or depletion of a GO category within a class of genes: which test? *Bioinformatics*, **23**, 401–407.

8 Nam, D. and Kim, S.Y. (2008) Gene-set approach for expression pattern analysis. *Brief. Bioinform.*, **9**, 189–197.

9 Mootha, V.K. et al. (2003) PGC-1 alpha-responsive genes involved in oxidative phosphorylation are coordinately down regulated in human diabetes. *Nat. Genet.*, **34**, 267–273.

10 Subramanian, A. et al. (2005) Gene set enrichment analysis: a knowledge-based approach for interpreting genome-wide expression profiles. *Proc. Natl Acad. Sci. USA*, **102**, 15545–15550.

11 Tian, L. et al. (2005) Discovering statistically significant pathways in expression profiling studies. *Proc. Natl Acad. of Sci. USA*, **102**, 13544–13549.

12 Chen, J.J. et al. (2007) Significance analysis of groups of genes in expression profiling studies. *Bioinformatics*, **2007**, **23**, 2104–2112.

13 Dinu, I. et al. (2007) Improving gene set analysis of microarray data by SAM-GS. *BMC Bioinformatics*, **8**, 242.

14 Adewale, A.J. et al. (2008) Pathway analysis of microarray data via regression. *J. Comput. Biol.*, **15**, 269–277.

15 Efron, B. and Tibshirani, R. (2007) On testing the significance of set s of genes. *Ann. Appl. Stat.*, **1**, 107–129.

16 Kong, S.W. et al. (2006) A multivariate approach for integrating genome wide expression data and biological knowledge. *Bioinformatics*, **22**, 2373–2380.

17 Tomfohr, J. et al. (2005) Pathway level analysis of gene expression using singular value decomposition. *BMC Bioinformatics*, **6**, 225.

18 Tsai, C.A. and Chen, J.J. (2009) Multivariate analysis of variance test for gene set analysis. *Bioinformatics*, **25**, 897–903.

19 Szabo, A. et al. (2003) Multivariate exploratory tools for microarray data analysis. *Biostatistics*, **4**, 555–567.

20 Kim, B.S. et al. (2005) Statistical methods of translating microarray data into clinically relevant diagnostic information in colorectal cancer. *Bioinformatics*, **21**, 517–528.

21 Lu, Y. et al. (2005) Hotelling's T^2 multivariate profiling for detecting differential expression in microarrays. *Bioinformatics*, **21**, 3105–3113.

22 Goeman, J.J. et al. (2004) A global test for groups of genes: testing association with a clinical outcome. *Bioinformatics*, **20**, 93–99.

23 Mansmann, U. and Meister, R. (2005) Testing differential gene expression in functional groups: Goeman's global test versus an ANCOVA approach. *Methods Inf. Med.*, **44**, 449–453.

24 Hummel, M. et al. (2008) GlobalANCOVA: exploration and assessment of gene group effects. *Bioinformatics*, **24**, 78–85.

25 Pavlidis, P. et al. (2004) Using the gene ontology for microarray data mining: a comparison of methods and application to age effects in human prefrontal cortex. *Neurochem. Res.*, **29**, 1213–1222.

26 Delongchamp, R. et al. (2006) A method for computing the overall statistical significance of a treatment effect among a group of genes. *BMC Bioinformatics*, **7** (Suppl. 2), S11.

27 Goeman, J.J. and Mansmann, U. (2008) Multiple testing on the directed acyclic graph of gene ontology. *Bioinformatics*, **24**, 537–544.

28 Marcus, R. et al. (1976) On closed testing procedures with special reference to ordered analysis of variance. *Biometrika*, **63**, 655–660.

29 Goeman, J.J. and Bühlmann, P. (2007) Analyzing gene expression data in terms of gene sets: methodological issues. *Bioinformatics*, **23**, 980–987.

30 Dinu, I et al. (2009) Gene set analysis and reduction. *Brief. Bioinform*, **10**, 24–34.

31 Tsai, C.A., Chen, Y.J., and Chen, J.J. (2003) Testing for differentially expressed genes with microarray data. *Nucl. Acids Res.*, **31**, e52.

32 O'Brien, P.C. (1984) Procedure for comparing samples with multiple endpoints. *Biometrics*, **40**, 1079–1087.

33 Läuter, J. (1996) Exact t and F tests for analyzing studies with multiple endpoints. *Biometrics*, **52**, 964–970.

34 Man, M.Z., Wang, Z., and Wang, Y. (2000) POWER_SAGE: comparing statistical tests for SAGE experiments. *Bioinformatics*, **16**, 953–959.

35 Al-Shahrour, F. *et al.* (2004) FatiGO: a web tool for finding significant associations of gene ontology terms with groups of genes. *Bioinformatics*, **20**, 578–580.

36 Beissbarth, T. and Speed, T.P. (2004) GOstat: find statistically overrepresented gene ontologies within a group of genes. *Bioinformatics*, **20**, 1464–1465.

37 Zeeberg, B.R. *et al.* (2003) GoMiner: a resource for biological interpretation of genomic and proteomic data. *Genome Biol.*, **4**, R28.

38 Schäfer, J. and Strimmer, K. (2005) A shrinkage approach to large-scale covariance matrix estimation and implications for functional genomics. *Stat. Appl. Genet. Mol. Biol.*, **4**, 32.

39 Dempster, A.P. (1960) A significance test for the separation of two highly multivariate small samples. *Biometrics*, **16**, 41–50.

40 Liu, Q., Dinu, I., Adewale, A.J., Potter, J.D., and Yasui, Y. (2007) Comparative evaluation of gene-set analysis methods. *BMC Bioinformatics*, **8**, 431.

41 Barry, W.T., Nobel, A.B., and Wright, F.A. (2005) Significance analysis of functional categories in gene expression studies: a structured permutation approach. *Bioinformatics*, **21**, 1943–1949.

42 Damian, D. and Gorfine, M. (2004) Statistical concerns about the GSEA procedure. *Nat. Genet.*, **36**, 663.

10
Differential Dependency Network Analysis to Identify Topological Changes in Biological Networks

Bai Zhang, Huai Li, Robert Clarke, Leena Hilakivi-Clarke, and Yue Wang

10.1
Introduction

Recent advances in high-throughput genomic technologies such as gene expression microarrays provide ample opportunities to study cellular activities at the individual gene expression and network levels. Microarray gene expression profiling measures simultaneously the expression levels of tens of thousands of genes under different experimental conditions, enabling studies on the phenotypic outcomes of certain treatment responses, disease progression, and developmental stages and the underlying gene expression patterns functionally associated with these phenotypes. These technologies also present new demands and challenges for data analysis to extract meaningful statistical and biological information from high throughput and high-dimensional data [1]. These data analysis tasks include signal pre-processing, clustering, visualization, classification, gene biomarker identification, and gene network modeling.

Gene network modeling and analysis attempts to explain the mechanisms that orchestrate the activities of genes and proteins in cells, and is one of the key goals in systems biology studies [2]. Several computational approaches have been proposed to model gene regulatory networks [3], such as Bayesian networks [4–6], probabilistic Boolean networks [7], state-space models [8], and network component analysis [9]. These methods attempt to construct a static network that can explain various gene regulation programs. While the inference of transcriptional networks using data from composite conditions could sometimes be contradictory due to changes in the underlying topology, most network learning algorithms assume an invariant network topology [5, 7, 8].

However, gene regulatory networks are context-specific and dynamic in nature [1, 10]. Under different conditions, different regulatory components and mechanisms are activated and the topology of the underlying gene regulatory network changes. For example, in response to diverse conditions in the yeast, transcription factors alter their interactions and rewire the signaling networks [11]. Therefore, some methods have been proposed to learn condition-specific transcriptional networks in yeast [12, 13]. It

---

Medical Biostatistics for Complex Diseases. Edited by Frank Emmert-Streib and Matthias Dehmer
Copyright © 2010 WILEY-VCH Verlag GmbH & Co. KGaA, Weinheim
ISBN: 978-3-527-32585-6

is important to focus on the topological changes in transcriptional networks between disease and normal conditions, or across different stages of cell development. For example, a deviation from normal regulatory network topology may reveal the mechanism of pathogenesis [14], and the genes that undergo the most network topological changes may serve as biomarkers for the disease state or as targets for drug discovery or therapeutic intervention.

Several methods have been proposed to utilize network topology information to carry out various bioinformatics tasks. Liu et al. have introduced a topology-based cancer classification method [15], where correlation networks were first constructed and later used to perform classification. Fuller et al. have developed weighted gene co-expression network analysis strategies, using single network analysis and differential network analysis, to identify physiologically relevant modules [16]. Qiu et al. have proposed an ensemble dependence model to detect the dependence changes of gene clusters between cancer and normal conditions for cancer classification, and further extended the dependence model to dependence networks [17, 18]. Wei and Li have introduced a Markov random field model for network-based analysis of genomic data that utilizes the known pathway structures to identify differentially expressed genes and subnetworks [19, 20]. Emmert-Streib has presented a comparative pathway analysis to study the chronic fatigue syndrome. The comparative pathway analysis identifies undirected dependency graphs, which represent biological processes according to the gene ontology database, using correlations and partial correlations of gene expression data. The structural comparison of undirected dependency graphs of sick versus non-sick patients is then used to make predictions about the modification of pathways due to pathogenesis [21].

In this chapter we discuss differential dependency network (DDN) analysis as a new method to model and detect the statistically significant topological changes in transcriptional networks between two conditions. This discussion is based on the work proposed in Reference [22]. We use local dependency models to characterize the dependencies of genes in the network and extract and represent local network substructures. Local dependency models decompose the entire network into a series of local networks, which serve as the basic network elements for subsequent statistical testing. Local dependency models select the number of dependent variables automatically by the Lasso method [23], and thereby learn the local network structures. Subsequently, we perform permutation tests on the local dependency models under two conditions and assign the *p*-values to the local structures. It may seem straightforward to construct an entire network under each condition and compare the differences between the two networks [16, 18]. However, in realistic applications this approach runs into the difficulty that the network structure learning can be inconsistent with a limited number of data samples.

When applied to the very high-dimensional data produced by gene expression microarrays, the properties of the data impose additional constraints and complications [1]. The detection procedure proposed here assures the statistical significance of the detected network topological changes by performing a permutation test on individual local structures. We also pinpoint "hot spots" in the network where the genes exhibit network topological changes between two conditions above a given significance level. Lastly, we extract and visualize the DDN, that is, the subnetworks exhibiting the most significant topological changes. We demonstrate the usefulness of the proposed method on both simulated and real microarray data. Tested on a simulation dataset, the proposed algorithm accurately captured the genes with network topological changes. When applied to the estrogen-dependent T-47D estrogen receptor-positive (ER+) breast cancer cell line dataset and normal adult rat mammary glands exposed to excess E2 *in utero* dataset, the DDN analysis obtained biologically meaningful and promising results.

10.2 Preliminaries

10.2.1 Probabilistic Graphical Models and Dependency Networks

Probabilistic graphical models are diagrammatic representations of probability distributions for a set of random variables. In a probabilistic graphical model, each node represents a random variable (or a group of random variables), and edges (either directed or undirected) express dependent relationships between these variables [24].

Probabilistic graphical models have been widely used to represent biological networks. Because microarray data are very noisy, the probabilistic nature of graphical models automatically takes into account the noise in the data and intrinsic uncertainties in the models. Further, diagrammatic representations of graphical models naturally visualize the relationships of genes, which can facilitate new insights and motivate new biological hypotheses. Typical examples of probabilistic graphical models are Bayesian networks, Markov networks, linear Gaussian networks, and dependency networks [24, 25].

Dependency networks were first proposed to encode and learn probabilistic relationships by Heckerman [26]. Unlike Bayesian networks, the graph of a dependency network can be cyclic, and dependency networks are considerably easier to learn from data. More specifically, given a set of random variables $\boldsymbol{X} = \{X_1, X_2, \ldots, X_M\}$, a dependency network for $\boldsymbol{X}$ is modeled by a set of local conditional probability distributions, one for each node given its parents, denoted as Z_i, which satisfies:

$$P(X_i|Z_i) = P(X_i|\boldsymbol{X}_{-i}) \tag{10.1}$$

where $\boldsymbol{X}_{-i} = \{X_1, X_2, \ldots, X_{i-1}, X_{i+1}, \ldots, X_M\}$ and $Z_i \subset \boldsymbol{X}_{-i}$. $P(X_i|Z_i)$ also represents the local structure of node X_i, that is, the relationship of node X_i and its parents Z_i on the graph. Dependency networks are constructed by learning each conditional probability distribution independently, resulting in significant efficiency gains when compared with Bayesian network approaches.

10.2.2
Graph Structure Learning and ℓ_1-Regularization

Efficiently learning the structure of graph models is often very challenging. It has been proved that learning the structure of a Bayesian network is a NP-hard problem [27]. In gene regulatory network modeling, the network structure is of great interest, but learning the network structure is especially difficult in this case because the samples are usually very limited and the random variables, for example, genes and proteins, are numerous.

Recently, ℓ_1-regularization has drawn great interest in the statistics and machine learning community [23, 28–32]. Penalty or constraint on ℓ_1-norm of the regression coefficients has two very useful properties: sparsity and convexity. The ℓ_1-norm constraint tends to make some coefficients exactly zeros, leading to a parsimonious solution, which naturally performs variable selection or sparse linear model estimation. Further, the convex nature of ℓ_1-norm constraint makes the problem computationally tractable, which can be solved readily by many existing convex optimization methods [33].

Lasso is a linear regression minimizing squared error loss with ℓ_1-norm constraint proposed by Tibshirani [23]. The theoretical analysis of Lasso shows that the sparsity pattern of the Lasso estimator is asymptotically identical to the true sparsity pattern under certain conditions [31]. On the algorithmic side, a very efficient algorithm, least angle regression (LARS), can be modified to solve Lasso problems. LARS has a nice geometric interpretation and also gives the whole solution path with the same computational complexity as ordinary least squares, making it computationally appealing.

The idea of ℓ_1-regularization has also been applied to graph structure learning. For instance, ℓ_1-regularization was used to learn the structures of linear Gaussian networks [29], Markov networks [34], and directed acyclic graphs [30].

10.3
Method

10.3.1
Local Dependency Model in DDN

Inspired by the formulation of dependency networks, we propose a local dependency model to describe the dependencies of genes in a transcriptional network. Unlike a conventional dependency network approach, where there is only one conditional probability distribution for each node given its parents, our local dependency model allows more than one conditional probability distributions for each node. Mathematically, suppose there are M genes in the network of interest, and the dependencies of gene i on other genes are formulated by a set of conditional probabilities:

$$\mathbb{P}_i = \{P(X_i|\mathbf{Z}_{i,1}), P(X_i|\mathbf{Z}_{i,2}), \ldots, P(X_i|\mathbf{Z}_{i,s_i})\}, \quad i = 1, 2, \ldots, M, \quad (10.2)$$

where $Z_{i,1}, Z_{i,2}, \ldots, Z_{i,s_i}$ are some subsets of X_{-i} and s_i is the number of conditional probabilities for random variable X_i. We use X_i to refer both to the expression values of gene i and to its corresponding node on the graph. This modification is primarily based on the following considerations. First, our goal is not to construct the entire network that represents the full joint distribution of all variables, rather we wish to model the local structures for further statistical testing. Second, many genes are highly correlated and the data points are very limited when extracting most biological networks. Through our experiments, we found that the conventional approach misses some meaningful dependency connections in data-sparse situations. For example, regulator genes R1 and R2 have the same target gene A, and the expression patterns of R1, R2 and A are highly correlated. When the data points are few, the standard approach may only select one of the dependencies, for instance, gene A on gene R1, even though the dependency of gene A on gene R2 is only slightly less significant than the dependency of gene A on gene R1. However, the dependencies of gene A on genes R1 and R2 are both important, and we want to keep the rich structural information for a later step to assess the topological changes. Therefore, to retain more meaningful local structure information, instead of selecting the best local structure, we select a set of sufficiently good local structures for further statistical testing. We achieve this goal by allowing each node to be modeled by more than one conditional probability distribution.

10.3.2
Local Structure Learning

Now the question is how to learn the local dependency models for DDN. We consider a linear regression model in which the variable X_i is predicted by a linear function of Z_i

$$X_i = \beta^T Z_i + \varepsilon_i \tag{10.3}$$

where

$Z_i \in \{Z_{i,1}, Z_{i,2}, \ldots, Z_{i,s_i}\}$ is a column vector of random variables,
β is a column vector of unknown parameters,
T represents matrix transpose.

The random error ε_i is independent of Z_i and is assumed to have a normal distribution $N(0, \sigma_i^2)$. The local conditional probability is, therefore:

$$P(X_i|Z_i) = N(\beta^T Z_i, \sigma_i^2) \tag{10.4}$$

Learning the structure of the local dependency model requires the selection of a Z_i that shows good predictability of X_i. Given a predefined maximum size of Z_i, K, we examine all C_{M-1}^K combinations of the elements in X_{-i} with size K. K can be empirically set to a positive integer between 1 and $M-1$. When $K = 1$, the proposed local dependency model only considers pairwise relationships. When $K = M-1$, the proposed local dependency model is equivalent to standard dependency networks.

Suppose one K-combination of $\mathbf{X}_{-i}$ is $\{X_{k_1}, X_{k_2}, \ldots, X_{k_K}\}$, where $k_1, \cdots k_K \in \{1, 2, \ldots, i-1, i+1 \ldots, M\}$, and there are N expression samples. Lower case letter $x_i(j)$ denotes the j-th sample value taken by the variable X_i, $j = 1, 2, \ldots, N$. We perform a ℓ_1 constrained regression of X_i on $\mathbf{Z}_i = \{X_{k_1}, X_{k_2}, \ldots, X_{k_K}\}$:

$$\hat{\beta}_{\text{Lasso}} = \arg\min \left\{ \sum_{j=1}^{N} \left(x_i(j) - \sum_{l=1}^{K} \beta_l x_{k_l}(j) \right)^2 \right\}, \text{ s.t. } \sum_{l=1}^{K} |\beta_l| \le t \quad (10.5)$$

The above equation is known as the Lasso estimator, which minimizes ℓ_2 norm loss with constraint on the ℓ_1 norm of $\beta = [\beta_1, \beta_2, \ldots, \beta_K]^T$. The nature of ℓ_1 constraint tends to make some coefficients in $\hat{\beta}_{\text{Lasso}}$ exactly zero, hence it automatically selects a subset of features and leads to a simpler model that avoids overfitting the data, and therefore usually has better generalization performance. The parameter $t \ge 0$ controls the amount of shrinkage that is applied to the estimates. In our software implementation, parameter t is determined by fivefold cross-validation. Solving the Lasso estimation is a convex optimization problem, and can be solved very efficiently. We adopt the LARS method to solve this problem; the detailed procedure of LARS can be found in Reference [28].

We also use a prescreening strategy to reduce the computational burden. We first regress X_i on $\mathbf{Z}_i = \{X_{k_1}, X_{k_2}, \ldots, X_{k_K}\}$, using the ordinary least-square method:

$$\hat{\beta}_{\text{OLS}} = \arg\min \left\{ \sum_{j=1}^{N} \left(x_i(j) - \sum_{l=1}^{K} \beta_l x_{k_l}(j) \right)^2 \right\} \quad (10.6)$$

If the corresponding mean square error (MSE) is above a predetermined threshold T, which means X_i cannot be accurately predicted by the subset $\{X_{k_1}, X_{k_2}, \ldots, X_{k_K}\}$, then subset $\{X_{k_1}, X_{k_2}, \ldots, X_{k_K}\}$ will be discarded. If the MSE is below T, we will then perform the ℓ_1 constrained regression of X_i.

We perform the above prescreening and local structure learning with the Lasso on each of K-combinations of $\mathbf{X}_{-i}$, and obtain predictor sets $\mathbf{Z}_{i,1}$, $\mathbf{Z}_{i,2}, \ldots, \mathbf{Z}_{i,S_i}$ and the conditional probability distributions $\mathbb{P}_i = \{P(X_i|\mathbf{Z}_{i,1}), P(X_i|\mathbf{Z}_{i,2}), \ldots, P(X_i|\mathbf{Z}_{i,S_i})\}$ for node X_i.

To measure how well variables $\mathbf{Z}_i$ can predict X_i, or how well the local dependency model fits gene expression microarray data, we further introduce the definition of the coefficient of determination (COD):

$$\text{COD} = \frac{\text{var}[X_i] - \text{var}[X_i - f_{X_i|\mathbf{Z}_i}(\mathbf{Z}_i)]}{\text{var}[X_i]} \quad (10.7)$$

where $\text{var}[\cdot]$ is the variance of the random variable and $f_{X_i|\mathbf{Z}_i}(\cdot)$ is the best function in a given function class that minimizes the residual variance. COD has been successfully used in nonlinear signal processing and probabilistic Boolean network inference [7, 35]. Here we only use linear functions, and $\text{var}[X_i - f_{X_i|\mathbf{Z}_i}(\mathbf{Z}_i)]$ is an estimate of σ_i^2.

10.3.3
Detection of Statistically Significant Topological Changes

To detect the statistically significant network topological changes between two experimental conditions, we assume there are M genes in the network of interest, and N_1 samples from condition 1 and N_2 samples from condition 2. We further denote the datasets from two conditions by:

$$D^{(m)} = [x^{(m)}(1), x^{(m)}(2), \cdots, x^{(m)}(N_m)]$$

where superscript (m) indicates condition m, $m = 1, 2$. The bold italic face lower case letter $x^{(m)}(j)$ denotes the column vector $[x_1^{(m)}(j), x_2^{(m)}(j), \cdots, x_M^{(m)}(j)]^T$, where lower case letter $x_i^{(m)}(j)$ denotes the j-th sample value taken by variable X_i under condition m, and the superscript T denotes matrix transpose.

By applying the learning procedure to datasets $D^{(1)}$ and $D^{(2)}$, respectively, we obtain:

$$\mathbb{P}_i^{(1)} = \{P(X_i|Z_{i,1}^{(1)}), P(X_i|Z_{i,2}^{(1)}), \cdots, P(X_i|Z_{i,S_i^{(1)}}^{(1)})\}$$

under condition 1 and:

$$\mathbb{P}_i^{(2)} = \{P(X_i|Z_{i,1}^{(2)}), P(X_i|Z_{i,2}^{(2)}), \cdots, P(X_i|Z_{i,S_i^{(2)}}^{(2)})\}$$

under condition 2 for each node i, $i = 1, 2, \ldots, M$. Then we take the union of the local structures learned under two conditions:

$$\mathbb{P}_i = \mathbb{P}_i^{(1)} \cup \mathbb{P}_i^{(2)}, \quad i = 1, 2, \ldots, M \tag{10.8}$$

for further statistical testing.

For each conditional probability distribution in $\mathbb{P}_i$, $i = 1, 2, \ldots, M$, for instance, $P(X_i|Z_i) \in \mathbb{P}_i$, we perform a permutation test to assess how significantly it differs between two conditions. Given samples:

$$\{[x_i^{(1)}(j^{(1)}), z_i^{(1)}(j^{(1)})]^T, j^{(1)} = 1, 2, \ldots, N_1\}$$

under the first condition and:

$$\{[x_i^{(2)}(j^{(2)}), z_i^{(2)}(j^{(2)})]^T, j^{(2)} = 1, 2, \ldots, N_2\}$$

under the second condition, we calculate $\text{COD}^{(1)}$ and $\text{COD}^{(2)}$, using Equation (10.7). A test statistic $\hat{\theta}$ is defined by the absolute difference of the coefficients of determination under two conditions:

$$\hat{\theta} = |\text{COD}^{(1)} - \text{COD}^{(2)}| \tag{10.9}$$

We want to test the null hypothesis, H_0, of no difference between $P^{(1)}(X_i|Z_i)$ and $P^{(2)}(X_i|Z_i)$. We first combine:

$$\{[x_i^{(1)}(j^{(1)}), z_i^{(1)}(j^{(1)})]^T, j^{(1)} = 1, 2, \ldots, N_1\}$$

and:

$$\{[x_i^{(2)}(j^{(2)}), z_i^{(2)}(j^{(2)})]^T, j^{(2)} = 1, 2, \ldots, N_2\}$$

and then randomly permute samples from two conditions and divide the data into two sets of N_1 and N_2 samples, respectively. We perform the above procedure B times, where B is set to 5000 in our software implementation, and calculate $\hat{\theta}_b^*$, $b = 1, 2, \ldots, B$ according to Equation (10.9). An estimate of the achieved significance level (ASL) of the test is:

$$\text{ASL} = \frac{\sum_{b=1}^{B} 1_{\{\hat{\theta}_b^* \geq \hat{\theta}\}}}{B} \tag{10.10}$$

where the random variable $\hat{\theta}_b^*$ is generated by permutation and $1_{\{\hat{\theta}_b^* \geq \hat{\theta}\}}$ denotes the indicator function, which takes 1 when $\hat{\theta}_b^* \geq \hat{\theta}$ and 0 otherwise. The smaller the ASL, the stronger the evidence is against H_0. Equation (10.10) is also an estimate of the p-value. The detailed permutation procedure is described elsewhere [36]. The detection procedure is performed on every local structure in $\mathbb{P}_i$, $i = 1, 2, \ldots, M$, and each local structure is assigned a p-value.

10.3.4
Identification of "Hot Spots" in the Network and Extraction of the DDN

Given a user defined p-value cutoff, we obtain a set of statistically significant differential local structures. The nodes in these differential local structures are identified as "hot spots" in the network, which are the genes undergoing topological changes defined by a specified significance level. These genes may correspond to the genes in disease- or process-related pathways.

DDN is the focused subnetwork that exhibits the topological changes. We consider a connection to exist from each element in Z_i to X_i under one specific condition if the variance of $P(X_i|Z_i)$ is below the user-defined threshold T for that condition. We use different colors to represent connections appearing under different conditions. DDN provides a way to visualize the topological changes, and when applied to disease studies, DDN extracts and focuses on the disease-related pathways that may contribute to the understanding of the mechanism of the disease.

Figure 10.1 summarizes the algorithm of differential dependency network analysis in a flowchart.

10.4
Experiments and Results

10.4.1
A Simulation Experiment

We first use a simulation experiment to illustrate the concept of differential dependency network and analyze the DDN algorithm using the known ground truth.

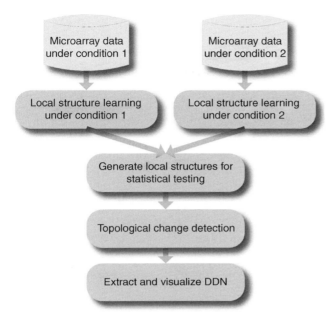

Figure 10.1 Flowchart of differential dependency network analysis.

10.4.1.1 Experiment Data

We used the software SynTReN [37] to generate one simulation dataset of a subnetwork drawn from an existing signaling network in *Saccharomyces cerevisiae*. Then we changed part of network topology and used SynTReN to generate another dataset according to this modified network. Figure 10.2 shows the network topology under two conditions. The network contains 20 nodes that represent 20 genes. The black lines indicate the regulatory relationships that exist under both conditions. The red and green lines are the regulatory relationships that exist only under condition 1 and condition 2, respectively. The subnetwork consisting of nodes MBP1_SWI6, CLB5, CLB6, PHO2, FLO1, FLO10 and TRP4 and green and red lines is the DDN that our algorithm tries to identify from expression data.

10.4.1.2 Application of DDN Analysis

The parameters for our algorithm are threshold T is 0.25, p-value cutoff is 0.01, and the maximum size of Z_i, K, is 2. Figure 10.3 shows the DDN between the two conditions extracted by the proposed algorithm. The DDN shows network topological changes and the genes involved therein. The red lines in Figure 10.3 represent the connections that exist only under condition 1, and the green lines represent the connections that exist only under condition 2. Compared with the known network topology shown in Figure 10.2, the proposed algorithm correctly identified and extracted all the nodes with topology changes and 9 of 10 differential connections, with only the connection between PHO2 and TRP4 under condition 1 falsely missed, and the connection between PHO2 and SWI4 under condition 1 and the connection

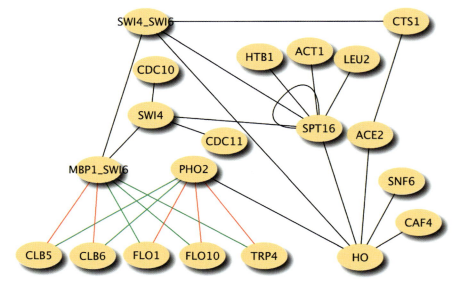

Figure 10.2 Network topology under two conditions in the simulation study. Nodes in the network represent genes. Lines in the network indicate regulatory relationships between genes. Black lines are the regulatory relationships that exist under both conditions. Red and green lines represent the regulatory relationships that exist only under condition 1 and under condition 2, respectively. The differential dependency network between the two conditions is the subnetwork that consists of nodes MBP1_SWI6, CLB5, CLB6, PHO2, FLO1, FLO10, and TRP4 and green and red lines.

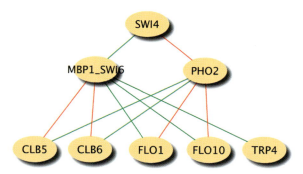

Figure 10.3 Differential dependency network extracted by the proposed algorithm in the simulation study. Red lines represent the connections (dependencies) that only exist under condition 1, and the green lines represent the connections (dependencies) that only exist under condition 2. The proposed differential dependency network analysis successfully detected 9 of 10 connections that are different between two conditions and all the genes involved in the network topology changes. The connections between PHO2 and SWI4 under condition 1 (red) and between MBP_SWI6 and SWI4 under condition 2 (green) were falsely detected and the connection between PHO2 and TRP4 under condition 1 (red) was falsely missed.

between MBP1-SWI6 and SWI4 under condition 2 falsely detected. Moreover, our algorithm picked up all genes involved in topological changes, including some genes that did not show a significant difference in fold-change or t-tests, such as CLB6, FLO1, and MBP1-SWI6. This indicates that our algorithm can successfully detect these interesting genes using their topological information, even though the means of their expressions did not change substantially between the two conditions. Therefore, this method is able to identify biomarkers that cannot be picked up by traditional gene ranking methods, providing a complementary approach for biomarker identification problem.

10.4.1.3 Algorithm Analysis

To investigate the effects of threshold T on the results of the proposed algorithm, we performed DDN analysis on the simulation data given different thresholds. In this simulation experiment, we know the ground truth, which is the underlying network topology and how the network topology changes between two conditions. We can demonstrate the effectiveness of this method by showing the precision–recall curves from the DDN analysis (Figures 10.4 and 10.5) [38]. In Figure 10.4, the precision and recall were calculated to assess the detection of the changes of gene–gene connections. In Figure 10.5, the precision and recall were calculated to assess the detection of the "hot spots", which are genes involved in topological changes; $T = 0.25$ was used in the simulation experiment. Figures 10.4 and 10.5 show that the DDN analysis can successfully retrieve most of the changes in the network between two conditions, while keeping the precision relatively high.

Another parameter in the DDN algorithm is the p-value cutoff. The local structures with p-values smaller than the user-defined p-value cutoff (0.01 in this experiment)

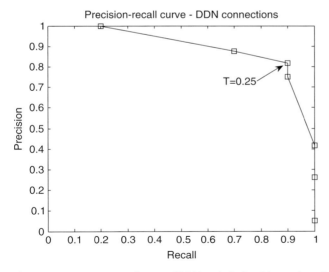

Figure 10.4 Precision–recall curve of DDN analysis. Precision and recall were calculated based on the detected changes in gene–gene connections between two conditions.

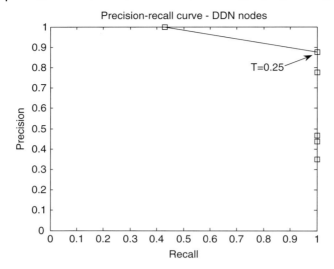

Figure 10.5 Precision–recall curve of DDN analysis. Precision and recall were calculated based on the detected "hot-spots" under two conditions.

are considered to be significant. A natural question is how many of the detected significant local structures are falsely discovered, in other words, are truly null features. To explore this question, we first need to distinguish two related but distinct concepts: false positive rate and false discovery rate (FDR). The false positive rate is the rate that truly null features are called significant, while the false discovery rate is the rate that significant features are truly null [39]. The p-value is a measure of significance in terms of the false positive rate; the q-value is a measure of the FDR. We adopted the q-value estimation algorithm detailed in Reference [39], to estimate the number of false discoveries in the DDN results. At the given p-value cutoff in this experiment, the estimated number of false discoveries is 1.

10.4.2
Breast Cancer Dataset Analysis

10.4.2.1 Experiment Background and Data
We further applied our method to the dataset from an estrogen receptor-positive (ER+) breast cancer cell line study by Lin et al. [40]. In this dataset, the estrogen-dependent T-47D ER+ breast cancer cell line was treated with 17β-estradiol (E2) and with E2 in combination with the pure antiestrogen ICI 182 780 (ICI, Faslodex, Fulvestrant). Samples were then harvested on an hourly basis for the first 8 h (0–8 h) and bi-hourly for the next 16 h (10–24 h) for a total of 16 time points under each condition. Experiments were performed on microarrays generated by spotting the Compugen 19 K human oligo library, made by Sigma-Genosys, on poly-L-lysine-coated glass slides. In this study, we are interested in the cellular response to the drug ICI, which inhibits E2 signaling through the ER [41].

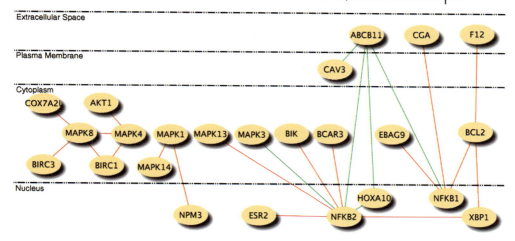

Figure 10.6 Differential dependency network between breast cancer cell line treated with E2 and cell line treated with E2 + ICI. Red lines represent the connections that exist only in breast cancer cell line treated with E2, and green lines represent the connections that exist only in breast cancer cell line treated with E2 + ICI.

10.4.2.2 Application of DDN Analysis

We first selected 55 genes that are reported in the literature (e.g., [42–44]) to be relevant to breast cancer and responsiveness to ICI. We then applied our differential dependency network analysis to the data under two conditions (E2 versus E2 + ICI). The parameters in our algorithm are threshold T is 0.25, p-value cutoff is 0.01, and K is 2.

Figure 10.6 shows the differential dependency network under these two conditions. In the figure, there are 18 red connections in the differential dependency network, which implies that these connections exist only under E2 condition and disappear after the addition of ICI. ICI 182 780 is an estrogen receptor antagonist, which works by both down-regulating and degrading the estrogen receptor alpha (ER-alpha) protein. Thus, it is plausible that these connections disappear because ICI is blocking or inactivating their connections. For example, as a transcription factor, XBP1 can directly regulate gene expression through binding to its responsive element [45], or it can act as a co-regulator of other transcription factors, most notably ER-alpha, to enhance their transcriptional activity [46, 47]. Because BCL2 contains response elements for both ER-alpha and XBP1 [48, 49], the connection between XBP1 and BCL2 in the differential dependency network may either be direct or involve ER-alpha as a latent variable, or intervening gene. In direct support of this predicted edge, it has been shown that constitutive overexpression of XBP1 in a different breast cancer cell line (MCF-7) led to significantly increased mRNA and protein expression of both ER-alpha and BCL2, and functionally conferred both antiestrogen resistance upon sensitive cells and estrogen-independence upon estrogen-dependent cells [48, 49].

Novel relationships between the genes identified by our differential dependency network analysis will also serve as useful guidance for future studies. For example, BCAR3 is a well-established effector of cell motility, estrogen independence, and antiestrogen resistance in ER + breast cancer cell lines [50–53]. Expression of NFKB2 and its activator BCL3 are also associated with estrogen independence in breast cancer cell lines [54]. Nuclear factor κB subunits appear to be selectively activated in clinical breast cancer [55]. However, there is no experimental evidence linking BCAR3 with NFKB2, so the suggestion that these two genes exhibit differential dependence under E2-treated conditions (Figure 10.6) provides a starting point for biological studies of their relationship.

Additional relationships that may be completely new to breast cancer are also identified by this method. For example, MAPK8 (also known as JNK1) has been shown to be activated by BIRC1 (also known as NAIP) during its inhibition of caspase-mediated cell death [56]. In chronic fatigue syndrome, growth factor receptor signaling can activate MAPK4, which via Ras and/or PI3K can subsequently increase AKT1 activity [57]. Finally, in B cells from patients with chronic lymphocytic leukemia NFKB1 (p50) homodimers are able to stimulate transcription from the BCL2 promoter through binding to another member of the BCL family (BCL3) [58].

10.4.3
In Utero Excess E2 Exposed Adult Mammary Glands Analysis

10.4.3.1 Experiment Background and Data

The level of estrogenicity of the *in utero* environment significantly affects the developmental programming of the mammary gland and its susceptibility to tumorigenesis later in life. An elevated *in utero* estrogenic environment may increase later susceptibility to develop breast cancer. The key transcription factors and signaling that mediates the effects of *in utero* estrogenic environment on later estrogen sensitivity and breast cancer risk are unknown. Transcriptome analysis of mRNA from normal adult rat mammary glands exposed to excess E2 *in utero* and vehicle controls may help to shed light on the important genes and pathways. In this gene expression dataset, there are five samples of normal adult rat mammary glands exposed to excess E2 *in utero* and five samples of vehicle controls.

10.4.4
Application of DDN Analysis

We applied our DDN analysis to this dataset. The parameters in our algorithm are threshold T is 0.4, p-value cutoff is 0.05, and K is 1. Figure 10.7 shows the differential dependency network of control group versus excess E2 *in utero* group. Since the exposure was *in utero*, but the differential transcriptome analysis done in adulthood, the altered expression of these genes over time could be, at least in part, a consequence of transcriptional reprogramming regulated by promoter methylation status. Many of these genes are known to be regulated by promoter methylation, for example, ER [59, 60], BCL2 [60, 61], LEP (leptin) [62], and EGR1 [63]. AKT1 can

10.5 Closing Remarks

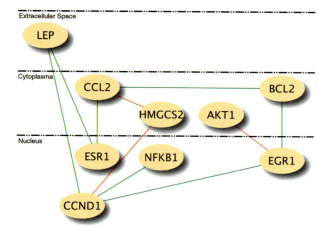

Figure 10.7 Differential dependency network between control group and excess E2 *in utero* group. Red lines represent the connections that exist only in the control group, and green lines represent the connections that exist only in the excess E2 *in utero* group.

regulate methylation patterns in some promoters, which may explain the nature of the AKT1-EGR1 edge present only in the control mammary glands, providing a testable hypothesis [64].

10.5
Closing Remarks

In this chapter we discuss a systematic approach to detect the statistically significant changes in transcriptional networks between two different experimental conditions. We tested our algorithm on simulation data and two real datasets. From the simulation study, we see that the proposed algorithm can efficiently and accurately capture the topological changes. This approach utilizes the network structure information and provides an alternative way for biomarker identification. In addition, as knowledge of cellular networks accumulates, many biological databases will expand to contain more useful information. The proposed approach is an open framework, into which biological knowledge in specific applications can be easily incorporated as the local structure learning constraints.

The high level of correlation among genes is a common feature of microarray data. Therefore, we propose a local dependency model that allows multiple predictor sets for each node. Accordingly, a local structure learning algorithm is also represented. Lasso is used to select features for the predictor sets [23], an approach that has been successfully applied to variable selection and graph structure learning [29]. In the linear Gaussian case, under certain conditions it is proved that the probability of estimating the correct neighborhood converges exponentially to 1. Consequently, it is possible to obtain a consistent estimation of the full edge set [29]. In microarray data, the so-called irrepresentable condition [31] or the neighborhood stability assumption [29] can easily be violated in the presence of highly correlated genes [1]. Some modified algorithms have been proposed to deal with the highly correlated cases, for example, elastic net [32] and network-constrained regularization [19], both of which tend to group highly correlated predictors in the regression process. However, neither of these two approaches is suitable for our problem because the grouping of highly correlated variables can be different under two conditions and this makes the later statistical testing problematic. The local structure learning algorithm proposed here attempts to alleviate the effects of highly correlated data and to preserve local structure information for further statistical testing.

Some issues are worth further exploration. Currently, only linear relationships are considered. How nonlinear relationships should be modeled efficiently and correctly remains a difficult problem. Second, since many cellular reactions take place in the genome, transcriptome, and proteome, it is essential to construct pathways by integrating data from heterogeneous sources.

In summary, DDN analysis presents a new approach to extract knowledge of a biological network by emphasizing the dynamic nature of cellular networks and utilizing a network's structural information. It also provides an alternative and promising approach to identifying possible biomarkers and drug targets.

References

1 Clarke, R., Ressom, H.W., Wang, A.T. et al. (2008) The properties of high-dimensional data spaces: implications for exploring gene and protein expression data. *Nat. Rev. Cancer*, **8** (1), 37–49.

2 Kitano, H. (2002) Systems biology: A brief overview. *Science*, **295** (5560), 1662–1664.

3 Li, H., Xuan, J., Wang, Y. et al. (2008) Inferring regulatory networks. *Front. Biosci.*, **13** (1), 263–275.

4 Friedman, N. (2004) Inferring cellular networks using probabilistic graphical models. *Science*, **303** (5659), 799–805.

5 Friedman, N., Linial, M., Nachman, I. et al. (2000) Using Bayesian networks to analyze expression data. *J. Comput. Biol.*, **7** (3–4), 601–620.

6 Husmeier, D. (2003) Sensitivity and specificity of inferring genetic regulatory interactions from microarray experiments with dynamic Bayesian networks. *Bioinformatics*, **19** (17), 2271–2282.

7 Shmulevich, I., Dougherty, E.R., Kim, S. et al. (2002) Probabilistic Boolean networks: a rule-based uncertainty model for gene regulatory networks. *Bioinformatics*, **18** (2), 261–274.

8 Rangel, C., Angus, J., Ghahramani, Z. et al. (2004) Modeling T-cell activation using gene expression profiling and state-space models. *Bioinformatics*, **20** (9), 1361–1372.

9 Liao, J.C., Boscolo, R., Yang, Y.L. et al. (2003) Network component analysis: reconstruction of regulatory signals in biological systems. *Proc. Natl. Acad. Sci. USA*, **100** (26), 15522–15527.

10 Beyer, A., Bandyopadhyay, S., and Ideker, T. (2007) Integrating physical and genetic maps: from genomes to interaction networks. *Nat. Rev. Genet.*, **8** (9), 699–710.

11 Luscombe, N.M., Babu, M.M., Yu, H.Y. et al. (2004) Genomic analysis of regulatory network dynamics reveals large topological changes. *Nature*, **431** (7006), 308–312.

12 Kim, H., Hu, W., and Kluger, Y. (2006) Unraveling condition specific gene transcriptional regulatory networks

in Saccharomyces cerevisiae. *BMC Bioinformatics*, **7**, 165.

13 Segal, E., Shapira, M., Regev, A. *et al.* (2003) Module networks: identifying regulatory modules and their condition-specific regulators from gene expression data. *Nat. Genet.*, **34** (2), 166–176.

14 Hood, L., Heath, J.R., Phelps, M.E. *et al.* (2004) Systems biology and new technologies enable predictive and preventative medicine. *Science*, **306** (5696), 640–643.

15 Liu, C.C., Chen, W.S.E., Lin, C.C. *et al.* (2006) Topology-based cancer classification and related pathway mining using microarray data. *Nucleic Acids Res.*, **34** (14), 4069–4080.

16 Fuller, T.F., Ghazalpour, A., Aten, J.E. *et al.* (2007) Weighted gene coexpression network analysis strategies applied to mouse weight. *Mamm. Genome*, **18** (6–7), 463–472.

17 Qiu, P., Wang, Z.J., and Liu, K.J. (2005) Ensemble dependence model for classification and prediction of cancer and normal gene expression data. *Bioinformatics*, **21** (14), 3114–3121.

18 Qiu, P., Wang, Z.J., Liu, K.J. *et al.* (2007) Dependence network modeling for biomarker identification. *Bioinformatics*, **23** (2), 198–206.

19 Li, C. and Li, H. (2008) Network-constrained regularization and variable selection for analysis of genomic data. *Bioinformatics*, **24** (9), 1175–1182.

20 Wei, Z. and Li, H. (2007) A Markov random field model for network-based analysis of genomic data. *Bioinformatics*, **23** (12), 1537–1544.

21 Emmert-Streib, F. (2007) The chronic fatigue syndrome: A comparative pathway analysis. *J. Comput. Biol.*, **14** (7), 961–972.

22 Zhang, B., Li, H., Riggins, R.B. *et al.* (2009) Differential dependency network analysis to identify condition-specific topological changes in biological networks. *Bioinformatics*, **25** (4), 526–532.

23 Tibshirani, R. (1996) Regression shrinkage and selection via the Lasso. *J. R. Stat. Soc. B Method.*, **58** (1), 267–288.

24 Bishop, C. (2006) *Pattern Recognition and Machine Learning*, Springer, pp. 359–418.

25 Airoldi, E.M. (2007) Getting started in probabilistic graphical models. *PLoS Comput. Biol.*, **3** (12), e252.

26 Heckerman, D., Chickering, D.M., Meek, C. *et al.* (2000) Dependency networks for inference, collaborative filtering, and data visualization. *J. Machine Learn. Res.*, **1** (1), 49–75.

27 Chickering, D. (1996) Learning Bayesian networks is NP-complete, in *Learning from Data: Artificial Intelligence and Statistics V*, Springer-Verlag, pp. 121–130.

28 Efron, B., Hastie, T., Johnstone, I. *et al.* (2004) Least angle regression. *Ann. Stat.*, **32** (2), 407–451.

29 Meinshausen, N. and Buhlmann, P. (2006) High-dimensional graphs and variable selection with the Lasso. *Ann. Stat.*, **34** (3), 1436–1462.

30 Schmidt, M.W., Niculescu-Mizil, A., and Murphy, K.P. (2007) Learning graphical model structure using L1-regularization paths, in *Proceedings of the Twenty-Second AAAI Conference on Artificial Intelligence*, (ed Anthony Cohn), AAAI Press, pp. 1278–1283.

31 Zhao, P. and Yu, B. (2006) On model selection consistency of Lasso. *J. Machine Learn. Res.*, **7**, 2541–2563.

32 Zou, H. and Hastie, T. (2005) Regularization and variable selection via the elastic net. *J. R. Stat. Soc. B*, **67**, 301–320.

33 Schmidt, M., Fung, G., and Rosales, R. (2007) Fast optimization methods for L1 regularization: a comparative study and two new approaches, in *Machine Learning: ECML 2007: 18th European conference on Machine Learning, Warsaw* (eds J.N. Kok, J. Koronacki, R. Lopez de Mantaras, S. Matwin, D. Mladenic, and A. Skowron), Lecture Notes in Artificial Intelligence, vol. **4701**, pp. 286–297.

34 Lee, S.-I., Ganapathi, V., and Koller, D. (2007) Efficient structure learning of Markov networks using L1 regularization, in *Advances in Neural Information Processing Systems 19* (eds B. Scholkopf,

35 Dougherty, E.R., Kim, S., and Chen, Y.D. (2000) Coefficient of determination in nonlinear signal processing. *Signal Process.*, **80** (10), 2219–2235.

36 Efron, B. and Tibshirani, R. (1993) *An Introduction to the Bootstrap*, Chapman & Hall, New York.

37 Van den Bulcke, T., Van Leemput, K., Naudts, B. et al. (2006) SynTReN: a generator of synthetic gene expression data for design and analysis of structure learning algorithms. *BMC Bioinformatics*, **7**, 43.

38 Hand, D.J., Mannila, H., and Smyth, P. (2001) *Principles of Data Mining*, MIT Press, Cambridge, MA., pp. 452–455.

39 Storey, J.D. and Tibshirani, R. (2003) Statistical significance for genomewide studies. *Proc. Natl. Acad. Sci. USA*, **100** (16), 9440–9445.

40 Lin, C.Y., Strom, A., Vega, V.B. et al. (2004) Discovery of estrogen receptor alpha target genes and response elements in breast tumor cells. *Genome Biol.*, **5** (9), R66.

41 Howell, A. (2006) Pure oestrogen antagonists for the treatment of advanced breast cancer. *Endocr. Relat. Cancer*, **13** (3), 689–706.

42 Kuo, M.T. (2007) Roles of multidrug resistance genes in breast cancer chemoresistance, *Breast Cancer Chemosensitivity, Advances in Experimental Medicine and Biology*, Springer-Verlag, Berlin, pp. 23–30.

43 Riggins, R.B., Bouton, A.H., Liu, M.C. et al. (2005) Antiestrogens, aromatase inhibitors, and apoptosis in breast cancer, in *Vitamins and Hormones - Advances in Research and Applications, Vitamins and Hormones-Advances in Research and Applications*, vol. **71**, Elsevier Academic Press Inc., San Diego, pp. 201–237.

44 Riggins, R.B., Schrecengost, R.S., Guerrero, M.S. et al. (2007) Pathways to tamoxifen resistance. *Cancer Lett.*, **256** (1), 1–24.

45 Iwakoshi, N.N., Lee, A.H., and Glimcher, L.H. (2003) The X-box binding protein-1 transcription factor is required for plasma cell differentiation and the unfolded protein response. *Immunol. Rev.*, **194** (1), 29–38.

46 Ding, L.H., Yan, J.H., Zhu, J.H. et al. (2003) Ligand-independent activation of estrogen receptor alpha by XBP-1. *Nucleic Acids Res.*, **31** (18), 5266–5274.

47 Fang, Y., Yan, J.H., Ding, L.H. et al. (2004) XBP-1 increases ER alpha transcriptional activity through regulation of large-scale chromatin unfolding. *Biochem. Biophys. Res. Commun.*, **323** (1), 269–274.

48 Gomez, B.P., Riggins, R.B., Shajahan, A.N. et al. (2007) Human X-Box binding protein-1 confers both estrogen independence and antiestrogen resistance in breast cancer cell lines. *FASEB J.*, **21** (14), 4013–4027.

49 Somai, S., Chaouat, M., Jacob, D. et al. (2003) Antiestrogens are pro-apoptotic in normal human breast epithelial cells. *Int. J. Cancer*, **105** (5), 607–612.

50 Felekkis, K.N., Narsimhan, R.P., Near, R. et al. (2005) AND-34 activates phosphatidylinositol 3-kinase and induces anti-estrogen resistance in a SH2 and GDP exchange factor-like domain-dependent manner. *Mol. Cancer Res.*, **3** (1), 32–41.

51 Riggins, R.B., Quilliam, L.A., and Bouton, A.H. (2003) Synergistic promotion of c-Src activation and cell migration by Cas and AND-34/BCAR3. *J. Biol. Chem.*, **278** (30), 28264–28273.

52 Schrecengost, R.S., Riggins, R.B., Thomas, K.S. et al. (2007) Breast cancer antiestrogen resistance-3 expression regulates breast cancer cell migration through promotion of p130(Cas) membrane localization and membrane ruffling. *Cancer Res.*, **67** (13), 6174–6182.

53 Van Agthoven, T., Veldscholte, J., Smid, M. et al. (2006) Functional identification of genes causing estrogen independence. *Breast Cancer Res. Treat.*, **100**, S37–S137

54 Pratt, M.A.C., Bishop, T.E., White, D. et al. (2003) Estrogen withdrawal-induced NF-kappa B activity and Bcl-3 expression in breast cancer cells: Roles in growth and hormone independence. *Mol. Cell Biol.*, **23** (19), 6887–6900.

55 Zhou, Y., Eppenberger-Castori, S., Marx, C. et al. (2005) Activation of nuclear factor-kB (NFkB) identifies a high-risk subset of

hormone-dependent breast cancers. *Int. J. Biochem. Cell Biol.*, **37** (5), 1130–1144.

56 Sanna, M.G., Correia, J.D., Ducrey, O. et al. (2002) IAP suppression of apoptosis involves distinct mechanisms: The TAK1/JNK1 signaling cascade and caspase inhibition. *Mol. Cell Biol.*, **22** (6), 1754–1766.

57 Englebienne, P. and Meirleir, K. (2002) *Chronic Fatigue Syndrome: A Biological Approach*, CRC Press.

58 Viatour, P., Bentires-Alj, M., Chariot, A. et al. (2003) NF-kappa B2/p100 induces Bcl-2 expression. *Leukemia*, **17** (7), 1349–1356.

59 Ferguson, A.T., Lapidus, R.G., Baylin, S.B. et al. (1995) Demethylation of the estrogen receptor gene in estrogen receptor-negative breast cancer cells can reactivate estrogen receptor gene expression. *Cancer Res.*, **55** (11), 2279–2283.

60 Widschwendter, M., Siegmund, K.D., Muller, H.M. et al. (2004) Association of breast cancer DNA methylation profiles with hormone receptor status and response to tamoxifen. *Cancer Res.*, **64** (11), 3807–3813.

61 Friedrich, M.G., Weisenberger, D.J., Cheng, J.C. et al. (2004) Detection of methylated apoptosis-associated genes in urine sediments of bladder cancer patients. *Clin. Cancer Res.*, **10** (22), 7457–7465.

62 Noer, A., Boquest, A., and Collas, P. (2007) Dynamics of adipogenic promoter DNA methylation during clonal culture of human adipose stem cells to senescence. *BMC Cell Biol.*, **8** (1), 18.

63 Seyfert, V., McMahon, S., Glenn, W. et al. (1990) Methylation of an immediate-early inducible gene as a mechanism for B cell tolerance induction. *Science*, **250** (4982), 797–800.

64 Cha, T.-L., Zhou, B.P., Xia, W. et al. (2005) Akt-mediated phosphorylation of EZH2 suppresses methylation of lysine 27 in histone H3. *Science*, **310** (5746), 306–310.

11
An Introduction to Time-Varying Connectivity Estimation for Gene Regulatory Networks

André Fujita, João Ricardo Sato, Marcos Angelo Almeida Demasi, Satoru Miyano, Mari Cleide Sogayar, and Carlos Eduardo Ferreira

11.1
Regulatory Networks and Cancer

Cellular behavior and phenotype, resulting from many biological processes, are dependent on complex interactions among numerous cell constituents. DNA, RNA, proteins, and small molecules act in concert in the cell through many interdependent interactions, generating large and complex cellular networks. Elucidating the structure and dynamics of these networks in different cellular contexts has become the main goal of systems biology [1–4]. In this chapter we illustrate the process of inferring the structure of gene regulatory networks from high-throughput gene expression data as well as to gain insights into their properties and dynamics in a specific pathological state, namely, cancer.

The hallmark of cancer cells is their uncontrolled cellular proliferation. During tumor development, cancer cells acquire additional capabilities, such as sustained blood supply, invasion of others tissues, and colonization of other parts of the body, with the latter being known as metastasis [5]. Cancer can be considered as a genetic disease since several genetic alterations (e.g., point mutations, chromosomal translocations, gene and chromosomal amplification or deletions) accumulate during tumor development and progression. These genetic alterations are related to functional disruption of classes of genes associated with regulatory circuits that control normal cell proliferation and homeostasis [5]. During the past two decades several cancer-associated genes have been identified [6]. Since these genes and the activity of their products ultimately underlie cancer susceptibility, onset, and progression, it is essential to understand how mutations in cancer genes affect their function in the context of complex cellular networks.

Data mining of high-throughput gene expression experiments has made it possible to study cellular biological states in unprecedented detail, by modeling gene regulatory networks. Gene regulatory networks describe the regulatory relationship of a class of genes, that is, those coding for transcription factors and regulatory RNAs, in controlling the expression of other genes.

Medical Biostatistics for Complex Diseases. Edited by Frank Emmert-Streib and Matthias Dehmer
Copyright © 2010 WILEY-VCH Verlag GmbH & Co. KGaA, Weinheim
ISBN: 978-3-527-32585-6

However, understanding the complex control of regulatory networks requires integrated theoretical descriptions of the dynamics of relationships and degree of interconnectivity among numerous cellular constituents.

Several studies using high-throughput biological data combined with mathematical concepts have shed light into the general cellular network structure and/or topology [7]. Determination of these topological properties and dynamics of cellular networks should provide important insights into cell cycle control and the onset of cancer.

The cell cycle consists of a sequential routine, which is required for cell division. This routine can be roughly divided into four phases, namely: G1, S, G2, and M [8]. DNA synthesis occurs during the S phase and the events of nuclear division and cytokinesis, yielding two identical daughter cells, takes place during the M phase. Upon completion of the M phase occurs the first gap in the cell cycle, also known as G1, which precedes the S phase. A second gap, known as G2, exists between the S and M phase [8]. It is during these gaps that eventual replication errors or DNA damage may be repaired. Additionally, it is during the G1 phase that multiple signals jointly act to influence the cell division process, especially in multicellular organisms. Thus, depending on the extra- and intracellular inputs, the cellular response may be (i) to proceed through the cell cycle and divide, (ii) to interrupt the cell cycle and enter a cell differentiation program, or (iii) to die . Disruption of the proper control of the cell cycle, by maintaining the cell in a continuous proliferative state, and avoiding terminal differentiation and cell death, are some of the basic mechanisms of tumorigenesis [5–9].

An ongoing challenge for biologists is to continue deciphering the intricate cell cycle process and improve the ability to predict the biological behavior associated with both physiological and pathological/cancerous states. A crucial point in this effort is to develop statistical and mathematical tools to extract reasonable molecular network structures and properties from the overwhelming amount of high-throughput biological data already available. One such approach is to reconstruct gene regulatory networks by using specific statistical tools from DNA microarrays gene expression data [10]. This approach is based on the assumption that, with sufficient gene expression data, it is possible to retrieve relevant gene networks by developing specific algorithms, although laboratory experiments are necessary to further validate the results obtained *in silico*.

In the last few years, several methods based on Vector Autoregressive (VAR) models have been developed to construct regulatory networks. The simplest one is the standard VAR model that identifies linear relationships between gene expression signals [11]. Since it is known that the relationship between gene expression signals may be nonlinear [12], a generalization of the standard VAR that can identify nonlinear associations was developed, namely, the nonlinear vector autoregressive (NVAR) model [13, 14]. Another problem in bioinformatics is the high dimensional characteristic of gene expression data, where the number of genes is higher than the number of microarrays. To overcome this limitation, the sparse vector autoregressive (SVAR) model was proposed [15–18]. However, none of these methods can identify time-varying connectivities. To identify networks whose structure dynamically change along the cell cycle the dynamic vector autoregressive (DVAR) model was proposed [19].

The next sections introduce the statistical background and present the DVAR model. DVAR is also illustrated by capturing the structural dynamics of two important cancer-associated gene regulatory networks that operate during the cell cycle.

11.2
Statistical Approaches

11.2.1
Causality and Granger Causality

Causality is a topic that has been generating numerous discussions over hundreds of years in several different fields of science, such as sociology [20], psychology [21], physics [22], and so on. Intuitively, causality may be understood as a relationship between a *cause* and an *effect*, where the occurrence of the effect depends on that of the cause. Moreover, the effect never occurs before its cause, and both cause and effect must be at least connected by a chain of intermediate events.

When experiments to detect causality are unfeasible, inference is generally carried out by using quantitative observational data and conditional probabilities. Pearl has developed the D-separation algorithm [23] to compute all the conditional independent relations, while Spirtes et al. [24] connected the work of Pearl to the problem of testing and discovering causal structures in behavioral sciences. Implementation of the algorithm of Spirtes et al. may be accessed by the TETRAD software [25] which is publicly available. The basic idea of Pearl consists of the distinction between three possible types of causal structures. Suppose three events X, Y, and Z and the following causal structures where the direction of causality is represented by arrows: (i) $X \rightarrow Y \rightarrow Z$; (ii) $X \leftarrow Y \rightarrow Z$ and (iii) $X \rightarrow Y \leftarrow Z$. Conditions (i) and (ii) are indistinguishable since X and Z are independent given Y. On the other hand, condition (iii) can be uniquely identified since X and Z are marginally independent and all other pairs are dependent. This structure (iii) is called, the v-structure. Unfortunately, the lack of this method is that it requires acyclic graphs and at least three nodes are necessary to infer causality since it is based on conditional independence and v-structure [23].

Another concept of causality that comes earlier than Pearl's work is Granger causality [26].

Clive W.J. Granger [26–28] has defined a concept of causality based solely on quantitative predictions of time series data. Owing to its simplicity and the intuitive idea that an effect never occurs before its cause, it has been widely used in several areas such as econometrics [29–31], neuroscience [32–34], and, more recently, in bioinformatics [11, 13, 15, 19]. The idea is that, if a variable x affects a variable y, past values of the former could be useful in generating predictions for the latter.

Intuitively, Granger causality may be illustrated as described in Figure 11.1. Consider two time series x_t and y_t for which the latter can be predicted by using

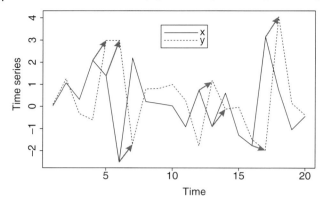

Figure 11.1 Illustration of a case where time series x_t Granger-causes time series y_t. The arrows indicate that past values of x_t contain information to predict future values of y_t.

x_{t-1}. In other words, past values of x_t contain information that may be useful to predict future values of y_t, that is, x_t Granger-causes y_t.

To formalize this concept, suppose that $\Im_t$ is a set containing all relevant information available up to and including time-point t. Let $y_t(h|\Im_t)$ be the optimal [i.e., the minimum mean squared error (MSE)] h-step predictor of the process y_t from the time point t, based on the information in $\Im_t$. The corresponding forecast MSE will be denoted by $\Omega_y(h|\Im_t)$. The process x_t is said to Granger-cause y_t if:

$$\Omega_y(h|\Im_t) < \Omega_y(h|\Im_t \setminus \{x_s|s \leq t\}) \quad \text{for at least one } h = 1, 2, \ldots \tag{11.1}$$

where $\Im_t \setminus \{x_s|s \leq t\}$ is the set containing all relevant information except by the information in the past and present of x_t. In other words, if y_t can be predicted more efficiently when the information in x_t is taken into account, then x_t is said to be Granger-causal for y_t.

Applying the idea of Granger causality in regulatory networks, a gene expression time series x_t Granger-causes another gene expression time series y_t, if x_t provides statistically more significant information about future values of y_t than considering only the past values of y_t. Thus, past gene expression values of x_t allow the prediction of more accurate gene expression values of y_t. Notice that, since this relationship is not reciprocal, Granger causality may be interpreted as information flow [35]. Moreover, it is important to highlight that Granger causality is not actually inferring effective causality, that is, interaction of gene products (or protein–protein interactions), since the former is based solely on prediction and quantitative criteria as described before; however, this concept may be useful in suggesting some insights into molecular interactions (effective causality) that may then be experimentally confirmed.

Vector autoregressive (VAR) models are often used to identify Granger causality due to their simplicity. In the following sections we describe the standard VAR model and also its extended version used to infer time-varying influence and structural changes in regulatory networks along the cell cycle, namely, the dynamic vector autoregressive (DVAR) model.

11.2.2
Vector Autoregressive Model – VAR

In most practical applications, Granger causality is usually identified by estimating vector autoregressive (VAR) models and by statistically testing their parameters.

The equations system of a k-dimensional VAR model of order p is as follows:

$$\begin{cases} y_{1,t} = v_1 + a_{11}^{(1)} y_{1,(t-1)} + \ldots + a_{11}^{(p)} y_{1,(t-p)} + \ldots + a_{k1}^{(1)} y_{k,(t-1)} + \ldots + a_{k1}^{(p)} y_{k,(t-p)} + \varepsilon_{1,(t)} \\ y_{2,t} = v_2 + a_{12}^{(1)} y_{1,(t-1)} + \ldots + a_{12}^{(p)} y_{1,(t-p)} + \ldots + a_{k2}^{(1)} y_{k,(t-1)} + \ldots + a_{k2}^{(p)} y_{k,(t-p)} + \varepsilon_{2,(t)} \\ \vdots \\ y_{k,t} = v_k + a_{1k}^{(1)} y_{1,(t-1)} + \ldots + a_{1k}^{(p)} y_{1,(t-p)} + \ldots + a_{kk}^{(1)} y_{k,(t-1)} + \ldots + a_{kk}^{(p)} y_{k,(t-p)} + \varepsilon_{k,(t)} \end{cases}$$

where

y contains the gene expression values,
k is the number of genes,
T is the time series length,
ε_t is a vector of random variables with zero mean and covariance matrix Σ.

Notice that each gene y_i ($i = 1, \ldots, k$) is represented by a linear combination of the past values of itself and by the past values of other genes.

Owing to simplicity and easier computational implementation, the above system of equations is usually represented in a matricial form, given by:

$$Y_t = v + A_1 Y_{t-1} + A_2 Y_{t-2} + \cdots + A_p Y_{t-p} + \varepsilon_t \quad t = 1, \ldots, T \tag{11.2}$$

where

$$Y_t = \begin{pmatrix} y_{1t} \\ \vdots \\ y_{kt} \end{pmatrix} \tag{11.3}$$

and:

$$\Sigma = \begin{pmatrix} \sigma_{11}^2 & \sigma_{21} & \ldots & \sigma_{k1} \\ \sigma_{12} & \sigma_{22}^2 & \ldots & \sigma_{k2} \\ \sigma_{13} & \sigma_{23} & \ldots & \sigma_{k3} \\ \vdots & \vdots & \ddots & \vdots \\ \sigma_{1k} & \sigma_{2k} & \ldots & \sigma_{kk}^2 \end{pmatrix} \tag{11.4}$$

is a $k \times k$ matrix, v and $A_l (l = 1, 2, \ldots, p)$ are an intercept vector and coefficient matrices, respectively, given by:

$$v = \begin{pmatrix} v_1 \\ v_2 \\ \vdots \\ v_k \end{pmatrix} \tag{11.5}$$

$$A_l = \begin{pmatrix} a_{11}^{(l)} & a_{21}^{(l)} & \cdots & a_{k1}^{(l)} \\ a_{12}^{(l)} & a_{22}^{(l)} & \cdots & a_{k2}^{(l)} \\ a_{13}^{(l)} & a_{23}^{(l)} & \cdots & a_{k3}^{(l)} \\ \vdots & \vdots & \ddots & \vdots \\ a_{1k}^{(l)} & a_{2l}^{(l)} & \cdots & a_{kk}^{(l)} \end{pmatrix}, \quad l = 1, \ldots, p \tag{11.6}$$

Note that the disturbances ε_t are serially uncorrelated, but may be contemporaneously correlated, that is, Σ may not necessarily be an identity matrix.

It is important to highlight that, in this multivariate model, each gene expression value may depend not only on its own past values but also on the past expression values of other genes.

Owing to its simplicity, the VAR model allows a simple way of identifying linear Granger causality in weakly stationary processes (see Definition 11.1). A necessary and sufficient condition for gene y_j being not Granger-causal for gene y_i is if and only if $a_{ij}^{(l)} = 0$ for all $l = 1, \ldots, p$. Thus, Granger-non-causality may be identified by analyzing the autoregressive matrices A_l of VAR models. The direction of Granger causality suggests the activation/repression of a gene product of another gene (if the coefficient a_{ij} is greater than zero, then gene y_j may be inducing the expression of gene y_i; if a_{ij} is negative, then gene y_j may be repressing the expression of gene y_i).

11.2.2.1 Estimation Procedure

The estimation procedure can be described in a matrix form as follows:

$$Y_t = \begin{pmatrix} y_{1,(p+1)} & y_{2,(p+1)} & \cdots & y_{k,(p+1)} \\ y_{1,(p+2)} & y_{2,(p+2)} & \cdots & y_{k,(p+2)} \\ \vdots & \vdots & \ddots & \vdots \\ y_{1,(T)} & y_{2,(T)} & \cdots & y_{k,(T)} \end{pmatrix} \tag{11.7}$$

$$Y_{t-l} = \begin{pmatrix} y_{1,(p-l+1)} & y_{2,(p-l+1)} & \cdots & y_{k,(p-l+1)} \\ y_{1,(p-l+2)} & y_{2,(p-l+2)} & \cdots & y_{k,(p-l+2)} \\ \vdots & \vdots & \ddots & \vdots \\ y_{1,(T-l)} & y_{2,(T-l)} & \cdots & y_{k,(T-l)} \end{pmatrix}, \quad l = 1, 2, \ldots, p, \tag{11.8}$$

$$B = \begin{pmatrix} v & A_1 & \cdots & A_p \end{pmatrix}. \tag{11.9}$$

Therefore, the model may be rewritten as:

$$Z = M\beta + E \quad E_i \sim N(0, \Sigma) \quad i = 1, \ldots, k \tag{11.10}$$

where:

$$Z = \text{vec}(Y_t) \tag{11.11}$$

$$\boldsymbol{\beta} = \text{vec}(\boldsymbol{B}) \tag{11.12}$$

$$\boldsymbol{M} = (\boldsymbol{Y}_{t-1}, \ldots, \boldsymbol{Y}_{t-p}) \tag{11.13}$$

and $\boldsymbol{E}_i$ follows a multivariate Gaussian distribution $N(0, \boldsymbol{\Sigma})$, with zero mean $\boldsymbol{0}_{(k \times 1)}$ and covariance matrix $\boldsymbol{\Sigma}$. For details about the vec operator, see Definition 11.3.

This model can be fitted by ordinary least-squares (OLS), whose estimator is given by:

$$\hat{\boldsymbol{\beta}} = (\boldsymbol{I}_k \otimes (\boldsymbol{M}'\boldsymbol{M})^{-1}\boldsymbol{M}')\boldsymbol{Z} \tag{11.14}$$

where $\boldsymbol{I}_k$ is the identity matrix of size k and $\otimes$ is the Kronecker product (see Definition 11.4).

Let Γ be the limit in probability of $\boldsymbol{M}'\boldsymbol{M}/T$ when $T \to \infty$. Therefore:

$$\sqrt{T}(\hat{\boldsymbol{\beta}} - \boldsymbol{\beta}) \xrightarrow{D} N(0, \boldsymbol{\Sigma} \otimes \Gamma^{-1}) \tag{11.15}$$

when $T \to \infty$. $\xrightarrow{D}$ denotes convergence in distribution [36].

11.2.2.2 Hypothesis Testing

Lemma 11.1 (Lütkepohl [36])

Let $\boldsymbol{y}_t$ be a VAR(p) process that satisfies the condition of stability (see Definition 11.2), and $a_{ij}^{(l)}$ be the element of the i-th row and j-th column of the autoregressive coefficients matrix of order l, A_l. The time series $\boldsymbol{y}_{jt}$ Granger causes the time series $\boldsymbol{y}_{it}$ if and only if $a_{ij}^{(l)} \neq 0$, for some l.

Thus, to verify whether there is Granger causality from gene y_{jt} to gene y_{it}, we may test whether the estimated autoregressive coefficients are statistically equal to zero or not. Therefore, suppose we are interested in testing whether $\boldsymbol{\beta} = \boldsymbol{0}_{k(k+1)}$. In other words, we may perform the following test:

$$H_0 : \boldsymbol{C}\boldsymbol{\beta} = \boldsymbol{0} \quad \text{against} \quad H_1 : \boldsymbol{C}\boldsymbol{\beta} \neq \boldsymbol{0} \tag{11.16}$$

where $\boldsymbol{C} = \boldsymbol{I}_{k(k+1)}$ is a matrix of contrasts, that is, the linear combination of the parameters and $\boldsymbol{0}$ is a $(k \times (k+1))$ matrix of zeros. The Wald test is given by:

$$W = (\boldsymbol{C}\hat{\boldsymbol{\beta}})' \left[\boldsymbol{C}\left[(\boldsymbol{M}'\boldsymbol{M})^{-1} \otimes \hat{\boldsymbol{\Sigma}}\right]\boldsymbol{C}'\right]^{-1}(\boldsymbol{C}\hat{\boldsymbol{\beta}}) \tag{11.17}$$

where W follows, under the null hypothesis, a chi-squared distribution with rank($\boldsymbol{C}$) degrees of freedom (see Definition 11.6) [37].

11.2.3
Dynamic Vector Autoregressive Model – DVAR

In this section we present the dynamic vector autoregressive (DVAR) model [19], a generalization of the VAR model, in which the parameters are a function of time, to model time-varying influences along the cell cycle.

The equations system DVAR(p) model is defined by:

$$\begin{cases} y_{1,t} = v_1(t) + a_{11}^{(1)}(t)y_{1,(t-1)} + \cdots + a_{11}^{(p)}(t)y_{1,(t-p)} + \cdots + a_{k1}^{(1)}(t)y_{k,(t-1)} + \cdots + a_{k1}^{(p)}(t)y_{k,(t-p)} + \varepsilon_{1,(t)} \\ \\ y_{2,t} = v_2(t) + a_{12}^{(1)}(t)y_{1,(t-1)} + \cdots + a_{12}^{(p)}(t)y_{1,(t-p)} + \cdots + a_{k2}^{(1)}(t)y_{k,(t-1)} + \cdots + a_{k2}^{(p)}(t)y_{k,(t-p)} + \varepsilon_{2,(t)} \\ \vdots \\ y_{k,t} = v_k(t) + a_{1k}^{(1)}(t)y_{1,(t-1)} + \cdots + a_{1k}^{(p)}(t)y_{1,(t-p)} + \cdots + a_{kk}^{(1)}(t)y_{k,(t-1)} + \cdots + a_{kk}^{(p)}(t)y_{k,(t-p)} + \varepsilon_{k,(t)} \end{cases}$$

where

Y_t contains the gene expressions,
k is the number of genes,
T is the time series length,
ε_t is a vector of random variables with zero mean and covariance matrix $\Sigma(t)$.

The matricial form of this system is given by:

$$Y_t = v(t) + A_1(t)y_{t-1} + A_2(t)y_{t-2} + \ldots + A_p(t)y_{t-p} + \varepsilon_t \quad t = 1, \ldots, T \quad (11.18)$$

where:

$$Y_t = \begin{pmatrix} y_{1t} \\ \vdots \\ y_{kt} \end{pmatrix} \quad (11.19)$$

$$\Sigma(t) = \begin{pmatrix} \sigma_{11}^2(t) & \sigma_{21}(t) & \cdots & \sigma_{k1}(t) \\ \sigma_{12}(t) & \sigma_{22}^2(t) & \cdots & \sigma_{k2}(t) \\ \sigma_{13}(t) & \sigma_{23}(t) & \cdots & \sigma_{k3}(t) \\ \vdots & \vdots & \ddots & \vdots \\ \sigma_{1k}(t) & \sigma_{2k}(t) & \cdots & \sigma_{kk}^2(t) \end{pmatrix} \quad (11.20)$$

$v(t)$ and $A_l(t)(l = 1, 2, \ldots, p)$ are an intercept vector and coefficient matrices, respectively, given by:

$$v(t) = \begin{pmatrix} v_1(t) \\ v_2(t) \\ \vdots \\ v_k(t) \end{pmatrix} \quad (11.21)$$

11.2 Statistical Approaches

$$A_l(t) = \begin{pmatrix} a_{11}^{(l)}(t) & a_{21}^{(l)}(t) & \cdots & a_{k1}^{(l)}(t) \\ a_{12}^{(l)}(t) & a_{22}^{(l)}(t) & \cdots & a_{k2}^{(l)}(t) \\ a_{13}^{(l)}(t) & a_{23}^{(l)}(t) & \cdots & a_{k3}^{(l)}(t) \\ \vdots & \vdots & \ddots & \vdots \\ a_{1k}^{(l)}(t) & a_{2k}^{(l)}(t) & \cdots & a_{kk}^{(l)}(t) \end{pmatrix}, \quad l = 1, \ldots, p \qquad (11.22)$$

Given this dynamic structure for the intercept (related to the time-varying mean gene expression level), autoregressive coefficients, and covariance matrices, it is possible to infer the regulatory network in a time-varying fashion, that is, to analyze the connectivity changes along the cell cycle.

Estimates of the time-variant functions $v(t)$, $A_l(t)$, and $\Sigma(t)$ may be obtained by wavelet expansions.

First, consider an orthonormal basis generated by a mother wavelet function $\psi(t)$ as:

$$\psi_{m,n}(t) = 2^{m/2}\psi(2^m t - n), \quad m, n \in Z \qquad (11.23)$$

and assume the following properties:

1) $\int_{-\infty}^{\infty} \psi(t)\, dt = 0$
2) $\int_{-\infty}^{\infty} |\psi(t)|\, dt < \infty$
3) $\int_{-\infty}^{\infty} \frac{|\psi(\omega)|^2\, d\omega}{|\omega|} < \infty$, where the function $\psi(\omega)$ is the Fourier transform of $\psi(t)$
4) $\int_{-\infty}^{\infty} t^m \psi(t)\, dt = 0$, $m = 0, 1, \ldots, r-1$ for $r \geq 1$ and $\int_{-\infty}^{\infty} t^m \psi(t)\, dt = 0$.

The main idea is that any function $f(t)$ with $\sum_{-\infty}^{\infty} f^2(t)\, dt < \infty$ may be expanded as:

$$f(t) = \sum_{m=-\infty}^{\infty} \sum_{n=-\infty}^{\infty} c_{m,n} \psi_{m,n}(t) \qquad (11.24)$$

Hence, a function $f(t)$ can be represented by a linear combination of wavelet functions $\psi_{m,n}(t)$, where the indexes m and n are related to scale and time-location, respectively. In other words, considering the wavelet expansion, an approximation to the autoregressive coefficient functions $a_{ji}^{(l)}(t)$ may be reformulated as:

$$a_{ji}^{(l)}(t) = \sum_{m=-1}^{D} \sum_{n=0}^{2^D-1} c_{m,n}^{(l)} \psi_{m,n}(t) \qquad (11.25)$$

where

T is the time series extension,
$c_{m,n}^{(l)}$ ($m = -1, 0, 1, \ldots, T-1$; $n = 0, 1, \ldots, 2^D-1$; $l = 1, 2, \ldots, p$) are the wavelet coefficients for the l-th autoregressive coefficient function $a_{ji}^{(l)}(t)$.

Since $\psi(t)$ is known, estimation of the wavelet dynamic autoregressive parameters consists of obtaining each of the wavelet coefficients $c_{m,n}^{(l)}$ for all the autoregressive functions in the matrices $A_l(t)$ ($l = 1, 2, \ldots, p$), the intercept functions in $v(t)$, and the covariance functions in $\Sigma(t)$.

An important point is the determination of the maximum resolution scale parameter D, which refers to the truncation of wavelet expansion. The larger the number of expansions D, the larger will be the variance of the estimated curve. An inherent problem in non-parametric curves estimation is that bias reduction implies in variance increase and vice versa. An objective criterion to select the optimum number D may be obtained by cross-validation. On the other hand, one may choose the maximum scale parameter according to the expected degree of smoothness based on expected changes, according to biological knowledge or desired level of detail.

11.2.3.1 Estimation Procedure

To estimate v, A, and Σ, consider the following matrices:

$$Y_t = \begin{pmatrix} y_{1,(p+1)} & y_{2,(p+1)} & \cdots & y_{k,(p+1)} \\ y_{1,(p+2)} & y_{2,(p+2)} & \cdots & y_{k,(p+2)} \\ \vdots & \vdots & \ddots & \vdots \\ y_{1,(T)} & y_{2,(T)} & \cdots & y_{k,(T)} \end{pmatrix} \tag{11.26}$$

$$Y_{t-l} = \begin{pmatrix} y_{1,(p-l+1)} & y_{2,(p-l+1)} & \cdots & y_{k,(p-l+1)} \\ y_{1,(p-l+2)} & y_{2,(p-l+2)} & \cdots & y_{k,(p-l+2)} \\ \vdots & \vdots & \ddots & \vdots \\ y_{1,(T-l)} & y_{2,(T-l)} & \cdots & y_{k,(T-l)} \end{pmatrix} \tag{11.27}$$

$$\Psi = \begin{pmatrix} \psi_{-1,0}(p+1) & \psi_{0,0}(p+1) & \cdots & \psi_{D,2^D-1}(p+1) \\ \psi_{-1,0}(p+2) & \psi_{0,0}(p+2) & \cdots & \psi_{D,2^D-1}(p+2) \\ \vdots & \vdots & \ddots & \vdots \\ \psi_{-1,0}(T) & \psi_{0,0}(T) & \cdots & \psi_{D,2^D-1}(T) \end{pmatrix} \tag{11.28}$$

and also:

$$Q = [1_{T-p} \otimes^R \Psi \, Y_{t-1} \otimes^R \Psi \ldots Y_{t-l} \otimes^R \Psi] \tag{11.29}$$

$$M = I_K \otimes Q \tag{11.30}$$

where

1_{T-p} is a column vector of $(T-p)$ ones,
I_k is the identity matrix of order k rows
$\otimes^R$ is the row-Kronecker product (see Definition 11.5).

Consider $Z = \text{vec}(Y_t)$, thus, the DVAR model can be written as:

$$Z = M\beta + E \tag{11.31}$$

11.2 Statistical Approaches

A vector of parameters $\boldsymbol{\beta}$ contains the wavelet coefficients $c_{m,n}^{(l)}$ for all intercept and connectivity functions (autoregressive functions). Let Θ to be the covariance matrix of $\boldsymbol{E}$.

Thus, the generalized least-squares (GLS) estimator for the parameters of the model is given by:

$$\hat{\boldsymbol{\beta}} = (\boldsymbol{M}'\Theta^{-1}\boldsymbol{M})^{-1}\boldsymbol{M}'\Theta^{-1}\boldsymbol{Z} \tag{11.32}$$

where Θ is the covariance matrix denoted by:

$$\Theta = \begin{pmatrix} \text{diag}[\sigma_{11}^2(t)] & \text{diag}[\sigma_{12}(t)] & \cdots & \text{diag}[\sigma_{1k}(t)] \\ \text{diag}[\sigma_{21}(t)] & \text{diag}[\sigma_{22}^2(t)] & \cdots & \text{diag}[\sigma_{2k}(t)] \\ \vdots & \vdots & \ddots & \cdots \\ \text{diag}[\sigma_{k1}(t)] & \text{diag}[\sigma_{k2}(t)] & \cdots & \text{diag}[\sigma_{kk}^2(t)] \end{pmatrix} \tag{11.33}$$

where $\text{diag}[f(t)]$ is a diagonal matrix with the main diagonal elements given by $f(t)$ for all $t = (p+1), (p+2), \ldots, T$.

11.2.3.2 Covariance Matrix Estimation

In practice, the covariance matrix Θ is unknown. Therefore, it is necessary to estimate it.

Sato et al. [34] have proposed an iterative generalized least-squares estimation that consists of a two-stage loop. The first stage consists of estimating the coefficients of wavelets expansions $A_l(t)$ and $v(t)$ using a generalized least-squares estimation. In the second stage, the squared residuals obtained in the previous stage are used to estimate the wavelets expansion functions in the covariance matrix $\Sigma(t)$. Details of this procedure are as follows:

- **Step 1**: estimate the DVAR model using an OLS procedure, that is, assume $\Theta = I$.
- **Step 2**: estimate the univariate variances and the covariance functions using an OLS.
- **Step 3**: re-estimate the DVAR model using a generalized least-squares (GLS) considering the estimated Θ in step 2.
- **Step 4**: Go to step 2 until convergence of the parameters.

Notice that this algorithm is an extension of the Cochrane–Orcutt procedure [38], which yields better estimates than using an OLS procedure by taking into account the errors covariance matrix.

11.2.3.3 Hypothesis Testing

The hypothesis of connectivity significance or any linear combination of parameters in β can be achieved simply by applying the Wald test, considering an adequate contrast matrix (see Definition 11.6) [37].

The statistics for the Wald test for contrasts are given by:

$$W = \frac{(C\hat{\beta})'[M'\Theta^{-1}M]^{-1}(C\hat{\beta})}{\text{rank}(C)} \qquad (11.34)$$

We would like to perform the following test of hypothesis:

$$H_0 : C\beta = \mathbf{0} \quad \text{against} \quad H_1 : C\beta \neq \mathbf{0} \qquad (11.35)$$

Under the null hypothesis, the W statistics follows a chi-squared distribution with rank (C) degrees of freedom.

To illustrate the matrix of contrasts C, suppose that one is interested in testing the presence of Granger causality from gene y_j to gene y_i in a DVAR model of order one. Therefore, assume:

$$C = (\mathbf{0}_{D_j D_0}, \mathbf{0}_{D_j D_1}, \ldots, \mathbf{0}_{D_j D_{j-1}}, I_{D_j D_j}, \ldots, \mathbf{0}_{D_j D_{j+1}}, \ldots, \mathbf{0}D_j D_k) \qquad (11.36)$$

where $\mathbf{0}_{D_j D_0}$ is a $(D_j \times D_0)$ matrix of zeros, D_0 is the number of wavelet expansions for the intercept, D_j for $j = 1, \ldots, k$ is the number of wavelet expansions for gene j and $I_{D_j D_j}$ is an identity matrix of size D_j.

11.3
Simulations

This section shows illustrative examples of DVAR modeling for simulated data. The variation sources are controlled, that is, all variables, parameters, time-varying functions, and random errors' distribution are known. In this respect, application of Monte Carlo simulation to generate outcomes from a specific DVAR model is useful to evaluate the feasibility and quality of the parameter estimation procedure. Importantly, despite the fact that asymptotic results [39] ensure estimator's consistency, these approximations may not be suitable for actual and finite samples.

Actually, time series data of gene expression are generally short, due to the high costs of data acquisition. This means that although the expression values of several genes are quantified, only a small number of observations in time are available. Considering this limitation, estimation of time-varying functions requires sampling of repeated or similar events throughout time. In other words, if one is interested in estimating time-varying vector autoregressive models for events consisting of only n time points (e.g., $n = 16$), the estimates will probably be poor. However, if one replicates this event R times, and assumes that the underlying process of interest is similar at each repetition, it is possible to use the $T = R \times n$ observations to estimate the time-varying function of length n, resulting in higher precision. The main idea of this approach is to consider that the function of interest is the same for each repetition (e.g., cell cycle). Thus, the wavelet expansion for this function consists of only n time points and is assumed to be the same for each event.

Considering the issues previously described, two sets of simulated data were generated using time-varying functions of length 16, which were replicated 3 and 6 times. Thus, these configurations will produce time series data with length $T = 48$

and 96, respectively, allowing an empirical evaluation of time series length effects on the estimates' variances. One thousand simulations were carried out for each time series length, assuming the following DVAR model:

$$\begin{cases} y_{1,t} = 0.25\sin\left(\frac{2\pi t}{16}\right) + 0.3 y_{1,t-1} - 0.2 y_{2,t-1} - 0.75\cos\left(\frac{2\pi t}{16} + \pi\right) y_{4,t-1} + \varepsilon_{1,t} \\ y_{2,t} = 0.25\sin\left(\frac{2\pi t}{16}\right) - 0.25\sin\left(\frac{2\pi t}{16} - \frac{\pi}{2}\right) y_{2,t-1} - 0.75\cos\left(\frac{2\pi t}{16} + \frac{\pi}{2}\right) y_{4,t-1} + \varepsilon_{2,t} \\ y_{3,t} = -0.3 + 0.75\cos\left(\frac{2\pi t}{16} + \frac{\pi}{2}\right) y_{2,t-1} + 0.4 y_{4,t-1} + \varepsilon_{3,t} \\ y_{4,t} = -0.2 + 0.25\sin\left(\frac{2\pi t}{16} + \pi\right) y_{2,t-1} + 0.75\cos\left(\frac{2\pi t}{16} + \frac{\pi}{2}\right) y_{3,t-1} + \varepsilon_{4,t} \end{cases}$$

with random errors given by:

$$\begin{cases} \varepsilon_{1,t} = 0.35\eta_{1,t} \\ \varepsilon_{2,t} = 0.35\left(1 + \frac{\cos\left(\frac{2\pi t}{16}\right)}{6}\right)\eta_{2,t} \\ \varepsilon_{3,t} = 0.5\left(0.7\eta_{3,t} - 0.5\varepsilon_{1,t}\right) \\ \varepsilon_{4,t} = 0.5\left(1 - \frac{\sin\left(\frac{2\pi t}{16}\right)}{3}\right)(0.7\eta_{4,t} + 0.5\varepsilon_{2,t}) \end{cases}$$

where $\eta_{i,t}(i=1,\ldots,4)$ are independent random variables following a Gaussian distribution with mean zero and variance one. The wavelet basis consisted of Daublets 16 functions [40], assuming periodic boundary conditions, since we are interested in modeling repeated events.

A diagram describing the Granger relationships between the four time series generated by this model is shown in Figure 11.2. Figure 11.3 shows the example generated by the specified model. Results of the simulations are illustrated in Figures 11.4 and 11.5, which show the mean and standard deviation for each estimated autoregressive and causality time-varying function.

The results suggest that the estimation algorithm is effective. The estimator seems to be unbiased and, as expected, the standard deviation of estimates decreases as time series length increases. In summary, we conclude that estimation of the DVAR model

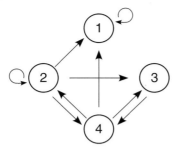

Figure 11.2 Diagram of relationships between the simulated time series. The arrows describe the presence of Granger causality.

for short-run events is feasible, if one assumes a repeated or periodic behavior of the function of interest. In addition, if long-run data is available, this assumption is not necessary and the time-varying functions may be estimated for a single event.

11.4
Application of the DVAR Method to Actual Data

The DVAR approach was applied to the analysis of the HeLa cell cycle gene expression data collected by Whitfield *et al.* [41]. HeLa is an immortal cell line, derived from a human epithelial cervical carcinoma, which is widely used as a cellular model in cancer research [42–44]. Its cell cycle is of approximately 16 hours. The gene

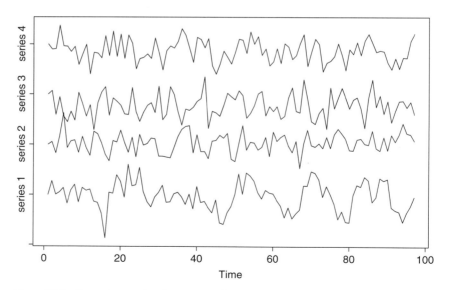

Figure 11.3 Illustrative simulated time series from a single realization of the DVAR model ($T = 96$).

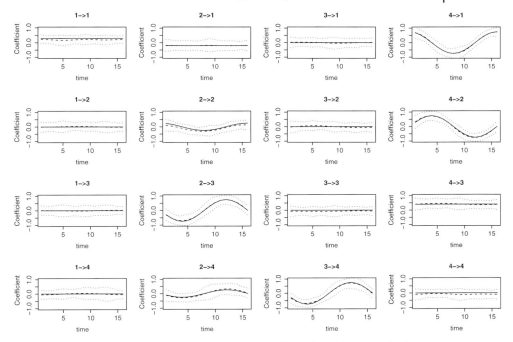

Figure 11.4 Simulations results for $T = 48$. The solid, dashed, and dotted lines describe the true time-varying connectivity function, the average of estimates (point-by-point), and one standard deviation interval, respectively.

expression data used in this study comprise three complete cell cycles, that is, 48 time points distributed at intervals of one hour; therefore, they were assumed as triplicates at each time point. The HeLa gene expression data is freely available at: http://genome-www.stanford.edu/Human-CellCycle/HeLa/.

To illustrate the application of DVAR to actual data, two regulatory networks were modeled: one composed by the *NFKB* (nuclear factor-kappa B), *IL1B* (interleukin-1 beta), *TNF* (tumor necrosis factor-alpha), and *BIRC2* (baculoviral IAP repeated-containing 2) genes (Figure 11.6) and the second by the *TP53* (tumor protein p53), *FAS* (TNF receptor superfamily, member 6) and *MASPIN* [serpin peptidase inhibitor, clade B (ovalbumin), member 5] genes (Figure 11.7).

To ensure that the power of the test will not be lost, networks composed of three or four genes were constructed, considering the available time series length. Notice that the larger is the network the lower is the statistical power. Owing to small sample size, networks composed of seven or more genes begin to display numeric computational problems, and *p*-values obtained by hypothesis tests may be strongly underestimated. Consequently, larger time series data are required. Therefore, if one is interested in constructing large networks, a solution is to perform a pairwise comparison and control the false positives rate by using the FDR (false discovery rate) [45].

DVAR of order one was applied due to the low number of time points in our time series data. Importantly, as the DVAR order increases, the power of the test decreases,

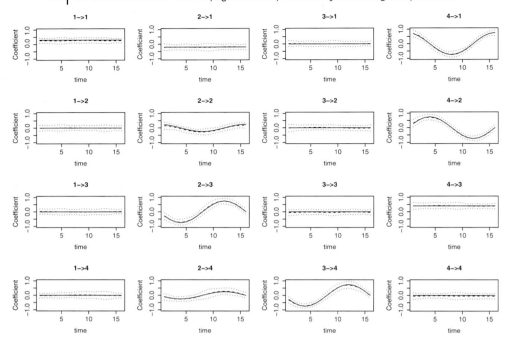

Figure 11.5 Simulations results for $T = 96$. The solid, dashed, and dotted lines describe the true time-varying connectivity function, the average of estimates (point-by-point), and one standard deviation intervals, respectively.

since the number of parameters to be estimated increases. In this application, the number of wavelet expansions D was set to four because it is known that regulatory connectivities vary along four different cell cycle phases (S, G2, M, G1). The wavelet used was the Daublets 16 function.

The direction of the edges in Figures 11.6 and 11.7 represents the direction of Granger causality, that is, the information flow. The graphics around the edges represent the time-varying connectivities (Granger causality) along the different cell phases. Positive connectivity suggests induction while negative connectivity suggests repression. Loops mean that there is a feedback process that may not be necessarily direct. For example, in Figure 11.6, there is a loop in the *BIRC2* gene. BIRC2 may be regulating a pathway while this pathway may be regulating BIRC2. Other regulatory events may also be indirect if there is an intermediate gene that is not in the model.

The two gene regulatory networks modeled in this chapter involve two highly connected signaling proteins with pivotal roles in various types of cancer, namely NFKB and TP53. Functional disruption of these two proteins may have important implications in pathways associated with cell cycle control and other cellular functions [6, 46].

Figures 11.6 and 11.7 represent the gene regulatory networks involving NFKB and TP53, respectively, obtained with DVAR analysis using HeLa cells gene expression data. The connections described in Figures 11.6 and 11.7 for the NFKB pathway:

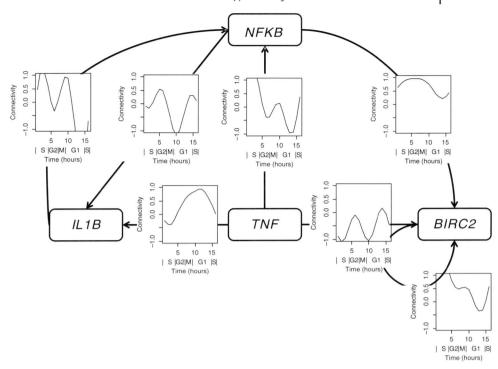

Figure 11.6 Application of the DVAR model to a network composed of the *NFKB, IL1B, TNF,* and *BIRC2* genes; p-values lower than 0.05 were considered as statistically significant. The connectivity functions are shown in each arrow. In each connectivity function, the x-axis represents the time in hours and the four cell cycle phase intervals (S, G2, M, and G1). The y-axis represents the connectivity intensity along the cell cycle.

NFKB and TNF, NFKB and IL1B, NFKB and BIRC2, TNF and IL1B, and TNF and BIRC2; and for the TP53 pathway: TP53 and MASPIN, and TP53 and FAS, are well established in the literature [46, 47].

The signaling cascade initiated by TNF binding to its cell surface receptors is one of the most classical signaling pathways leading to NFKB pathway activation [48]. Once activated, NFKB, a transcription factor, controls the expression of various target genes. One of these genes is *IL1B*, a cytokine involved in immune and inflammatory response [46], and also linked to the carcinogenesis process [49]. BIRC2 is an anti-apoptotic regulator and an important mediator of TNF activation of NFKB [50]. BIRC2 has also been described to have a role in some types of cancers [46].

The *TP53* gene encodes a transcription factor, playing a pivotal role in the etiology of numerous tumors [51]. The connection of TP53 with MASPIN – a protease inhibitor and tumor suppressor associated with growth blockage, invasion, and metastatic properties of some tumors – and with FAS, a protein associated with cell death signaling, have already been described in the literature [47].

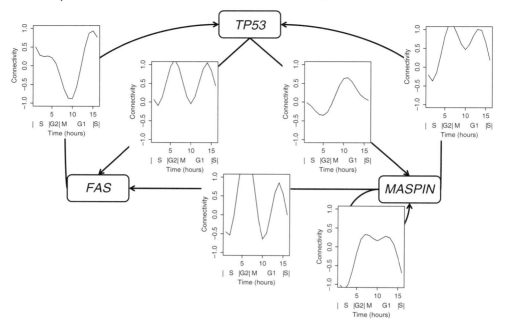

Figure 11.7 Application of the DVAR model to a network composed of the *TP53*, *FAS*, and *MASPIN* genes; p-values lower than 0.05 were considered as statistically significant. The connectivity functions are shown in each arrow. In each connectivity function, the x-axis represents the time in hours and the four cell cycle phase intervals (S, G2, M, and G1). The y-axis represents the connectivity intensity along the cell cycle.

Notably, the above-described connections for the NFKB and TP53 pathways are very important for understanding the functional relationships between the proteins that are part of these networks. However, these functional connections are a somewhat static view of these networks. In other words, it is well established that these NFKB or TP53 pathways connections exist, but little is known about their dynamics during certain cellular processes, such as the cell cycle. Moreover, it seems possible to capture these dynamics from gene expression datasets using specific algorithms, such as DVAR. These results are indicative of the fact that the connectivity between those members of NFKB and TP53 signaling pathways is dependent on the cell cycle phase.

The DVAR method suggests that new experiments focusing on the dynamics in connectivity may be performed to validate these results and to investigate their functional role.

11.5
Final Considerations

Understanding gene regulatory networks is crucial to uncover biological processes and, consequently, to find new treatments for several diseases, such as cancer.

Nevertheless, the complexity and time-varying properties of gene expression data along the cell cycle are obstacles for the application of standard mathematical models, because different cell phases demand different circuitries. Hence, adoption of probably unwarranted stationarity assumptions may lead to spurious results.

DVAR allows the analysis of different network topologies for each time point, being useful to suggest which gene is going to be activated/repressed and when this event occurs. In other words, instead of providing only one regulatory structure for the entire data set such as the standard VAR model (and other regulatory network models), DVAR provides different structures for each cell phase or time point. DVAR may be useful to provide insights on the pathways that are operating and when they are activated/repressed and, also, to compare the networks taking place under different experimental conditions, such as the response to drugs and antigens or comparison between normal versus diseased cells and tissues to identify potential targets for treatment.

DVAR measures partial time-varying Granger causalities, that is, it measures the Granger causality between two genes, removing the effect of a set of controlling genes.

Since DVAR is based on the standard VAR model, it does not require model prespecification, unlike the structural equation modeling (SEM) [52], in which the connectivity and directionality are given *a priori*. Therefore, DVAR may infer new connections, being useful to design experiments to find new targets for a specific gene product. Differently from graphical Gaussian models (GGMs) [53], which operate with partial correlations, that is, no directionality at the edges, DVAR infers information flow based on the Granger causality concept. Another advantage when compared to classical models, such as the Boolean network [54–56], is the fact that discretization of gene expression data to Boolean variables is not necessary for DVAR. Therefore, there is no loss of information. In addition, it is naturally applied to networks containing cycles, an advantage relative to models that assume DAGs (directed acyclic graphs) such as Bayesian networks [57–61] and structural equation models [52], since it is well known that genetic networks maintain their control and balance through a number of positive/negative feedbacks (cycles).

Although DVAR (and other VAR-based models) have several advantages over other regulatory network models, as described above, these techniques are limited for the application of time series data. Since it is known that there are several nonlinear relationships between genes and that most gene expression data are not in the time series format, more studies are required to model these complex characteristics. One possible solution for this case is to infer contagion [65]. Contagion was first introduced in finances [62–64] and subsequently applied to the analysis of gene expression signals [65] to define directionality even in pairwise non-time series data. Contagion can be interpreted as a switch system where the correlation appears in the tails of the distribution. Although contagion is not causality, since statistical interpretations are different, it is useful to identify asymmetries between gene expression signals and, thus, directionality at the edges of a regulatory network.

Work with the VAR model is proceeding in several directions, one of which is analyzing gene expression in the frequency domain, by identifying Granger causalities using partial directed coherence (PDC) [35, 66]. Although the use of PDC is quite straightforward, identification of Granger causality in the frequency domain currently is a challenge due to the short time series length. Another crucial research area is the interpretation of Granger causality in a biological sense, that is, to identify what kind and how much information is being transferred from one gene to another. This is a challenging task, since several problems must be tackled, the first of which is the curse of dimensionality. Although, with the advance of microarrays, the expression levels of tens of thousands of genes may be measured, only a few (tens in the case of time series data or hundreds in the case of independent data) microarrays are available. Therefore, improved estimators based on L1 penalization [67], for example, must be developed. The second problem is the observational data accuracy and bias caused by measurement errors. Gene expression signals measured by microarrays are masked by several sources of errors, such as probe design, background signal, scanner detection, data pre-processing algorithms, and so on. One potential solution to estimate measurement error for each experiment is by using technical replicates [68].

At the moment, we are working towards three independent goals. The first consists of correcting VAR models for measurement errors. It is well known that the ordinary least-squares estimator is biased under the presence of measurement errors [69]. Therefore, we are improving VAR models to incorporate latent variables and consequently diminishing/eliminating the bias caused by measurement errors. The second goal is generalizing the definition of Granger causality between *sets* of time series data, that is, extending the concept of Granger causality between m and n time series. We hope that this generalization may help biomedical researchers to identify yet unknown cross-talks between pathways. The third goal is to better understand the meaning of Granger causality from a biological point of view. In other words, by simulating *in silico* the whole cells, protein–protein interactions, signal transduction pathways, and so on using software such as Cell Illustrator [70] we believe it will be possible to uncover what kind of information we are obtaining upon analyzing gene expression signals.

11.6
Conclusions

In this chapter we have presented both the mathematical concept of Granger causality and its identification method in time series data. Demonstrations were carried out using both simulated and actual biological data to illustrate the main advantages of the wavelet-based DVAR method, that is, its ability to identify time-varying influences and the fact that, at the edges, the direction has a statistical interpretation, that is, it is based on the Granger causality concept.

Acknowledgments

This work has been supported by grants from RIKEN, Japan, and by Brazilian research agencies (FAPESP, CNPq, FINEP, and CAPES).

11.A
Appendix

Definition 11.1
Weakly stationary process
A stochastic process is *weakly stationary* if its first and second moments are time invariant, that is, a stochastic process y_t is stationary if:

$$E(y_t) = \mu < \infty \quad \text{for all } t \qquad (11.A.1)$$

and:

$$E[(y_t-\mu)(y_{t-h}-\mu)'] = \Gamma_y(h) = \Gamma_y(-h)' \quad \text{for all } t \text{ and } h = 0, 1, 2, \ldots \qquad (11.A.2)$$

In other words, *weak stationarity* means that all y_t have the same finite mean vector μ and that the auto-covariances of the process do not depend on t but only on the time interval h for which the two vectors y_t and y_{t-h} are apart.

Definition 11.2
Stability condition
A VAR(p) is said to be stable if all eigenvalues of A have modulus less than one. This is equivalent to:

$$\det(I_K - Az) \neq 0 \quad \text{for} \quad |z| \leq 1 \qquad (11.A.3)$$

Definition 11.3
The vec operator
Let $A = (a_1, \ldots, a_n)$ be an $(m \times n)$ matrix with $(m \times 1)$ columns a_i. The vec operator transforms A into an $(nm \times 1)$ vector by stacking the columns, that is:

$$\text{vec}(A) = \begin{pmatrix} a_1 \\ \vdots \\ a_n \end{pmatrix} \qquad (11.A.4)$$

Definition 11.4
The Kronecker product
Let $A = (a_{ij})$ and $B = (b_{ij})$ be $(m \times n)$ and $(p \times q)$ matrices, respectively. The $(mp \times nq)$ matrix:

$$A \otimes B \begin{pmatrix} a_{11}B & \cdots & a_{1n}B \\ \vdots & & \vdots \\ a_{m1}B & \cdots & a_{mn}B \end{pmatrix} \qquad (11.A.5)$$

is the *Kronecker product* or *direct product* of A and B.

Definition 11.5
The row-Kronecker product
This is defined by:

$$\begin{pmatrix} a_1 \\ a_2 \\ \vdots \\ a_n \end{pmatrix} \otimes^R \begin{pmatrix} b_1 \\ b_2 \\ \vdots \\ b_n \end{pmatrix} = \begin{pmatrix} a_1 \otimes b_1 \\ a_2 \otimes b_2 \\ \vdots \\ a_n \otimes b_n \end{pmatrix} \tag{11.A.6}$$

Definition 11.6
The Wald Test [37]
This is a classical statistical approach for hypothesis testing in linear regression models. The main difference between the Wald and conventional z or t statistics of estimated coefficients is that the former allows testing linear combinations of regression parameters. Take the following linear model:

$$y = X\beta + \varepsilon \tag{11.A.7}$$

where:

$$y = \begin{pmatrix} y_1 \\ y_2 \\ \vdots \\ y_N \end{pmatrix}, \quad X = \begin{pmatrix} X_{11} & X_{21} & \cdots & X_{1k} \\ X_{21} & X_{22} & \cdots & X_{2k} \\ \vdots & \vdots & \ddots & \vdots \\ X_{N1} & X_{N2} & \cdots & X_{Nk} \end{pmatrix}, \quad \begin{pmatrix} \varepsilon_1 \\ \varepsilon_2 \\ \vdots \\ \varepsilon_N \end{pmatrix} \tag{11.A.8}$$

and:

$$\beta = \begin{pmatrix} \beta_1 \\ \beta_2 \\ \vdots \\ \beta_k \end{pmatrix} \tag{11.A.9}$$

Suppose we are interested in testing the following hypothesis:

$$H_0 : C\beta = 0 \quad \text{against} \quad H_1 : C\beta \neq 0 \tag{11.A.10}$$

where C is a matrix of contrasts of the parameters we wish to test. The Wald statistics is given by:

$$W = (C\hat{\beta})'[C((X'X)^{-1} \otimes \hat{\Sigma})C']^{-1}(C\hat{\beta}) \tag{11.A.11}$$

where $\hat{\beta}$ is the estimated parameters and $\hat{\Sigma}$ is the estimated covariance matrix of errors in e. The null hypothesis can then be tested, since under H_0, W follows a chi-square distribution with rank (C) degrees of freedom. For an illustrative example, suppose that we have a linear model with $k = 4$ and we would like to test the hypothesis that $\beta_1 + \beta_3$ and $\beta_2 - \beta_4$ are equal to zero. The contrast matrix can then be tested by specifying C matrix as:

$$C = \begin{pmatrix} 1 & 0 & 1 & 0 \\ 0 & 1 & 0 & -1 \end{pmatrix} \tag{11.A.12}$$

In this case, under H_0, W follows a chi-square distribution with two degrees of freedom. Thus, the *p*-value can be computed by calculating the probability $P(W > W_{\text{obs}})$, where W_{obs} is the observed Wald statistic.

References

1 Ideker, T., Galitski, T., and Hood, L. (2001) A new approach to decoding life: systems biology. *Annu. Rev. Genomics Hum. Genet.*, **2**, 343–372. doi: 10.1146/annurev.genom.2.1.343

2 Hood, L., Heath, J.R., Phelps, M.E., and Lin, B. (2004) Systems biology and new technologies enable predictive and preventative medicine. *Science*, **306**, 640–643. doi: 10.1126/science.1104635

3 Aderem, A. (2005) Systems biology: its practice and challenges. *Cell*, **121**, 511–513. doi: 10.1016/j.cell.2005.04.020

4 Butcher, E.C., Berg, E.L., and Kunkel, E.J. (2004) Systems biology in drug discovery. *Nat. Biotechnol.*, **22**, 1253–1259. doi: 10.1038/nbt1017

5 Hanahan, D. and Weinberg, R.A. (2000) The hallmarks of cancer. *Cell*, **100**, 57–70. doi: 10.1016/S0092-8674(00)81683-9

6 Vogelstein, B. and Kinzler, K.W. (2004) Cancer genes and the pathways they control. *Nat. Med.*, **10**, 789–799. doi: 10.1038/nm1087

7 Albert, R., Jeong, H., and Barabasi, A.L. (2000) Error and attack tolerance of complex networks. *Nature*, **406**, 378–382. doi: 10.1038/35019019.

8 Massagué, J. (2004) G1 cell-cycle control and cancer. *Nature*, **432**, 298–306. doi: 10.1038/nature03094

9 Albert, R. (2005) Scale-free networks in cell biology. *J. Cell Sci.*, **118**, 4947–4957. doi: 10.1242/10.1242/jcs.02714

10 Wang, E., Lenferink, A., and O'Connor-McCourt, M. (2007) Cancer systems biology: exploring cancer-associated genes on cellular networks. *Cell. Mol. Life Sci.*, **64**, 1752–1762. doi: 10.1007/s00018-007-7054-6

11 Mukhopadhyay, N.D. and Chatterjee, S. (2007) Causality and pathway search in microarray time series experiment. *Bioinformatics*, **23**, 442–449. doi: 10.1093/bioinformatics/btl598

12 Fujita, A., Sato, J.R., Demasi, M.A.A., Sogayar, M.C., Ferreira, C.E., and Miyano, S. (2009) Comparing Pearson, Spearman and Hoeffding's D measure for gene expression association analysis. *J. Bioinform. Comput. Biol.*, **7**, 663–684. doi: 10.1142/S0219720009004230

13 Fujita, A., Sato, J.R., Garay-Malpartida, H.M., Sogayar, M.C., Ferreira, C.E., and Miyano, S. (2008) Modeling nonlinear gene regulatory networks from time series gene expression data. *J. Bioinform. Comput. Biol.*, **6**, 961–979. doi: 10.1142/S0219720008003746

14 Kojima, K., Fujita, A., Shimamura, T., Imoto, S., and Miyano, S. (2008) Estimation of nonlinear gene regulatory networks via L1 regularized NVAR from time series gene expression data. *Genome Informatics*, **20**, 37–51. doi: 10.1142/9781848163003_0004

15 Fujita, A., Sato, J.R., Garay-Malpartida, H.M., Yamaguchi, R., Miyano, S., Sogayar, M.C., and Ferreira, C.E. (2007) Modeling gene expression regulatory networks with the sparse vector autoregressive model. *BMC Syst. Biol.*, **1**, 39. doi: 10.1186/1752-0509-1-39

16 Shimamura, T., Imoto, S., Yamaguchi, R., Fujita, A., Nagasaki, M., and Miyano, S. (2009) Recursive regularization for inferring gene networks from time-course gene expression profiles. *BMC Syst. Biol.*, **3**, 41. doi: 10.1186/1752-0509-3-41

17 Opgen-Rhein, R. and Strimmer, K. (2007) Learning causal networks from systems biology time course data: an effective model selection procedure for the vector autoregressive process. *BMC Syst. Biol.*, **8**, S3. doi: 10.1186/1471-2105-8-S2-S3

18 Lozano, A.C., Abe, N., Liu, Y., and Rosset, S. (2009) Grouped graphical Granger modeling for gene expression regulatory networks discovery. *Bioinformatics*, **25**,

i110–i118. doi: 10.1093/bioinformatics/btp199

19 Fujita, A., Sato, J.R., Garay-Malpartida, H.M., Morettin, P.A., Sogayar, M.C., and Ferreira, C.E. (2007) Time-varying modeling of gene expression regulatory networks using the wavelet dynamic vector autoregressive method. *Bioinformatics*, **23**, 1623–1630. doi: 10.1093/bioinformatics/btm151

20 Goldthorpe, J.H. (2001) Causation, statistics, and sociology. *Eur. Sociol. Rev.*, **17**, 1–20.

21 Piaget, J., Garcia, R., Miles, D., and Miles, M. (1974) *Understanding Causality*, Norton, New York.

22 Bohm, D. (1984) *Causality and Change in Modern Physics*, Routledge, London.

23 Pearl, J. (1988) *Probabilistic Reasoning in Intelligent Systems*, Morgan and Kauffman, San Mateo.

24 Spirtes, P., Glymour, C., and Scheines, R. (1993) *Causation, Prediction and Search*, 2nd edn, Springer-Verlag, MIT Press, New York.

25 Spirtes, P., Glymour, C., and Scheines, R. (1990) Simulation studies of the reliability of computer aided model specification using the TETRAD, EQS and LISREL programs. *Sociol. Methods Res.*, **19**, 3–66.

26 Granger, C.W.J. (1969) Investigating causal relationships by econometric models and cross-spectral methods. *Econometrica*, **37**, 424–438.

27 Granger, C.W.J. (1980) Testing for causality: A personal viewpoint. *J. Economet. Dynam. Control*, **2**, 329–352.

28 Granger, C.W.J. (2001) *Essays in Econometrics: The Collected Papers of Clive W.J. Granger*, Cambridge University Press, Cambridge.

29 McCrorie, J.R. and Chambers, M.J. (2006) Granger causality and the sampling of economic process. *J. Econometrics*, **132**, 311–336. doi: 10.1016/j.jeconom.2005.02.002

30 Wong, T. (2006) Granger causality tests among openness to international trade, human accumulation and economic growth in China: 1952–1999. *Int. Econom. J.*, **20**, 285–302. doi: 10.1080/10168730600879356

31 McCracken, M.W. (2007) Asymptotics for out of sample tests of Granger causality. *J. Econometr.*, **140**, 719–752. doi: 10.1016/j.jeconom.2006.07.020

32 Brovelli, A., Mingzhou, D., Ledberg, A., Chen, Y., Nakamura, R., and Bressler, S.L. (2004) Beta oscillations in a large-scale sensorimotor cortical network: directional influences revealed by Granger causality. *Proc. Natl. Acad. Sci. USA*, **101**, 9849–9854. doi: 10.1073/pnas.0308538101

33 Roebroeck, A., Formisano, E., and Goebel, R. (2006) Mapping directed influence over the brain using Granger causality and fMRI. *NeuroImage*, **25**, 230–242. doi: 10.1016/j.neuroimage.2004.11.017

34 Sato, J.R., Amaro, E. Jr., Takahashi, D.Y., de Maria Felix, M., Brammer, M.J., and Morettin, P.A. (2006) A method to produce evolving functional connectivity maps during the course of an fMRI experiment using wavelet-based time-varying Granger causality. *Neuroimage*, **32**, 187–196. doi: 10.1016/j.neuroimage.2005.11.039

35 Baccala, L.A. and Sameshima, K. (2001) Partial directed coherence: a new concept in neural structure determination. *Biol. Cybern.*, **84**, 463–474. doi: 10.1007/PL00007990

36 Lütkepohl, H. (2006) *New Introduction to Multiple Time Series Analysis*, Springer-Verlag, New York.

37 Graybill, F.A. (1976) *Theory and Application of the Linear Model*, Duxbury Press, North Scituate, MA.

38 Cochrane, D. and Orcutt, H. (1949) Application of least squares regression to relationships containing autocorrelated error terms. *J. Am. Stat. Assoc.*, **44**, 32–61.

39 Sato, J.R., Morettin, P.A., Arantes, P.R., and Amaro, E. Jr. (2007) Wavelet based time-varying vector autoregressive modelling. *Comput. Stat. Data Anal.*, **51**, 5847–5866. doi: 10.1016/j.csda.2006.10.027

40 Daubechies, I. (2004) Ten Lectures on Wavelets, CBMS-NSF Regional Conference Series in Applied Mathematics, 61, Society for Industrial and Applied Mathematics.

41 Whitfield, L., Perou, C., Hurt, M., Brown, P., and Botstein, D. (2002) Identification of

genes periodically expressed in the human cell cycle and their expression in tumors. *Mol. Biol. Cell.*, **13**, 1977–2000. doi: 10.1091/mbc.02-02-0030

42 Beausoleil, S.A., Jedrychowski, M., Schwartz, D., Elias, J.E., Villń, J., Li, J., Cohn, M.A. *et al.* (2004) Large-scale characterization of HeLa cell nuclear phosphoproteins. *Proc. Natl. Acad. Sci. USA*, **101**, 12130–12135. doi: 10.1073/pnas.0404720101

43 Koehler, J.A., Yusta, B., and Drucker, D.J. (2005) The HeLa cell glucagon-like peptide-2 receptor is coupled to regulation of apoptosis and ERK1/2 activation through divergent signalling pathways. *Mol. Endocrinol.*, **19**, 459–473. doi: 10.1210/me.2004-0196

44 Yasuda, S., Taniguchi, H., Oceguera-Yaneza, F., Ando, Y., Watanabe, S., Monypenny, S., and Narumiya, S. (2006) An essential role of Cdc42-like GTPases in mitosis of HeLa cells. *FEBS Lett.*, **580**, 3375–3380. doi: 10.1016/j.febslet.2006.05.009

45 Benjamini, Y. and Hochberg, Y. (1995) Controlling the false discovery rate: a practical and powerful approach to multiple testing. *J. R. Stat. Soc. B*, **57**, 289–300.

46 Karin, M. (2006) Nuclear factor-kappaB in cancer development and progression. *Nature*, **441**, 431–436. doi: 10.1038/nature04870

47 Vogelstein, B., Lane, D., and Levine, A.J. (2000) Surfing the p53 network. *Nature*, **408**, 307–310. doi: 10.1038/35042675

48 Beg, A.A. and Baltimore, D. (1996) An essential role for NF-κB in preventing TNF-α induced cell death. *Science*, **274**, 782–784. doi: 10.1126/science.274.5288.782

49 El-Omar, E.M., Carrington, M., Chow, W.H., McColl, K.E., Bream, J.H., Young, H.A., Herrera, J. *et al.* (2000) Interleukin-1 polymorphisms associated with increased risk of gastric cancer. *Nature*, **404**, 398–402. doi: 10.1038/35006081

50 Varfolomeev, E., Goncharov, T., Fedorova, A.V., Dynek, J.N., Zobel, K., Deshayes, K., Fairbrother, W.J., and Vucic, D. (2008) c-IAP1 and c-IAP2 are critical mediators of TNFalpha-induced NF-kappaB activation. *J. Biol. Chem.*, **283**, 24295–24299. doi: 10.1074/jbc.C800128200

51 Sherr, C.J. and McCormick, F. (2002) The RB and p53 pathways in cancer. *Cancer Cell*, **2**, 103–112. doi: 10.1016/S1535-6108(02)00102-2

52 Xiong, M., Li, J., and Fang, X. (2004) Identification of genetic networks. *Genetics*, **166**, 1037–1052.

53 Schäffer, J. and Strimmer, K. (2005) An empirical Bayes approach to inferring large-scale gene association networks. *Bioinformatics*, **21**, 754–764.

54 Akutsu, T., Miyano, S., and Kuhara, S. (2000) Algorithms for identifying Boolean networks and related biological networks based on matrix multiplication and fingerprint function. *J. Comput. Biol.*, **7**, 331–343. doi: 10.1089/106652700750050817

55 Pal, R., Datta, A., Bittner, M.L., and Dougherty, E.R. (2005) Intervention in context-sensitive probabilistic Boolean networks. *Bioinformatics*, **21**, 1211–1218. doi: 10.1093/bioinformatics/bti131

56 Shmulevich, I., Dougherty, E.R., and Zhang, W. (2002) Gene perturbation and intervention in probabilistic Boolean networks. *Bioinformatics*, **18**, 1319–1331.

57 Dojer, N., Gambim, A., Mizera, A., Wilczyński, B., and Tiuryn, J. (2006) Applying dynamic Bayesian networks to perturbed gene expression data. *BMC Bioinformatics*, **7**, 249. doi: 10.1186/1471-2105-7-249

58 Friedman, N., Linial, M., Nachman, I., and Pe'er, D. (2000) Using Bayesian networks to analyze expression data. *J. Comput. Biol.*, **7**, 601–620.

59 Friedman, N. (2004) Inferring cellular networks using probabilistic graphical models. *Science*, **303**, 799–805. doi: 10.1089/106652700750050961

60 Imoto, S., Goto, T., and Miyano, S. (2002) Estimation of genetic networks and functional structures between genes by using Bayesian networks and nonparametric regression. *Pacific Symp. Biocomput.*, **7**, 175–186.

61 Tamada, Y., Kim, S.Y., Bannai, H., Imoto, S., Tashiro, K., Kuhara, S., and Miyano, S. (2003) Estimating gene networks from

gene expression data by combining Bayesian network model with promoter element detection. *Bioinformatics*, **19**, ii227–ii236. doi: 10.1093/bioinformatics/btg1082

62 Bradley, B.O. and Taqqu, M.S. (2004) Framework for analyzing spatial contagion between financial markets. *Finance Lett.*, **2**, 8–15.

63 Bradley, B.O. and Taqqu, M.S. (2005) How to estimate spatial contagion between financial markets. *Finance Lett.*, **3**, 64–76.

64 Bradley, B.O. and Taqqu, M.S. (2005) Empirical evidence on spatial contagion between financial markets. *Finance Lett.*, **3**, 77–86.

65 Fujita, A., Sato, J.R., Demasi, M.A.A., Yamaguchi, R., Shimamura, T., Ferreira, C.E., Sogayar, M.C., and Miyano, S. Inferring contagion in regulatory networks. *IEEE/ACM Trans. Comput. Biol. Bioinformatics*, (in press).

66 Sato, J.R., Takahashi, D.Y., Arcuri, S.M., Sameshima, K., Morettin, P.A., and Baccala, L.A. (2009) Frequency domain connectivity identification: an application of partial directed coherence in fMRI. *Hum. Brain Mapp.*, **30**, 452–461. doi: 10.1002/hbm.20513

67 Tibshirani, R. (1996) Regression shrinkage and selection via the lasso. *J. R. Stat. Soc. B*, **58**, 267–288.

68 Fujita, A., Sato, J.R., da Silva, F.H.L., Galvão, M.C., Sogayar, M.C., and Miyano, S. (2009) Quality control and reproducibility in DNA microarray experiments. *Genome Informatics*, **23**, 21–31.

69 Fuller, W. (1987) *Measurement Error Models*, Wiley-Interscience, New York.

70 Nagasaki, M., Doi, A., Matsuno, H., and Miyano, S. (2003) Genomic Object Net: a platform for modeling and simulating biopathways. *Appl. Bioinformatics*, **2**, 181–184.

12
A Systems Biology Approach to Construct A Cancer-Perturbed Protein–Protein Interaction Network for Apoptosis by Means of Microarray and Database Mining

Liang-Hui Chu and Bor-Sen Chen

12.1
Introduction

Cancer is among the most deadly and complex diseases worldwide. Tumorigenesis in human is a multistep process that reflects genetic alterations that drive the progressive transformation of normal human cells into highly malignant derivatives. Cancer is caused by genetic abnormalities, such as mutations of oncogenes or tumor-suppressor genes, which alter downstream signal transduction pathways and protein–protein interactions (PPIs). Integrated multilevel data sets encompassing genomics and proteomics are required to determine fully the contributions of genome alterations, host factors, and environmental exposures to tumor growth and progression [1, 2]. At the molecular level, genetic mutations, translocations, amplifications, deletions, and viral gene insertions can alter translated proteins and thereby disrupt signal transduction pathways and PPIs that are essential for apoptosis and other important cellular processes [3]. Although inactivated pro-apoptotic proteins or up-regulated expressions of anti-apoptotic proteins can result in unchecked growth of a tumor and inability to respond to cellular stress and DNA damage, deregulation of apoptosis that disrupts the delicate balance between cell proliferation and cell death can lead to cancer [4]. Cancer is recognized as a systems-biology disease that is mainly caused by malfunctions of perturbed protein interaction networks in the cell [5–7].

Apoptosis is necessary for human development and survival, with millions of cells committing suicide to prevent uncontrolled growth [8]. Once the decision is made, proper execution of the apoptotic program requires activation and execution of multiple subprograms through regulated PPIs. Apoptotic response is mediated through either (i) an intrinsic pathway that is triggered by death stimuli within a cell such as DNA damage or oncogene activation or (ii) an extrinsic pathway that is initiated by binding of an extracellular death ligand. The extrinsic pathway can link to the intrinsic pathway, which then triggers release of mitochondrial proteins through PPIs [9]. Evading apoptosis is an acquired capability of cancer cells, and anticancer treatment using cytotoxic drugs is considered to mediate cell death by activating key

Medical Biostatistics for Complex Diseases. Edited by Frank Emmert-Streib and Matthias Dehmer
Copyright © 2010 WILEY-VCH Verlag GmbH & Co. KGaA, Weinheim
ISBN: 978-3-527-32585-6

elements of the apoptosis program and the cellular stress response [10]. Comprehensive PPIs provide a framework for understanding the biology of cancer as an integrated system.

Most gene products mediate their functions within complex networks of interconnected macromolecules, forming a dynamic topological interactome [11–14]. Yeast-two-hybrid experiments [15, 16] and several web sites, such as BIND [17], Himap [18], HPRD (Human Protein Reference Database) [19], and Intact [20], enable analysis of the global topologies of human PPIs. BIND [17] provides information about protein sequences, pathways, binary PPIs, and protein complexes. Owing to the lack of results of complex experiments such as mass spectrometry on human proteins, description of cooperative interactions of protein complexes with a target protein are obtainable mainly from the BIND database. Himap [18] combines two datasets of yeast-two-hybrid experiments [15, 16] and a HPRD [19] with shared references to functions and predictions. HPRD [19] provides detailed data including protein sequences, localization, domains and motifs, and thousands of PPIs. Intact [20] contains descriptions of the enrichment of PPIs, lists of related literature, and experiments.

However, both experiments and databases exhibit some degree of false positives [21]. The yeast-two-hybrid experiments based on transactivation of reporter genes require the presence of auto-activators, in which the bait activates gene expression in the absence of any prey [11]. The yeast-two-hybrid technique can yield false positives (spurious interactions detected because of the high-throughput nature of the screening process) and false negatives (undetected interactions) [21, 22]. Therefore, reliable computational methods are needed to refine PPI networks and reduce false positives. Owing to the complex nature of the interactomes, such as those observed in the apoptosome complex during caspase formation [8], a nonlinear mathematical model provides a better characterization than a linear model. Besides nonlinear effects, intrinsic and extrinsic molecular noise results in stochastic variations in transcription and translation because molecules are subject to significant thermal fluctuations and noise [23, 24]. This study describes a nonlinear stochastic model that characterizes dynamic PPI networks for apoptosis in cancerous and normal cells.

In this work, a nonlinear stochastic model is constructed to truncate fake PPIs from a rough PPI network using a statistical method called the Akaike information criterion (AIC) by means of high-throughput protein-interaction data. This research considers mainly linear individual (or binary) protein interactions and nonlinear cooperative protein–complex memberships, ignoring other relationships such as DNA–protein or biochemical interactions. Other missing interactions are considered as basal interactions in the model developed here. Cancer-perturbed PPI networks for apoptosis of normal cells are obtained by means of comparisons of gain-of-function and loss-of-function networks. Because a drug designed to induce apoptosis is intended to kill cancer cells within unaffected normal cells, these cancer-perturbed PPI networks will provide identification and prediction of apoptosis drug targets.

12.2
Methods

12.2.1
Microarray Experimental Data

Microarray datasets were obtained from Reference [25], which compares the genomic expression of HeLa cervical cancer carcinoma cells with that of normal primary human lung fibroblasts under several stresses such as endoplasmic reticulum (ER) stress. Because the endoplasmic reticulum is recognized as a third subcellular compartment that controls apoptosis in addition to mitochondria and membrane-bound death receptors [8], this research considered the genomic expressions of HeLa cells and fibroblasts, both of which were treated with 2.5 mM DTT (dithiothreitol) under ER stress, as microarray sources. Samples are taken at 0, 0.5, 1, 2, 4, 6, 8, 16, 24, and 30 h in cancer cells and 0, 0.5, 1, 2, 3, 4, 6, 8, 12, 16, 24, and 36 h in normal cells under ER stress.

12.2.2
Construction of Initial Protein–Protein Interaction (PPI) Networks

Two systematic experimental mappings of human interactomes include yeast-two-hybrid systems [15, 16]. Several web sites and databases also provide fundamental global topologies for human PPIs, including BIND [17], Himap [18], HPRD [19], and Intact [20]. Because the union of these various databases can maximize the likelihood of a precise estimation of parameters as a basis for constructing rough PPIs [11], a rough PPI network was first constructed from the union of two yeast-two-hybrid experiments and web-site data to draw the general PPI map.

12.2.3
Nonlinear Stochastic Interaction Model

Although studies using large-scale PPIs can describe the overall landscape of protein-interaction networks, all large-scale experiments and databases contain high false-positive rates [26]. Therefore, an efficient computational method for integrating different databases and experiments is essential to refine the network with confidence. Microarray data were used to truncate fake interactions and reduce high false-positive rates after constructing a rough PPI network.

In recent years, some systems and computational biologists have used a dynamic perspective concept to describe biological functions because of their inherently dynamic nature [27–29]. The authors regard all proteins in an organism as a large dynamic interaction system and PPIs are considered as nonlinear stochastic processes with several expression profiles having interactive protein partners as input and the expression profile of a target protein as output. Owing to random noise and uncertainty during experiments, the PPIs were described using stochastic discrete nonlinear dynamic equations. Only two types of PPIs were considered, binary protein interactions and protein–complex memberships, regardless of other relationships that may exist such as DNA–protein or biochemical interactions. These missing interactions were considered as a single basal interaction, denoted as k, in the model, with $\varepsilon[t]$ representing stochastic molecular events such as fluctuations in interactions with the target protein [23].

In this study, "individual PPIs" were defined as the binary PPIs, and "cooperative PPIs" as the membership of the protein complex with the target protein; $x[t]$ was used to denote the expression profile of the target protein at time t, a the degree of influence of the target protein at time t on the target protein at time $t + 1$, b_i the individual or binary interactive ability of protein i with target protein $x[t]$, and c_{ij} as the cooperative ability of protein i and protein j to interact with and affect the target protein. Readers can also refer to Reference [30] for the basis of the mathematical modeling approach used here, although missing data and stochastic events have been considered in this study. Figure 12.1 shows the interactions of five individual proteins ($x_1[t]$, $x_2[t]$, $x_3[t]$, $x_4[t]$, and $x_5[t]$) with the target protein $x[t]$ and one cooperative

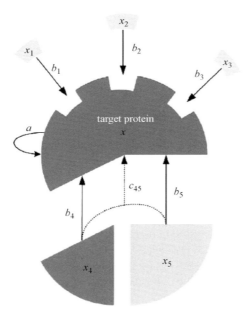

Figure 12.1 Graphical representation of individual protein interactions and cooperative protein interactions. The dynamic protein interaction equation developed here includes five individual proteins ($x_1[t]$, $x_2[t]$, $x_3[t]$, $x_4[t]$, and $x_5[t]$) interacting with a target protein ($x[t]$) and one cooperative interaction involving protein $x_4[t]$ and $x_5[t]$ with the target protein $x[t]$; a denotes the degree of influence of a target protein at one point in time on the target protein at the next point in time; b_i denotes the individual or binary interaction of protein i with target protein $x[t]$; and c_{ij} denotes the cooperative interaction of protein i and protein j with the target protein $x[t]$.

interaction involving proteins $x_4[t]$ and $x_5[t]$ with the target protein $x[t]$. Considering the basal interactions k and stochastic events $\varepsilon[t]$, it is possible to express the dynamic model of the target-protein-interaction profile as a function of t as follows:

$$x[t+1] = ax[t] + b_1x_1[t] + b_2x_2[t] + b_3x_3[t] + b_4x_4[t] + b_5x_5[t] + c_{45}x_{45}[t] + k + \varepsilon[t]$$

Therefore, for N interactive proteins, dynamic interactive behaviors between upstream interactive proteins and their target protein can be written in the following form according to [30–33]:

$$x[t+1] = ax[t] + \sum_{i=1}^{N} b_i x_i[t] + \sum_{i=1}^{N}\sum_{j=1}^{N} c_{ij}x_{ij}[t] + k + \varepsilon[t] \quad (12.1)$$

Remark: The discrete-time dynamic model in Equation (12.1) is based on discrete sampling of the continuous differential model:

$$\dot{x}[t] = -\lambda x[t] + \sum_{i=1}^{N} b_i x_i[t] + \sum_{i=1}^{N}\sum_{j=1}^{N} c_{ij}x_{ij}[t] + k + \varepsilon[t]$$

where $\dot{x}(t) = dx(t)/dt$ denotes the derivative of $x(t)$ with respect to continuous time t, and λ denotes the decay rate of $x[t]$. By unit sampling and with $\dot{x}[t] \cong x[t+1] - x[t]$, the following discrete model [34] can be obtained:

$$x[t+1] - x[t] = -\lambda x[t] + \sum_{i=1}^{N} b_i x_i[t] + \sum_{i=1}^{N}\sum_{j=1}^{N} c_{ij}x_{ij}[t] + k + \varepsilon[t]$$

or:

$$x[t+1] = (1-\lambda)x[t] + \sum_{i=1}^{N} b_i x_i[t] + \sum_{i=1}^{N}\sum_{j=1}^{N} c_{ij}x_{ij}[t] + k + \varepsilon[t]$$

$$= ax[t] + \sum_{i=1}^{N} b_i x_i[t] + \sum_{i=1}^{N}\sum_{j=1}^{N} c_{ij}x_{ij}[t] + k + \varepsilon[t]$$

where a denotes the influence of $x[t]$ on $x[t+1]$ and is dependent on the decay rate λ.

Iteratively, one target protein at a time and using Equation (12.1), it is possible to construct the whole PPI network, which is interconnected through the protein interactions $\sum_{i=1}^{N} b_i x_i(t)$ and $\sum_{i}^{N}\sum_{j=1}^{N} c_{ij}x_{ij}(t)$ in Equation (12.1) for all proteins. In (12.1), $x[t]$ represents the expression profile of the target protein at the molecular level at time t, which could be calculated from the corresponding mRNA expression profiles using a translational sigmoid function [31, 32]:

$$x[t] = f(y[t]) = \frac{1}{1 + \exp[-r(y[t] - M)]} \quad (12.2)$$

In Equation (12.2), r denotes the transition rate of the sigmoid function, and M denotes the mean of the mRNA expression level of the corresponding protein. $\sum_{i=1}^{N} x_i[t]$ represents all possible individual interactive functions, that is, all possible binary PPIs, of N interactive protein candidates of the target protein in the rough PPI network, a denotes the degree of influence of the current-time target protein on the next-time target protein, and b_i indicates the individual interactive ability of protein i with target protein $x[t]$. $\sum_{i=1}^{N} \sum_{j=1}^{N} c_{ij}x_{ij}[t]$ denotes all possible interactive functions of cooperative protein partners, that is, protein–complex memberships, with the target protein in the rough PPI network, where $x_{ij}[t]$ denotes a nonlinear cooperative interaction involving protein x_i and protein x_j with the target protein, that is, $x_{ij}[t] = f(y_i[t]) \cdot f(y_j[t])$, and c_{ij} denotes the cooperative interaction ability of protein i and protein j with the target protein. All possible cooperative interactions $\sum_{i=1}^{N} \sum_{j=1}^{N} c_{ij}x_{ij}[t]$ are obtained from high-throughput protein-interaction datasets and web sites containing putative protein complexes within the network. If the multiprotein complex is composed of more than three proteins or their equivalents, it is impossible to create directly a multiple expression profile for each protein. It is then necessary to add all combinations of two cooperative proteins from the protein complex because of the nonlinear property that one extreme value in the equation can lead to serious deviations in other estimated parameters. The basal interaction k in Equation (12.1) represents unknown PPIs resulting from other possible interactive proteins or other influences, for example, mRNA–protein interactions and protein synthesis. The term $\varepsilon[t]$ represents random noise due to model uncertainty and fluctuations of protein interactions with the target protein [23, 24].

12.2.4
Identification of Interactions in the Initial Protein–Protein Interaction Network

Before modification of the initial network, the interaction parameters of the initial network were estimated using maximum likelihood estimation. These parameters represent the interactions of all possible protein candidates in the initial network. After further rearrangement, Equation (12.1) can be rewritten as:

$$x[t+1] = \begin{bmatrix} x[t] & x_1[t] & \cdots & x_N[t] & x_{12}[t] & \cdots & x_{(N-1)N}[t] & 1 \end{bmatrix} \cdot \begin{bmatrix} a \\ b_1 \\ \vdots \\ b_N \\ c_{12} \\ \vdots \\ c_{(N-1)N} \\ k \end{bmatrix} + \varepsilon[t]$$

$$\equiv \phi[t] \cdot \theta + \varepsilon[t]$$

(12.3)

where $\phi[t]$ denotes the regression vector composed of elements that represent the expression levels of protein candidates in the initial network at time t.

Using the cubic spline method to interpolate microarray data makes it possible to obtain as many data points as needed [28, 29, 35]. In general, the number of data points should be at least five times the number of parameters to be estimated. The cubic spline method yields the following values: $\{x[t] \quad x_i[t_l] \quad x_j[t_l]\}$ for $l \in \{1\,2\,\cdots\,M\}$ and $i \in \{1\,2\,\cdots\,N\}$, $j \in \{1\,2\,\cdots\,S\}$, where M denotes the number of microarray data points, N the number of possible protein interactions for the target protein, and S the number of protein complexes in the network. These data points are used as the basis of a regression vector $\phi[t]$. By computing Equation (12.3) at different points in time, the following vector equation can be constructed:

$$\begin{bmatrix} x[t_2] \\ x[t_3] \\ \vdots \\ x[t_{M-1}] \\ x[t_M] \end{bmatrix} = \begin{bmatrix} \phi[t_1] \\ \phi[t_2] \\ \vdots \\ \phi[t_{M-2}] \\ \phi[t_{M-1}] \end{bmatrix} \cdot \theta + \begin{bmatrix} \varepsilon[t_1] \\ \varepsilon[t_2] \\ \vdots \\ \varepsilon[t_{M-2}] \\ \varepsilon[t_{M-1}] \end{bmatrix} \quad (12.4)$$

For simplicity, this can be represented as:

$$X = \Phi \cdot \theta + v \quad (12.5)$$

In Equation (12.4), the random noise term $\varepsilon[t_k]$ is regarded as white Gaussian noise with zero mean and unknown variance σ^2, that is, $E\{v\} = 0$ and $\Sigma_v = E\{vv^T\} = \sigma^2 I$. Next, a maximum likelihood estimation method [33, 34] was used to estimate θ and σ^2 using regression data obtained from the microarray data for the target protein and the proteins with which it interacts. Under the assumption that v is a Gaussian noise vector with $M-1$ elements, its probability density function can be written as follows:

$$p(v) = \left[(2\pi)^{M-1} \det\Sigma_v\right]^{-1/2} \exp\left(-\tfrac{1}{2} v^T \Sigma_v^{-1} v\right) \quad (12.6)$$

Because $v = X - \Phi \cdot \theta$ (12.5), Equation (12.6) can be rewritten as:

$$p(\theta, \sigma^2) = (2\pi\sigma^2)^{-(M-1)/2} \exp\left\{-\frac{(X-\Phi\cdot\theta)^T(X-\Phi\cdot\theta)}{2\sigma^2}\right\} \quad (12.7)$$

Maximum likelihood parameter estimation involves finding θ and σ^2, which maximize the likelihood function in Equation (12.7). To simplify the computation, it is practical to take the logarithm of Equation (12.7), which yields the following log-likelihood function:

$$\log L(\theta, \sigma^2) = -\frac{M-1}{2}\log(2\pi\sigma^2) - \frac{1}{2\sigma^2}\sum_{k=1}^{M-1}[x[t_k]-\phi[t_k]\cdot\theta]^2 \quad (12.8)$$

In Equation (12.8), $x[t_k]$ and $\phi[t_k]$ are the k-th elements of X and Φ, respectively. Here, the log-likelihood function can be expected to have maxima at $\theta = \hat{\theta}$ and $\sigma^2 = \hat{\sigma}^2$. The necessary conditions for determining the maximum likelihood estimates $\hat{\theta}$ and $\hat{\sigma}^2$ are [33, 34]:

$$\begin{aligned} \frac{\partial \log L(\theta, \sigma^2)}{\partial \theta} &= 0 \\ \frac{\partial \log L(\theta, \sigma^2)}{\partial \sigma^2} &= 0 \end{aligned} \quad (12.9)$$

After some computational manipulations based on Equation (12.9), the estimated parameters $\hat{\theta}$ and $\hat{\sigma}^2$ can be written as:

$$\hat{\theta} = (\Phi^T \Phi)^{-1} \Phi^T X \tag{12.10}$$

$$\hat{\sigma}^2 = \frac{1}{M-1} \sum_{k=1}^{M-1} [x[t_k] - \phi[t_k] \cdot \hat{\theta}]^2 = \frac{1}{M-1} (X - \Phi \cdot \hat{\theta})^T (X - \Phi \cdot \hat{\theta}) \tag{12.11}$$

After obtaining the estimate of $\hat{\theta}$, the estimated protein–protein interaction (12.1) can be rewritten as:

$$x[t+1] = \hat{a}x[t] + \sum_{i=1}^{N} \hat{b}_i x_i[t] + \sum_{i=1}^{N} \sum_{j=1}^{N} \hat{c}_{ij} x_{ij}[t] + \hat{k} \tag{12.12}$$

The interactions of all candidate proteins were quantified by the process described above. In Equation (12.12), the estimated parameter $\hat{a}$ denotes the estimated target protein residual, the estimated parameter $\hat{b}_i$ denotes the rate of individual interaction or binary protein–protein interaction between protein i and the target protein, and the estimated parameter $\hat{c}_{ij}$ denotes the cooperative interaction rate or the degree of protein–complex membership between protein i and protein j, that is, protein complex ij, with the target protein. A positive value implies positive interaction, a negative value implies negative interaction, and the interactions become more likely as the parameters get larger.

12.2.5
Modification of Initial PPI Networks

Although the maximum likelihood estimation method can help quantify the interactive abilities of all possible candidates with the target protein, it is still not known at what level of significance the interactive ability can be regarded as a true interaction. To achieve the goal of determining whether a protein interaction is significant, a statistical approach involving model validation is proposed for evaluating the significance of interactive abilities and for pruning the rough PPI network. In this study, a statistical approach called the Akaike information criterion (AIC) is used to validate the model order (the number of model parameters) to determine the significant interactions in the PPI network [33, 34].

The AIC, which attempts to include both the estimated residual variance and the model complexity in one statistic for model order detection in system identification, decreases as the residual variance $\hat{\sigma}^2$ decreases and increases as the number P of parameters increases. Because the expected residual variance decreases with increasing P for inadequate model complexities, the criterion should reach a minimum at approximately the correct number P of interaction parameters in the network. For fitting a protein-interaction model with P interaction parameters and with data from N samples, the AIC can be written as follows [33, 34]:

$$\text{AIC}(p) = \log\left(\frac{1}{N}(X - \hat{X})^T (X - \hat{X})\right) + \frac{2P}{N} \tag{12.13}$$

where $\hat{X}$ denotes the estimated expression profile of the target protein, that is, $\hat{X} = \phi \cdot \hat{\theta}$. After the statistical selection of P parameters by minimizing the AIC, that is, $\min_P \text{AIC}(P)$, it can easily be determined whether a protein interaction is a significant one or just a false positive, and thereby a refined PPI network can be constructed.

In the AIC detection results obtained in this study, protein i interacts with protein j if the protein interaction is within P significant interactions, and protein i does not interact with protein j if the interaction is outside P significant interactions. However, PPI networks represent a mutual binding relationship: if protein i binds to protein j, then protein j also binds to protein i. To determine mutual relationships in high-false-positive yeast-two-hybrid experiments, an algorithm was used that specifies that two proteins interact only if each protein binds to the other protein. In other words, an interaction is considered only if AIC detection results are both within P significant interactions when each partner is considered as the target protein. If an interaction exists in cancer cells but not in normal cells, the interaction is called "gain-of-function." If the interaction exists in normal cells but not in cancer cells, it is called "loss-of-function." Protein complexes are considered only once due to the incompleteness of the information from web sites. Iteratively, interactions can be pruned one protein at a time in the rough protein network using a similar procedure. Finally, a refined PPI network of human cancer or normal cells can be constructed.

All MATLAB programs can be downloaded [33]. Readers can simulate other target proteins using a similar procedure.

12.3
Results

12.3.1
Construction of a Cancer-Perturbed PPI Network for Apoptosis

Comprehensive protein–protein interactions in an organism provide a framework for understanding biology as an integrated system, and human-perturbed PPI networks offer insight into disease mechanisms such as cancer at a systems level [6, 11]. Before cancer-perturbed PPI networks can be investigated to determine their roles in the mechanisms of cancer, PPI networks for both cancer and normal cells must first be constructed and compared.

Available PPI datasets were downloaded from various web sites, including yeast-two-hybrid experiments, literature, and predictions, and used to construct a rough network. Well-known proteins involved in apoptosis were selected as the core nodes in the PPI network, including BAX (BCL2-associated X protein), BCL2 (B-cell CLL/lymphoma 2), BID (BH3-interacting domain death agonist), CASP3 (caspase-3), BIRC4 (baculoviral IAP repeat-containing 4), CASP9 (caspase-9), CYCS (cytochrome c, somatic), and DIABLO (diablo homolog, *Drosophila*). A rough PPI network for apoptosis was then constructed, containing 207 protein nodes and 841 PPI edges, to investigate the apoptosis mechanism and differential PPIs between human HeLa cervical carcinoma cells and primary lung fibroblasts. Each protein interaction was calculated twice, once when each partner was considered as the target protein. The

PPI networks for apoptosis in cancer and normal cells contain, respectively, 183 protein nodes and 552 edges, and 175 nodes and 547 edges, as drawn in Osprey 1.2.0 [36]. If an interaction does not exist in normal cells, but does exist in cancer cells, it is called "gain of function;" if the interaction exists in normal cells, but not in cancer cells, it is called "loss of function." Among 841 interactions, 157 interactions were classified as "gains of function" and 162 as "losses of function," or 18.7% and 19.3%, respectively, of all interactions. As can be seen, about 38% of all PPIs involved in apoptosis provide blueprints for finding possible drug targets.

To confirm these truncated PPI networks and to gain confidence in the results, false-positive and false-negative rates were calculated among the 85 BCL2-interactive proteins shown as a representative example in Figure 12.2. The BCL2-interactive proteins in normal cells were compared with the HPRD [19] and with the literature. The 85 BCL2-interactive proteins included 18 BCL2-interactive proteins found only in the literature (CAMLG, MAPK3, TGM2, ADM, CDH2, KITLG, EGFR, CEBPB, SERPINB9, TP53, PCNA, MITF, ABCB1, PPP2CA, BCL6, ZNF384, CEBPA, and VEGF), 14 found only in the HRPD (TOMM20, NRAS, FKBP8, BNIP1, PPP3CA, PKMYT1, SMN1, TEGT, HRK, HRAS, RTN4, PSEN1, PPP2R5A, and BNIP3), one found only in the present research (BAG5), four found in the HPRD and in the literature (BAK1, PIN1, BNIP2, and BAD), 30 found in the present research and in the literature (TNF, IGFBP3, CCR5, WT1, DEK, GRN, NPM1, MYC, ALK, DAPK1, CD69, NFKB2, BCR, MSH2, BCL2L1, FGFR1, TERT, CAPN2, TNFRSF6, CDH1, GHR, ERBB2, MKI67, IGF1, CSF1R, CDKN1B, MAPK1, TGFB1, MAP3K1, and

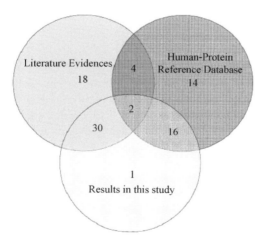

Figure 12.2 Eighty-five BCL2-interacting proteins identified from the results of this research, from the HPRD (Human Protein Reference Database), and from the literature. The 85 BCL2-interactive proteins include 18 found only in the literature, 14 found only in the HRPD (false negative), one found only in the results of this research (false positive), four found in the HPRD and in the literature (false negative), 30 found in the results of this research and in the literature, 16 found in the results of this research and in the HPRD, and two found in the results of this research, in the HPRD, and in the literature.

CLC), 16 found in the present research and in the HPRD (BAG3, BAG4, BCL2L14, ADPRT, BAG1, RAF1, BLK, RASD1, BID, ITM2B, HSPA1A, CYCS, KRAS2, BCL2L11, BNIP3L, and BIK), and two found in the present research, in the HPRD, and in the literature (CASP3 and BAX).

After refinement by the authors' algorithms, the false-positive rate was reduced to 1.16%, which indicates the success of the refinement procedure used. However, the false-negative rate was 41.87%, meaning that the construction of the network from current experiments and databases was incomplete. Therefore, the compensation using k in Equation (12.1) plays an important role in parameter estimation, because the current human PPIs are far from saturation.

12.3.2
Prediction of Apoptosis Drug Targets by Means of Cancer-Perturbed PPI Networks for Apoptosis

Systems-based drug design, which constructs disease-perturbed PPI networks and identifies drug targets by comparing cancer and normal networks, is one of the major applications of systems biology [6, 37, 38]. Several cancer therapies that reflect the traditional scientific approach of reducing cellular processes to their individual components or signal transduction pathways are targeted towards a specific molecule or signaling pathway to inhibit tumor growth. However, the behaviors of most biological systems, including those affected in cancer, cannot be attributed to a single molecule or pathway; rather, they emerge as a result of interactions at multiple levels and among many components [37]. Therefore, it is possible to construct a disease-perturbed gene regulatory network from these disease-perturbed microarray data. Moreover, through a comparison with the normal gene regulatory network derived from normal microarray data, it is possible to deduce drug targets through a process of systems biology-based cancer drug target discovery. By summing the degrees of perturbation, the perturbed protein hubs of the PPI network for cancer cells can be determined from a systematic perspective (Table 12.1). Once the target proteins of inhibitors or activators have been identified, a new level of knowledge will be needed about how a drug target is wired into the control circuitry of a complex cellular network [39]. Figure 12.3 illustrates a flow chart for identification and prediction of apoptosis drug targets in cancer drug discovery. Protein candidates with a degree of perturbation ≥ 5 were chosen, as shown in Figure 12.3, which represents the number of links associated with nodes that have been perturbed.

Once rough PPI networks had been built from large-scale experiments and databases, each microarray dataset of human HeLa cervical carcinoma cells and primary lung fibroblasts was used to prune the established PPI networks using the nonlinear stochastic model and the Akaike information criteria (AIC) to construct more precise PPI networks for cancer and normal cells. Then it was possible to compare cancer and normal networks, to derive gain- and loss-of-function networks, and to identify protein hubs with a high degree of perturbation in the network as apoptosis drug targets. Because scale-free networks are extremely sensitive to removal of targeted hubs, that is, they have high attack vulnerability [11, 40], the

Table 12.1 Gain- and loss-of-function proteins ranked by the sum of the degree of perturbation ≥9.

Protein targets	Sum of degree of perturbation	Gain-of-function proteins	Loss-of-function proteins	Agents
BCL2	35	ABCB1, ADM, BAD, BAG2, BCL6, CCND1, EGFR, HRK, KITLG, MAPK3, MCL1, MITF, PCNA, PKMYT1, PPP2R5A, TP53, VEGF, ZNF384	BAG4, BAG5, BCL2L14, BLK, BNIP3L, CAPN2, CDKN1A, CDKN1B, CLC, DEK, GHR, GRN, MAP3K1, RAF1, RTN4, TNF, WT1	G3139 (Genasense), ABT-737
CASP3	22	BAK1, BID, CASP2, CTSC, DFFA, GORASP1, GSK3B, HSPB2, SERPINB9	BIRC5, CFLAR, DEDD, HCLS1, HSPE1, IGF1, DE5A, PICALM, PRKCD, SREBF2, TGM2, TRAF1, TRAF3	Synthetic activators of caspases/apoptin/surviving
BAX	17	BCL2L1, BCL2L10, MFN2, TP53	ADPRT, APC, APP, BCL2A1, CASP2, CDKN1A, MAPK11, MCL1, RARG, RNF36, PRKCE, TGFBR2, TNFRSF5	Gene therapy through Bax vectors
TP53	17	BAX, BCL2, BID, CCND1, ERBB2, MYC, PEG3, TNFRSF6	APC, BIRC5, CDC42, CDH1, EGFR, GHR, MSH2, PML, PSEN1	ONY-015/INGN201/MDM2 inhibitors
BCL2L1	13	AVEN, BAG2, BAG4, BAX, BCL2L11, HRK, MCL1	BAK1, CASP9, CYCS, PSEN1, MAP3K1, RTN4, BCL2L14	Antisense BCL-xL
CDKN1A	13	BAD, IGF1, SP1, ZNF384	BAX, BCL2, CCND1, CDKN1B, CEBPA, IFNG, MAPK8, MCL1, TGFB1	
TNF	10	IKBKB, MMP1, PRKCD, PTEN	BCL2, BID, CASP7, MAPK3, MAPK8, MMP9	
EGFR	9	BCL2, CASP1, PTEN, VEGF	BCL2L11, CDH1, TP53, MAP3K14, TP53	Trastuzumab (Herceptin)
MAPK1	9	IGF1, NFKB1, PRKCD, SREBF2	CASP9, KRAS2, PEA15 PRKCE, SP1	CI-1040/PD0 325 901/ARRY-142 886
MAPK3	9	BIRC3, CEBPA, MAPK1, MAPK3, TNF	CASP9, EGFR, SREBF2, TNF	CI-1040/PD0 325 901/ARRY-142 886
MYC	9	ALK, CCND1, CDC6, TP53	CAMLG, CEBPA, CLC, DAPK1, ERBB2	Bortezomib (proteosome inhibitors)

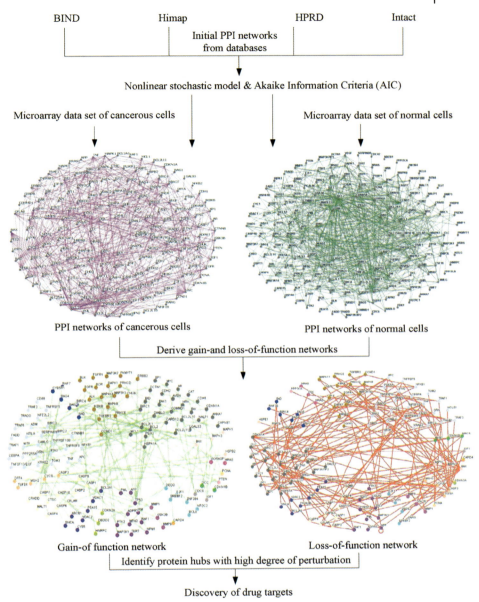

Figure 12.3 Flow chart for drug target identification from a cancer-perturbed protein–protein interaction network by means microarray data. The apoptotic PPI networks show 183 nodes and 552 edges, and 175 nodes and 547 edges, for HeLa cancerous cells and normal primary lung fibroblasts, respectively. The "gain-of-function" network shows 140 nodes and 157 edges, and the "loss-of-function" network shows 126 nodes and 162 edges. All protein–protein interaction networks in this study were constructed using Osprey version 1.2.0.

degree of perturbation (i.e., connectivity) of each node in the cancer-perturbed PPI network was summed to identify these perturbed hubs. The proteins with a degree of perturbation ≥9 were listed, as shown in Table 12.1, to identify the perturbed protein hubs that differentiate cancer and normal interactomes, which would be the most promising apoptosis-drug target proteins based on robustness-oriented drug design [5, 37]. Eleven possible drug target proteins in Table 12.1 could be grouped into six categories: common pathway: CASP3; extrinsic pathway: TNF; intrinsic pathway: BCL2, BAX, and BCL2L1; apoptosis regulators: TP53, MYC, and EGFR; stress-induced signaling: MAPK1 and MAPK3; and others: CDKN1A.

12.3.2.1 Common Pathway: CASP3

Caspases are the central components of the apoptotic response as a conserved family of enzymes that irreversibly commit a cell to die. An effector caspase such as caspase-3 is activated by an initiator caspase such as caspase-9, and the initiator caspase is activated through regulated PPIs [9, 41]. Targeting inhibitors of caspases can activate caspases and then lead a cancer cell to apoptosis. These agents include synthetic activators of caspases, apoptin, and IAP (inhibitor of apoptosis) targets such as survivin [42, 43]. Caspase-3 is subject to inhibition by IAPs such as Livin [9]. Like BCL-2 inhibitors, XIAP inhibitors must block PPIs. When released from mitochondria, Smac binds with XIAP and inactivates it, triggering apoptosis [44].

12.3.2.2 Extrinsic Pathway and Cross-Talk: TNF

The extrinsic pathway activated by death receptors including FAS (TNFRSF6/APO-1/CD95) and other TNF receptor family members provides the role of apoptosis in maintaining tissue homeostasis [8]. Although the death receptors of TNF (tumor-necrosis factor) superfamily members represent potential drug targets for promoting apoptosis in cancer, soluble TNF and agonistic anti-FAS antibodies and toxic side effects have been observed with these agents, and this has limited their therapeutic use [4].

12.3.2.3 Intrinsic Pathway: BCL2, BAX, and BCL2L1

Defective apoptosis in human cancers often results from overexpression or inhibition of BCL2 protein family members, which regulate the mitochondrial permeability transition by inhibiting (as with BCL2 and BCL2L1) or promoting (as with BAX and BID) the release of cytochrome c (CYCS) [43, 45]. BCL2 and several pro-survival or anti-apoptotic relatives such as BCL2L1 associate with the mitochondrial outer membrane and the endoplasmic reticulum nuclear membrane and maintain their integrity. Initiation of apoptosis requires not only pro-apoptotic family members such as BAX that closely resemble BCL2, but also distant cousins that are related only by the small BH3 protein-interaction domain [46]. In the results of this research, proteins with gain-of-function interactions with BCL2 include CCND1, BAD, MCL1, MAPK3, ADM, KITLG, EGFR, BAG2, PKMYT1, TP53, PCNA, MITF, ABCB1, BCL6, ZNF384, HRK, PPP2R5A, and VEGF, while proteins with loss-of-function interactions with BCL2 include CDKN1A, TNF, WT1, BAG4, BCL2L14, DEK, GRN, RAF1, BLK, BAG5, CAPN2, GHR, CDKN1B, RTN4, BNIP3L, MAP3K1, and CLC

(Table 12.1). BCL2 can be predicted to be the most promising apoptosis drug target because of its specificity to cancer cells based on systems-biology-based drug design, because BCL2 primarily differentiates PPI networks between cultured cancer and normal cells [6, 37, 45].

The present results agree with previous studies that BCL2 protein family members are drug targets for cancer therapy in apoptosis pathways such as BCL2 antisense Genasense [4, 42]. The activation of pro-apoptotic Bax protein can be induced by gene therapy through delivery of Bax vectors, and this approach has been successful in inducing apoptosis in cancer cell lines. Antisense BCL2L1 (BCL-xL) downregulates the expression of BCL2 and BCL2L1, induces apoptosis, and inhibits growth of different tumor types both *in vitro* and *in vivo* [42]. The biggest question about targeting BCL-2 is side effects, because many normal cells are dependent on BCL-2 family members to maintain mitochondrial function. The deficiency of antisense as a delivery system is also a problem in Genasense targeting BCL-2 [44].

12.3.2.4 Apoptosis Regulators: TP53, MYC, and EGFR

One of the most dramatic responses to p53 is induction of apoptosis and regulation of the intrinsic pathway [47]. The key contribution of p53 to apoptosis is the induction of the expression of genes that encode apoptotic proteins, functioning in both extrinsic and intrinsic pathways. Trials to target p53 as a cancer therapy include gene therapy involving ONYX-015 and INGN201 and antisense therapy to the target protein that controls p53 activity by nutlins which blocks p53/MDM2 interaction [4, 42]. The proto-oncogene c-MYC encodes a transcription factor that is implicated in various cellular processes, including cell growth, proliferation, loss of differentiation, and apoptosis. The induction of cell-cycle entry sensitizes the cell to apoptosis; in other words, cell-proliferative and apoptotic pathways are coupled [48]. Some agents, for example, agent ZD1839 for EGFR (epidermal growth factor receptor) inhibitors, do not primarily target apoptosis, but modulate apoptosis indirectly [42].

12.3.2.5 Stress-Induced Signaling: MAPK1 and MAPK3

Cells are continuously exposed to various environmental stresses and have to decide on survival or death depending on the types and strength of stress. MAPK family members are crucial for the maintenance of cells among many signaling pathways [49]. Three MEK (MAPK kinase) inhibitors, CI-1040, PD0 325 901, and ARRY-142 886, have been significantly developed in clinical trials [50]. Although some drug targets inhibit MAPK (mitogen-activated protein kinase), MAPK1 (ERK or p38) and MAPK3 (ERK1) are not the main drug targets in the apoptotic pathway [42].

12.3.2.6 Others: CDKN1A

CDKN1A (p21) (cyclin-dependent kinase inhibitor-1) plays a role in cell-cycle arrest and induction of apoptosis. The activities of cyclin D- and cyclin E-dependent kinases are linked through the Cip/Kip family of Cdk inhibitors, including p27 and p21 [51]. CCND1 is cyclin D1 in the G1/S transition of the cell cycle and is controlled by the tumor suppressor gene RB through cdk-cyclin D complexes [52].

12.3.3
Prediction of More Apoptosis Drug Targets by Decreasing the Degree of Perturbation

12.3.3.1 Prediction of More Cancer Drug Targets by Decreasing the Degree of Perturbation

In addition to identifying several apoptosis drug targets and comparing these targets with other studies, the method developed here can be used to predict more possible drug targets by decreasing the threshold of the degree of perturbation. For example, if the threshold of the degree of perturbation is set equal to 8 in Table 12.1, there are six more proteins among the predicted apoptosis drug targets: BID, CASP9, CCND1, CFLAR, CYCS, and TNFRSF6. If the threshold is set to 7, there are seven more proteins among the predicted apoptosis drug targets: BAK1, CASP2, BCL2A1, IGF1, PRKCD, NFKB1, and PCNA. Caspase-3 and caspase-9 are subject to inhibition by IAPs such as Livin [9]. Like BCL-2 inhibitors, XIAP inhibitors must block PPIs. When released from mitochondria, Smac binds XIAP and inactivates it, triggering apoptosis [44]. NFKB1 has both anti- and pro-apoptotic functions depending on the nature of the death stimulus, and the drug PS11 445 targets the NFKB1 inhibitor IKKβ [42]. Besides NFKB1, some possible drug targets are indicated above, such as BAK1 (BAX family, pro-apoptosis), BCL2A1 (Bcl-2 family, pro-survival), CASP2 (caspase 2, initiator caspase), and IGF1 (insulin-like growth factor, anti-apoptosis).

12.3.3.2 Prediction of New GO Annotations of the Four Proteins: CDKN1A, CCND, PRKCD, and PCNA

If all 24 proteins with the sum of their degrees of perturbation ≥ 7 are listed, there are four proteins, CDKN1A, CCND1, PRKCD, and PCNA (proliferating cell nuclear antigen), which are not inferred for apoptosis by gene ontology (GO) annotations. If the function of any one protein in the network is known, identification of its interacting partners will predict the function of some or all of the partners [11]. Therefore, the four proteins, CDKN1A, CCND, PCNA, and PRKCD, can be predicted using new gene ontology annotations for apoptosis. However, two proteins, PCNA and PRKCD, have been identified in DNA-damage-induced apoptosis. The protein PCNA is ubiquitinated and involved in the RAD6-dependent DNA repair pathway in response to DNA damage. If DNA damage is too significant, a cell may opt for apoptosis instead of repair of lesions [53]. The other protein, PRKCD (protein kinase C, delta), has been identified in association with DNA-damage-induced apoptosis that acts both upstream and downstream [54], whereas gene-ontology annotations of PRKCD do not contain apoptosis.

This research has provided not only efficient and precise methods to predict cancer drug targets but also a way to specify these target proteins using detailed gene-ontology annotations, which should help researchers explore more drug targets using other mechanisms such as the cell cycle. However, current time-series microarray datasets for cancer and normal cells are still insufficient, which limits the methods developed here to comparing different protein hubs among different cancer cell types. Side effects and problems in drug delivery also cannot be predicted by this method. Therefore, more genomic time-series microarray experiments and clinical research should be performed in future.

12.4
Apoptosis Mechanism at the Systems Level

This section investigates the apoptosis mechanism at the systems level and elucidates the cancer-perturbed PPI network topology (Figure 12.4). Evading apoptosis is one of the acquired capabilities of cancer cells. In many cancers, pro-apoptotic proteins are inactivated or anti-apoptotic proteins are up-regulated, leading to unchecked growth of tumors and inability to respond to cellular stress, harmful mutations, and DNA damage [4]. These gain- and loss-of-function mutations in cancer cells lead to aberrances in PPI networks. The correlations of interactome and genomic data developed in this work should provide a clearer understanding of the functional relationships underlying biological processes [7, 11].

12.4.1
Caspase Family and Caspase Regulators

The final execution of the death signal is activated through a series of protease caspases, including initiator caspase-2, -8, -9, -10 and effector caspase-3, -6, -7, which are all produced in cells as catalytically inactive zymogens and must undergo proteolytic activation during apoptosis [9, 41]. Most caspases, including CASP1, CASP2, CASP4, CASP7, CASP9, and CASP10, are found in both gain-of-function and loss-of-function networks, except for CASP6, which is present only in gain-of-function networks. Seven

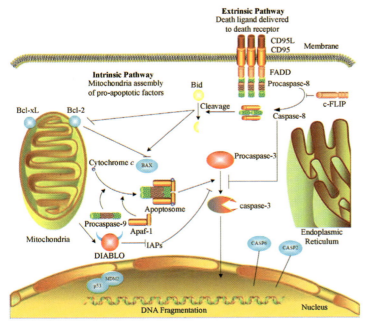

Figure 12.4 Global apoptosis mechanism.

caspase activators, inhibitors, and activity regulators – BAX, TP53, CFLAR, CYCS, CARD4, BIRC4, and DIABLO – are present both in gain- and loss-of-function networks. Proteins of caspase regulators in gain-of-function networks include CARD12, TNFRSF10B, AVEN, BCL2L10, MALT1, DFFA, NALP1, and CRADD, while proteins of caspase regulators in loss-of-function networks are BIRC5 and HSPE1, revealing the differential roles of caspase regulators between cancer and normal cells.

12.4.2
Extrinsic Pathway, Intrinsic Pathway, and Cross-Talk

The extrinsic pathway (death-receptor pathway) is triggered by members of the death receptor superfamily using extracellular signals that initiate apoptosis when death receptors recruit caspase-8 through the adapter protein FAS (TNFRSF6)-associated death domain (FADD) [8]. Binding of a death ligand to a death receptor triggers formation of a death-inducing signaling complex and leads to caspase-8 or caspase-10 activation and subsequent caspase-3 activation and cell death [55]. The intrinsic pathway (mitochondrial pathway) is triggered extensively in response to extracellular and internal stress where these diverse response pathways converge on mitochondria through activation of pro-apoptotic members of the Bcl-2 family which arbitrate the life-or-death decision [41, 45]. Cross-talk between extrinsic and intrinsic pathways is provided by Bid, a pro-apoptotic Bcl-2 family member [56]. Three subfamilies of Bcl-2 related proteins include anti-apoptotic proteins (such as BCL2 and BCL2L1), pro-apoptotic multidomain proteins (such as BAX and BAK), and members of the pro-apoptotic BH3-only protein family (such as BID and BIM) [9, 10, 46].

12.4.3
Regulation of Apoptosis at the Systems Level

Besides Bcl-2 and caspase family members, the proteins involved in apoptosis regulation include BIRC3, PTEN, CARD12, MAP3K7, DEDD2, MITF, MALT1, BCL6, NALP1, and CRADD, as seen in the gain-of-function network, as well as RTN4, PSEN1, IGFBP3, BNIP3L, and RARG, as seen in the loss-of-function network, and CFLAR, TRAF3, TRAF1, MCL1, CARD4, TRAF6, VEGF, BIRC2, FGFR1, PEA15, DEDD, MMP9, HRK, and TP53, as seen in both gain- and loss-of-function networks. Therefore, 29 proteins other than Bcl-2 family and caspase family members also regulate apoptosis at the systems level, creating a process like a tug of war in a cell between survival and death.

12.5
Conclusions

Construction of cancer-perturbed PPIs for apoptosis has shed light on the disease mechanisms at a systems level, generating results that could be applied for drug target discovery. In this study, a nonlinear stochastic model was used to describe individual and cooperative protein interactions with a target protein. This model is more precise in PPI computation compared with the linear models presented in previous literature. Microarray and proteome datasets have been successfully integrated to delineate the cancer-perturbed PPI apoptosis networks, which illustrate the apoptosis mechanism at the systems level and which can predict apoptosis drug targets using data from the literature. The predictions of cancer apoptosis drug targets developed here are highly coordinated with the current apoptosis cancer drug discovery process, which should help researchers find more possible drug targets for other mechanisms in future work.

References

1 Hanash, S. (2004) Integrated global profiling of cancer. *Nat. Rev. Cancer*, **4**, 638–644.
2 Rhodes, D.R., Kalyana-Sundaram, S., Mahavisno, V., Barrette, T.R., Ghosh, D., and Chinnaiyan, A.M. (2005) Mining for regulatory programs in the cancer transcriptome. *Nat. Genet.*, **37**, 579–583.
3 Hahn, W.C. and Weinberg, R.A. (2002) Modelling the molecular circuitry of cancer. *Nat. Rev. Cancer*, **2**, 331–341.
4 Fesik, S.W. (2005) Promoting apoptosis as a strategy for cancer drug discovery. *Nat. Rev. Cancer*, **5**, 876–885.
5 Kitano, H. (2007) A robustness-based approach to systems-oriented drug design. *Nat. Rev. Drug Discovery*, **6**, 202–210.
6 Hood, L., Heath, J.R., Phelps, M.E., and Lin, B. (2004) Systems biology and new technologies enable predictive and preventative medicine. *Science*, **306**, 640–643.
7 Hornberg, J.J., Bruggeman, F.J., Westerhoff, H.V., and Lankelma, J. (2006) Cancer: a systems biology disease. *Biosystems*, **83**, 81–90.
8 Danial, N.N. and Korsmeyer, S.J. (2004) Cell death: critical control points. *Cell*, **116**, 205–219.
9 Riedl, S.J. and Shi, Y. (2004) Molecular mechanisms of caspase regulation during apoptosis. *Nat. Rev. Mol. Cell Biol.*, **5**, 897–907.
10 Herr, I. and Debatin, K.M. (2001) Cellular stress response and apoptosis in cancer therapy. *Blood*, **98**, 2603–2614.
11 Cusick, M.E., Klitgord, N., Vidal, M., and Hill, D.E. (2005) Interactome: gateway into systems biology. *Hum. Mol. Genet.*, **14** (Spec No. 2), R171–R181.
12 Han, J.D., Bertin, N., Hao, T., Goldberg, D.S., Berriz, G.F., Zhang, L.V., Dupuy, D., Walhout, A.J., Cusick, M.E., Roth, F.P., and Vidal, M. (2004) Evidence for dynamically organized modularity in the yeast protein-protein interaction network. *Nature*, **430**, 88–93.
13 Huber, W., Carey, V.J., Long, L., Falcon, S., and Gentleman, R. (2007) Graphs in molecular biology. *BMC Bioinformatics*, **8** (Suppl. 6), S8.
14 Levy, E.D. and Pereira-Leal, J.B. (2008) Evolution and dynamics of protein interactions and networks. *Curr. Opin. Struct. Biol.*, **18**, 349–357.
15 Rual, J.F., Venkatesan, K., Hao, T., Hirozane-Kishikawa, T., Dricot, A., Li, N., Berriz, G.F., Gibbons, F.D., Dreze, M., Ayivi-Guedehoussou, N. et al. (2005) Towards a proteome-scale map of the human protein-protein interaction network. *Nature*, **437**, 1173–1178.
16 Stelzl, U., Worm, U., Lalowski, M., Haenig, C., Brembeck, F.H., Goehler, H., Stroedicke, M., Zenkner, M., Schoenherr, A., Koeppen, S. et al. (2005) A human protein-protein interaction network: a resource for annotating the proteome. *Cell*, **122**, 957–968.
17 Bader, G.D., Betel, D., and Hogue, C.W. (2003) BIND: the Biomolecular Interaction Network Database. *Nucleic Acids Res.*, **31**, 248–250.

18 Rhodes, D.R. and Chinnaiyan, A.M. (2005) Integrative analysis of the cancer transcriptome. *Nat. Genet.*, **37** (Suppl.), S31–S37

19 Peri, S., Navarro, J.D., Amanchy, R., Kristiansen, T.Z., Jonnalagadda, C.K., Surendranath, V., Niranjan, V., Muthusamy, B., Gandhi, T.K., Gronborg, M. *et al.* (2003) Development of human protein reference database as an initial platform for approaching systems biology in humans. *Genome Res.*, **13**, 2363–2371.

20 Hermjakob, H., Montecchi-Palazzi, L., Lewington, C., Mudali, S., Kerrien, S., Orchard, S., Vingron, M., Roechert, B., Roepstorff, P., Valencia, A. *et al.* (2004) IntAct: an open source molecular interaction database. *Nucleic Acids Res.*, **32**, D452–D455.

21 Carter, G.W. (2005) Inferring network interactions within a cell. *Brief. Bioinformatics*, **6**, 380–389.

22 Bader, J.S., Chaudhuri, A., Rothberg, J.M., and Chant, J. (2004) Gaining confidence in high-throughput protein interaction networks. *Nat. Biotechnol.*, **22**, 78–85.

23 Chen, B.S., Chang, C.H., and Chuang, Y.J. (2008) Robust model matching control of immune systems under environmental disturbances: dynamic game approach. *J. Theor. Biol.*, **253**, 824–837.

24 Chen, B.S. and Wang, Y.C. (2006) On the attenuation and amplification of molecular noise in genetic regulatory networks. *BMC Bioinformatics*, **7**, 52.

25 Murray, J.I., Whitfield, M.L., Trinklein, N.D., Myers, R.M., Brown, P.O., and Botstein, D. (2004) Diverse and specific gene expression responses to stresses in cultured human cells. *Mol. Biol. Cell*, **15**, 2361–2374.

26 Gandhi, T.K., Zhong, J., Mathivanan, S., Karthick, L., Chandrika, K.N., Mohan, S.S., Sharma, S., Pinkert, S., Nagaraju, S., Periaswamy, B. *et al.* (2006) Analysis of the human protein interactome and comparison with yeast, worm and fly interaction datasets. *Nat. Genet.*, **38**, 285–293.

27 Hood, L. (2003) Systems biology: integrating technology, biology, and computation. *Mech. Ageing Dev.*, **124**, 9–16.

28 Chen, H.C., Lee, H.C., Lin, T.Y., Li, W.H., and Chen, B.S. (2004) Quantitative characterization of the transcriptional regulatory network in the yeast cell cycle. *Bioinformatics*, **20**, 1914–1927.

29 Lin, L.H., Lee, H.C., Li, W.H., and Chen, B.S. (2005) Dynamic modeling of cis-regulatory circuits and gene expression prediction via cross-gene identification. *BMC Bioinformatics*, **6**, 258.

30 Alon, U. (2007) *An Introduction to Systems Biology: Design Principles of Biological Circuits*, Chapman & Hall/CRC, Boca Raton, FL.

31 Klipp, E.H.R., Kowald, A., Wierling, C., and Lehrach, H. (2005) *Systems Biology in Practice. Concepts, Implementation and Application*, Wiley-VCH Verlag GmbH, Weinheim.

32 Chang, Y.H., Wang, Y.C., and Chen, B.S. (2006) Identification of transcription factor cooperativity via stochastic system model. *Bioinformatics*, **22**, 2276–2282.

33 Chu, L.H. and Chen, B.S. (2008) Construction of a cancer-perturbed protein-protein interaction network for discovery of apoptosis drug targets. *BMC Syst. Biol.*, **2**, 56.

34 Johansson, R. (1993) *System Modeling and Identification*, Prentice Hall, Englewood Cliffs, NJ.

35 Chen, B.S., Yang, S.K., Lan, C.Y., and Chuang, Y.J. (2008) A systems biology approach to construct the gene regulatory network of systemic inflammation via microarray and databases mining. *BMC Med. Genomics*, **1**, 46.

36 Breitkreutz, B.J., Stark, C., and Tyers, M. (2003) Osprey: a network visualization system. *Genome Biol.*, **4**, R22.

37 Chen, B.S. and Li, C.H. (2007) Analysing microarray data in drug discovery using systems biology. *Exp. Opin. Drug Discov.*, **2**, 755–768.

38 Hood, L. and Perlmutter, R.M. (2004) The impact of systems approaches on biological problems in drug discovery. *Nat. Biotechnol.*, **22**, 1215–1217.

39 Araujo, R.P., Liotta, L.A., and Petricoin, E.F. (2007) Proteins, drug targets and the mechanisms they control: the simple truth

about complex networks. *Nat. Rev. Drug Discovery*, **6**, 871–880.

40 Pieroni, E., de la Fuente van Bentem, S., Mancosu, G., Capobianco, E., Hirt, H., and de la Fuente, A. (2008) Protein networking: insights into global functional organization of proteomes. *Proteomics*, **8**, 799–816.

41 Youle, R.J. and Strasser, A. (2008) The BCL-2 protein family: opposing activities that mediate cell death. *Nat. Rev. Mol. Cell Biol.*, **9**, 47–59.

42 Ghobrial, I.M., Witzig, T.E., and Adjei, A.A. (2005) Targeting apoptosis pathways in cancer therapy. *CA Cancer J. Clin.*, **55**, 178–194.

43 Andersen, M.H., Becker, J.C., and Straten, P. (2005) Regulators of apoptosis: suitable targets for immune therapy of cancer. *Nat. Rev. Drug Discovery*, **4**, 399–409.

44 Garber, K. (2005) New apoptosis drugs face critical test. *Nat. Biotechnol.*, **23**, 409–411.

45 Adams, J.M. and Cory, S. (2007) The Bcl-2 apoptotic switch in cancer development and therapy. *Oncogene*, **26**, 1324–1337.

46 Cory, S. and Adams, J.M. (2002) The Bcl2 family: regulators of the cellular life-or-death switch. *Nat. Rev. Cancer*, **2**, 647–656.

47 Vousden, K.H. and Lane, D.P. (2007) p53 in health and disease. *Nat. Rev. Mol. Cell Biol.*, **8**, 275–283.

48 Pelengaris, S., Khan, M., and Evan, G. (2002) c-MYC: more than just a matter of life and death. *Nat. Rev. Cancer*, **2**, 764–776.

49 Wada, T. and Penninger, J.M. (2004) Mitogen-activated protein kinases in apoptosis regulation. *Oncogene*, **23**, 2838–2849.

50 Sebolt-Leopold, J.S. and Herrera, R. (2004) Targeting the mitogen-activated protein kinase cascade to treat cancer. *Nat. Rev. Cancer*, **4**, 937–947.

51 Sherr, C.J. and McCormick, F. (2002) The RB and p53 pathways in cancer. *Cancer Cell*, **2**, 103–112.

52 Lewin, B. (2004) *Genes VIII*, Pearson Prentice Hall, Upper Saddle River, NJ.

53 Hoeijmakers, J.H. (2001) Genome maintenance mechanisms for preventing cancer. *Nature*, **411**, 366–374.

54 Basu, A. (2003) Involvement of protein kinase C-delta in DNA damage-induced apoptosis. *J. Cell Mol. Med.*, **7**, 341–350.

55 Riedl, S.J. and Salvesen, G.S. (2007) The apoptosome: signalling platform of cell death. *Nat. Rev. Mol. Cell Biol.*, **8**, 405–413.

56 Kaufmann, T., Tai, L., Ekert, P.G., Huang, D.C., Norris, F., Lindemann, R.K., Johnstone, R.W., Dixit, V.M., and Strasser, A. (2007) The BH3-only protein bid is dispensable for DNA damage- and replicative stress-induced apoptosis or cell-cycle arrest. *Cell*, **129**, 423–433.

13
A New Gene Expression Meta-Analysis Technique and Its Application to Co-Analyze Three Independent Lung Cancer Datasets

Irit Fishel, Alon Kaufman, and Eytan Ruppin

13.1
Background

The following section briefly reviews microarray technology and basic concepts in machine learning. These are the main pillars on which this work resides.

13.1.1
DNA Microarray Technology

The living cell is a dynamic complex system continuously changing through its developmental pathways and in response to various environmental stimuli. Although all cells in a particular organism have identical genome, only some of the genes are expressed (transcribed into mRNA) and in turn translated into proteins according to cell type and functional needs.

Microarray technology has provided researchers with the ability to measure the expression levels of thousands of genes simultaneously. It provides a unique snapshot of the genes in a particular cell type, at a particular time, under particular conditions. A DNA microarray consists of thousands of gene-specific probes embedded orderly at defined positions on an inert surface. RNA molecules extracted from tissue of interest (called *targets*) are labeled with fluorescent dyes and applied to the array for hybridization. After removing non-hybridized material, laser light is used to excite the fluorescent dye and the intensity of hybridization is represented by the fluorescent emission [1].

There are two main types of commercial microarrays, cDNA arrays and oligonucleotide arrays (Affymetrix).

13.1.1.1 cDNA Microarray
cDNA microarrays use cDNA molecules (synthesized DNA that contains only coding part of the sequence, complementary to its corresponding mRNA transcript) as probes to be spotted on the array. The experiment involves the extraction of mRNA molecules from two sample populations: test tissue (e.g., cancerous tissue)

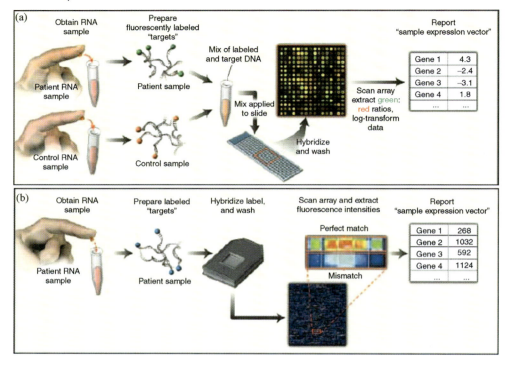

Figure 13.1 Overview of DNA microarray experiment. (a) cDNA microarray experiment: target samples obtained from test (patient samples) and control samples are labeled with distinguishable fluorescent dyes and hybridized to a single DNA microarray. Relative levels of gene expression in the two samples are estimated. (b) Oligonucleotide microarray experiment: labeled target samples are hybridized to a single microarray. Gene-expression levels are estimated by measuring the hybridization intensity for a series of "perfect match" probes corrected by the use of a corresponding set of "mismatch" probes. This figure was taken from Ref. [3].

and control tissue (e.g., normal tissue). The mRNA molecules are reverse-transcribed and simultaneously labeled (each labeled with a different dye). For example, the test samples may be labeled with a green fluorescing dye called Cy3 while the control samples are labeled with a red fluorescing dye called Cy5. The samples are mixed and hybridized in a competitive manner to the probes of the same array. If there are genes up-regulated in the test samples, more Cy3 bind to the complementary probes and the spot will fluoresce green. Conversely, genes with decreased expression in the test sample will fluoresce red. When the two samples have the same amount of expression, the dyes merge and the spot will appear yellow (Figure 13.1a). Importantly, the expression levels of genes evaluated in this method are not absolute but relative compared to a control sample tissue. The expression measurements are reported as the logarithm of the ratio of RNA intensity in a test sample compared to that in a control sample [1–3].

13.1.1.2 Oligonucleotide Microarray

In the oligonucleotide microarrays each gene on the array is represented by 11–16 different oligonucleotides of length 25 base pairs. Each of the oligonucleotide probes is perfect complement to a 25-base-long sub-sequence of the target gene. These probes are selected to have little homology with other genes so that non-specific hybridization will be minimized. To further increase specificity, for each probe on the array a second probe is added. The second probe is identical to the first probe except for a mismatched base at its center. The perfect match/mismatch probe strategy is used for specificity control, enabling the subtraction of background noise and evaluation of unspecific hybridization.

Unlike in cDNA microarrays, the experiment is performed for a single population of samples. Each target mRNA sample is converted into fluorescent cRNA and these are fragmented into sections of average length of 50 base pairs. The targets are hybridized to the array and bound by the various oligonucleotide probes (Figure 13.1b). The level of expression of each target gene is reported as a single fluorescence intensity that represents an estimation of the amount of mRNA in the cell [3, 4].

13.1.2
Machine Learning Background

We start by providing basic definitions and terms in machine learning, we then turn to focus on supervised learning in the context of gene-expression data. We conclude by briefly describing a state-of-the-art algorithm for classification (support vector machines) and for feature selection (support vector machine recursive feature elimination).

13.1.2.1 Basic Definitions and Terms in Machine Learning

The goal of machine learning is to program computers to use example data or past experience to solve a given problem. There are two major paradigms of learning: *supervised* and *unsupervised*. Supervised learning makes use of prior knowledge about the data to be learned whereas unsupervised learning does not require additional information about the data. In the case of supervised learning, *training samples* of known classification *labels* are given in advance to make an *induction algorithm* learn from these samples and produce a *classifier* in the form of a function. The classifier is designed to assign a correct label when applied to unseen data samples. A common procedure in supervised learning is to divide the data samples into a *training set* and a *test set*, construct a classifier based on the training set, and evaluate its *performance or generalization* (i.e., the ability to correctly classify data not in the training set) on the test set. Unsupervised learning techniques do not make use of class labels and the learning task is to gain some understanding of the process that generated the data. This type of learning includes clustering methods which aggregate the data into classes by a similarity measure that defines how close two data objects are [5]. Unsupervised methods are not considered in this work, and we focus our attention on supervised learning methodology.

13.1.2.2 Supervised Learning in the Context of Gene Expression Data

A typical gene expression analysis is based on data originating from a set of microarrays comprising a gene expression dataset. Gene expression datasets are usually displayed as a matrix in which rows correspond to genes and columns to biological samples or experimental conditions. Each element in the gene expression matrix represents the expression level of a single gene in a specific sample. The row vector of a gene is called the expression pattern of that gene. A column vector is called the expression profile of the sample or the condition.

Supervised machine learning techniques aim to obtain a function or a rule that uses a set of genes and their expression pattern to classify the class label of new unseen samples. The class labels, for example, can be normal versus cancerous tissues. The first step to build a classifier is to select an algorithm for classification (e.g., support vector machines) and "train" it on available data. The algorithm uses the expression profiles and the class labels of the samples to learn and build a computational rule that can be applied to a new sample (given its expression profile) and assign it to a biologic class label. Ideally, the trained classifier is applied to a test set of unseen samples to assess its performance.

13.1.3
Support Vector Machines

Support vector machines (SVMs) are supervised methods extensively used in various biological classification tasks, including in gene expression microarray data [6]. SVMs are presently one of the best known classification techniques and have been shown to outperform other classification methods [7].

We shall first formalize the classification task (we restrict ourselves to binary classification) and then introduce the SVMs approach.

The input for supervised algorithms is a training set of samples and their corresponding class labels $S = \{(x_1, y_1), \ldots, (x_l, y_l)\}$, $x_i \in R^n$, $y_i \in (+1, -1)$ (i.e., the training set is made up of "positive" and "negative" samples). The training set is used to build a decision function $f : X \subseteq R^n \rightarrow R$ that is a scalar function of an input sample $x \in X$. New samples are classified according to the sign of the decision function (decision rule):

$$f(x) \geq 0 \quad \text{label}(x) = +1$$
$$f(x) < 0 \quad \text{label}(x) = -1$$

We consider the case where $f(x)$ is a linear function of x, so that it can be written as:

$$f(x) = \langle w \cdot x \rangle + b = \sum_{i=1}^{n} w_i \cdot x_i + b, \quad \text{where} \quad w \in R^n \quad \text{and} \quad b \in R$$

$\langle w \cdot x \rangle + b = 0$ defines a hyperplane that splits the input space X into two parts. We wish to find a hyperplane direction w and an offset scalar b such that $\langle w \cdot x \rangle + b \geq 0$ for positive examples and $\langle w \cdot x \rangle + b < 0$ for negative examples (Figure 13.2).

Assuming the training data is linearly separable, there is more than one separating hyperplane for a given problem (Figure 13.3a). Which among the possible solutions

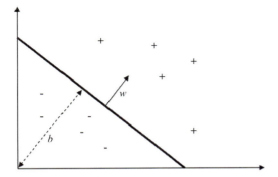

Figure 13.2 A separating hyperplane (w,b) for a two-dimensional training set. The hyperplane (dark line) separates two classes ($+,-$). The vector w defines a direction perpendicular to the hyperplane, while the value of b moves the hyperplane parallel to itself.

has the best generalization properties? The goal is to construct a learning machine that does well on unseen samples. We should note that doing well on the training set does not necessarily guarantee good performance on the test set, thus choosing a decision boundary that lies close to some of the training samples is less likely to generalize well since it is susceptible to small perturbations of those samples. We define the distance between the separating hyperplane and the closest training samples of each class (positive and negative) on both sides the *margin induced by the hyperplane*.

The objective is, therefore, to find a separating hyperplane that maximizes the margin of the training set samples in order to minimize the generalization error (Figure 13.3b). This task can be formulated as the following optimization problem.

Given a linearly separable training set $S = \{(x_1, y_1), \ldots, (x_l, y_l)\}$, the hyperplane ($w, b$) that solves the optimization problem is:

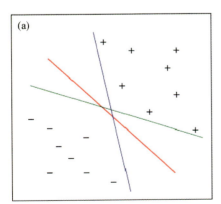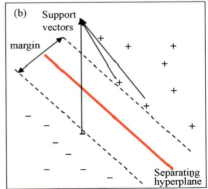

Figure 13.3 (a) There are many possible separating hyperplanes for a given problem. The lines represent the different hyperplanes separating the training set into two classes ($+,-$). (b) The SVM solution aims to find a separating hyperplane that maximizes the margin.

$$\min_{w,b} \langle w \cdot w \rangle$$
subject to $y_j(\langle w \cdot x_j \rangle + b) \geq 1$
$j = 1, \ldots, l$

The weight vector w can also be written as a linear combination of the training samples: $w = \sum_{j=1}^{l} \alpha_j y_j x_j$, where the α_j are Lagrange multipliers (which result from the optimization). Most weights α_j are a zero. The training samples with non-zero weights are called support vectors. Therefore, the resulting linear function $f(x)$ is a linear combination of support vectors only: $f(x) = \langle w \cdot x \rangle + b = \sum_{j=1}^{l} \alpha_j y_j \langle x_j \cdot x \rangle + b$

As noted before this solution requires the training data to be linearly separable. This condition is not always realistic. To allow some flexibility in separating the samples there are SVMs called soft-margin that incorporate a cost parameter that controls the tradeoff between allowing training errors and forcing rigid margins [8].

13.1.4
Support Vector Machine Recursive Feature Elimination

In this work we adopted the SVM-based recursive feature elimination (SVM-RFE) algorithm. SVM-RFE was first proposed by Guyon et al. [9] as a gene selection method that utilizes SVMs for the classification of gene expression data. In each step of the algorithm the least important gene (according to a ranking score) is removed and the remaining genes are re-evaluated. The process terminates when all genes are removed. The absolute values of the components of the weight vector w from a linear SVM are used to determine the importance of the genes. The least important gene refers to the one with the smallest weight value. Genes with high weight values are the most informative and influence significantly the classification decision. The SVM-RFE eliminates gene redundancy and thus yields more compact predictors.

The SVM-RFE procedure used in [9, 10] is as follows:

1) **Inputs**: Training samples with their corresponding class labels: $S = \{(x_1, y_1), \ldots, (x_l, y_l)\}$
2) **Initialization**:

    The gene ranked list : R = [ ]

    Subset of the genes : S = $[1, 2, \ldots, n]$

3) **Repeat**: until S = [ ] (all genes are ranked):
    a. train a linear SVM with all the training samples and genes in S [this step results in output w of length(S)];
    b. compute the ranking scores of genes in S: $c_i = (w_i)^2$;
    c. find the gene with the smallest ranking score $e = \arg \min(c)$;
    d. update R = [S(e),R];
    e. update S = S[1 : (e − 1),(e + 1): length(S)];
4) **Output**: ranked gene list R.

13.2
Introduction

Microarray technology has provided researchers with the ability to measure the expression levels of thousands of genes simultaneously. The development of high-throughput screening techniques has been used with great success for molecular profiling in diverse biological systems, including cancer research [11]. Supervised machine learning approaches for the analysis of gene expression profiling have proven to be a powerful tool in the prediction of cancer diagnosis [10, 12], prognosis [13], and treatment outcome [14]. Since most of the genes are not informative for the prediction task, feature selection methods, also known as gene selection, are applied prior to prediction. Such gene selection techniques aim to identify a small subset of genes that can best serve to correctly predict the class membership of unseen samples (e. g., normal versus cancerous tissues). A common step in gene selection methods is to rank the genes according to some importance measure and then select the genes with the highest score for further analysis [9, 10]. By excluding irrelevant genes it is hoped that prediction accuracy is enhanced and cancer-related genes are highlighted.

However, several microarray studies addressing similar prediction tasks report different sets of predictive genes [15, 16]. For example, two prominent studies have aimed to predict development of distant metastases within five years, van't Veer et al. [13] and Wang et al. [17]. Both studies came up with successful predictive gene sets (70 and 76 genes, respectively), yet with only three common overlapping genes. These findings raise the obvious question: What is the reason for this discordance between independent experiments? The trivial answer attributes this lack of agreement to biological differences among samples of different studies (e.g., age, disease stage), heterogeneous microarray platforms (spotted cDNA arrays versus synthesized oligonucleotide arrays), differences in equipment and protocols for obtaining gene expression measurements (e.g., washing, scanning, image analysis), and differences in the analysis methods [18, 19].

Recently, Ein-Dor et al. [20] argued that even if the differences mentioned above are eliminated, the discrepancies between studies remain. They limited themselves to a single dataset [13] and showed that random divisions of the data into training and test sets yield unstable ranked gene lists and, consequently, different predictive genes sets are produced. Michiels et al. [21], by reanalyzing data from seven published studies that attempted to predict prognosis of cancer patients, observed that within each dataset there are many optimal predictive gene sets that are strongly dependent on the subset of samples chosen for training. These findings indicate that low reproducibility occurs even within a microarray dataset (and not only among multiple datasets) and thus the disparity between datasets is not surprising.

For those interested primarily in high accuracy predictive results it is acceptable to have several different predictors. Yet, from a biological perspective, the inconsistency, or instability, of predictive gene sets may lead to disturbing interpretation difficulties. Moreover, the lack of transferability of these predictors (i.e., when one predictor generated by one study suffers from a marked decrease in its performance when tested on data of another study), as reported in Reference [15], implies a lack of reliability in terms of robustness, undermining the generalization power of the predictor in hand.

The reason for this instability phenomenon, according to Reference [22], is the combination of the "curse of dataset sparsity" (the limited number of samples) with the "curse of dimensionality" (the number of genes is very large). Microarray datasets are sensitive to both "curses" since a typical microarray experiment includes thousands of genes but only a limited number of samples. Ein-Dor et al. [15] have assessed that several thousands of patients are required, for the dataset of van't Veer, to obtain an overlap of 50% between two predictive gene sets. Unfortunately, obtaining such a large number of samples is currently prohibitive due to limited tissue availability and financial constraints.

A more ready way to increase sample size is to integrate microarray datasets obtained from different studies addressing the same biological question. Several transformation methods have been proposed to translate gene expression measurements from different studies into a common scale and thus allow the unification of these studies [19, 23]. Nevertheless, there is no consensus, or clear guidelines, as to the best way to perform such a data transformation. An alternative approach for integrating gene expression values into one large dataset is to combine the analysis results of different studies that address similar goals. In principle, the utilization of such meta-analysis methods can lead to the identification of reproducible biomarkers, eliminating study-specific biases. Such a comparison can reduce false positives (i.e., genes that are differentially expressed but do not underlie the observed phenomenon) and lead to more valid and more reliable results. Following this line, previous studies have applied meta-analysis methods to the analysis of cancer microarray data. These methods aimed at both identifying robust signatures of differentially expressed genes in a single cancer type [24, 25] and finding commonly expressed gene signatures in different types of cancer, across multiple datasets [26].

This study presents a meta-analysis of two publicly available cancer microarray datasets of normal and cancerous lung tissues [27, 28]. The analysis identifies a robust predictive gene set by jointly analyzing the two datasets and produces a transferable accurate classifier. From a methodological perspective we propose a new predictor-based approach to overcome the instability of ranked gene lists. Based on these stable lists we demonstrate that the subset of genes identified by our meta-analysis method is superior in terms of transferability to a third unseen dataset [29], compared with the outcome of analyzing each dataset separately. The end result is, hence, a predictive gene set that is able to better distinguish normal from cancerous lung tissues.

13.3
Methods

13.3.1
Overview and Definitions

A common task in gene expression analysis usually involves the selection of relevant genes for sample classification. Since most of the genes are not related to the classification problem, gene selection methods are used to rank the genes according to their importance to the biological question underlying the experiment and generate *ranked genes lists*. The genes eventually selected for classification are small subsets of the genes at the top of the ranked gene lists which we refer to as *predictive gene sets*. It has been previously shown [20] that the ranked gene lists are unstable and strongly depend on the training samples from which they were produced. We refer to the latter as the *instability phenomenon*, which leads to an inconsistency of these predictive sets.

The meta-analysis method presented in this work aims to identify a robust predictive gene set by jointly analyzing two independent gene expression datasets. The first stage of our method is to create stable ranked gene lists for each of the datasets separately. This is achieved by producing many different predictive gene sets (using different random partitions of the data and cross-validation) and ranking the genes according to their *repeatability frequency* in the ensemble of predictive gene sets (i.e., the frequency of appearance of each gene in the different predictive gene sets). The resulting aggregated ranked gene list is denoted the *repeatability-based gene list* (RGL). The *gene core-set* of the dataset includes all genes with a non-zero repeatability score (i.e., appearing in at least one predictive gene set). The core-set genes are ranked based on their repeatability frequency in the RGL.

The second stage of our method addresses the integration of two microarray experiments originating from different studies. This stage generates the *joint core* of genes, which includes genes that appear in the intersection of the gene core-sets of both datasets. The genes in the joint core are ranked such that genes with relatively high repeatability frequencies in both datasets are positioned at the top of the *ranked joint core*.

13.3.2
A Toy Example

To make the definitions and overview of our method more clear consider the following toy example (Figure 13.4). In this example we refer to two different datasets, dataset A and dataset B (Figure 13.4, A1 and A2 respectively), both investigating a common theme (e.g., the expression levels of genes in cancerous versus normal tissues). In each dataset the expression levels of the same 20 genes were measured from the same tissue of interest (e.g., lung tissue). The sample group of patients is different between the datasets.

The first stage in our method is to produce predictive gene sets for each of the datasets (Section 13.3.7). In our example ten different predictive gene sets were generated for dataset A and for dataset B (Figure 13.4, B1 and B2). For example, using genes G1, G4, G9, and G17 in a predefined predictive model achieves high results of prediction in dataset A (e.g., SVM classifier for normal and cancerous lung tissues). The genes that participate in the different predictive gene sets compose the gene core-set of the dataset. For example, the genes in the core set of datasets A and B are: (G1, G2, G4, G5, G8, G9, G11, G12, G17) and (G1, G2, G3, G6, G8, G9, G12, G13, G19, G20), respectively. From the predictive gene sets we produce the RGLs for each

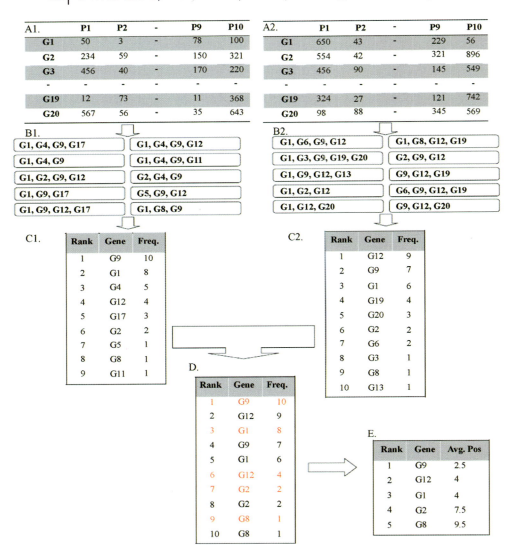

Figure 13.4 Toy example that overviews the meta-analysis method presented in this chapter. Dataset A (A1) and dataset B (A2) present two different datasets that investigate a similar theme. Each row presents a gene and each column presents a patient. The numbers in the table present the expression levels of a certain gene in a certain patient. For each dataset ten sets of predictive genes were generated (B1 and B2). From the predictive gene sets RGLs are generated (C1 and C2). From the RGLs of both datasets a joint ranked list is generated. First an intermediate list is produced (D) were the joint core genes are ranked according to their frequency of appearance in each RGL (each gene appears twice in the list, in red genes from core set A, in black genes from core set B). The genes are then re-ranked by averaging their positions in the intermediate list in decreasing order to produce the ranked joint core (E).

dataset. The RGL is simply a list of the genes in the core set ranked by their frequency of appearance in the predictive gene sets (Section 13.3.9). The RGLs produced for each dataset are presented in Figure 13.4, C1 and C2. The genes that appear in the intersection of both core sets are called the joint core genes. In our example the joint core is composed of five genes: G1, G2, G8, G9, and G12.

The second stage of our method combines the ranked core set genes into one ranked list called the ranked joint core; this is done in two phases. All five genes in the joint core are unified to a single list, where each gene appears twice and ranked according to its frequency of appearance in both datasets (Figure 13.4, D). In the next phase each gene is scored by averaging its ranks in the unified list. For example, gene G9 has a frequency of appearance of ten in dataset A and of seven in dataset B. In the unified list it is ranked in positions 1 and 4, and hence is scored 2.5 (Figure 13.4, E). The genes are then sorted in decreasing order according to their score. This means that the gene that is most frequent in both datasets will be positioned at the top of the list.

13.3.3
Datasets

The study includes three lung cancer microarray datasets [27–29]. All datasets were downloaded from publicly available supporting web sites. Table 13.1 summarizes the content of the datasets, naming them according to the university in which they were performed. Only adenocarcinoma tumors and normal lung samples are included in the analysis.

13.3.4
Data Pre-processing

We apply the following pre-processing procedure to the Michigan and Harvard datasets:

1) **Thresholding**: all expression values lower than 32 are set to 32 and all expression values higher than 16 000 are set to 16 000, creating a range of 32–16 000.
2) **Filtering**: genes with (max/min) $\Leftarrow$ 2 and (max-min) $\Leftarrow$ 50 are excluded, where max and min refer to the maximum and minimum expression values of a particular gene across all samples [30].

Table 13.1 Details of the datasets used in the analysis.

Dataset	Microarray platform	Number of probe sets	Number of cancer samples	Number of normal samples
Michigan [27]	Affymetrix (Hu6800)	7 127	86	10
Harvard [28]	Affymetrix (HG_U95Av2)	12 600	139	17
Stanford [29]	Spotted cDNA	24 000	41	5

3) **Logarithmic transformation**: base 2 logarithm is taken for each expression value.
4) **Normalization**: each gene is normalized to have a mean expression of 0 and standard deviation of 1.

For the Stanford dataset missing values are replaced by zeros and the genes are normalized.

13.3.5
Probe Set Reduction

The DAVID database [31] is used to convert probe sets into gene symbols. Only probe sets with unique gene symbols that appear in both the Michigan and of Harvard datasets are retained. After the pre-processing stage and the probe set reduction stage we remain with 5457 and 6164 probe sets in the Michigan and Harvard datasets, respectively. These probe sets represent 4579 unique gene symbols.

The Stanford dataset contains 24 000 cDNA clones that represent 8401 unique gene symbols. In the Stanford dataset, for each sample the expression values of all clones that correspond to the same gene symbol are given as the average expression value of the clones. Some 3509 gene symbols are common to all three datasets.

13.3.6
Constructing a Predictive Model

The data is randomly divided into two sets: 80% of the samples are assigned into a "working" set and 20% of the samples are assigned into a validation set. The proportion of normal and cancer samples in the working and validation sets is adjusted to the proportion in the complete dataset. The working set is used to identify a predictive gene set (as described in the subsequent section) and based on it a predictive model is constructed by training a support vector machine (SVM) classifier. The classification performance of the model is then evaluated on the validation set.

13.3.7
Constructing Predictive Gene Sets

This section explains in detail how a predictive gene set is constructed. An example is provided below (Figure 13.5) and we will refer to it throughout the method description.

Predictive gene sets are produced by two main stages: defining the number of genes required for classification and selecting the genes involved in the classification.

In the first stage, as described in the previous section, the entire data samples are randomly divided into two sets: 80% of the samples are assigned into a working set (marked in white and purple in Figure 13.5) and 20% of the samples are assigned into a validation set (marked in green).

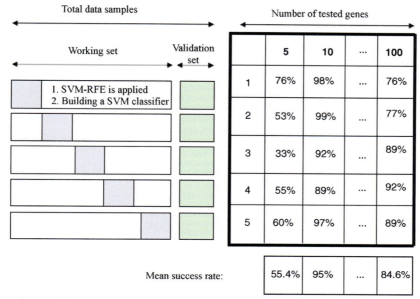

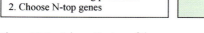

Second stage: Selecting the genes involved in the classification

Figure 13.5 Schematic view of the construction of a predictive gene set. The data samples are randomly divided into working set (marked in white and purple) and into validation set (marked in green). The working set is further randomly divided into five disjoint subsets. A fivefold cross-validation procedure is applied. In each iteration one of the five subsets functions as a testing set (marked in purple), while the other four subsets function as a training set (marked in white). In each iteration the SVM-RFE procedure is applied to the training set (resulting in a ranked gene list) and the success rate of various numbers of genes from the top of the list (ranging from 5 to 100 in increments of 5) are tested on the test set (right most table). The mean success rate is calculated. The number of genes chosen for classification, N, is the one that maximizes the success rate over the cross-validation iteration. To select the genes that participate in the gene set, SVM-RFE is applied to the working set and the N top genes are selected.

The working set is further divided into five random disjoint subsets. A fivefold cross-validation procedure is used to choose the optimal number of genes to be used in the classification. The cross-validation procedure is repeated five times; in each iteration one of the subsets is held out as test set (marked in purple). The remaining four subsets are used as training set (marked in white).

In each iteration a SVM-RFE ranking procedure is applied using the training set only. This stage results in a ranked gene list in which the top ranked genes are the most important for classification. After the ranking is completed, we examine the success rate obtained by using an increasing number of genes, starting from the top of the ranked list in increments of 5. An SVM classifier with a linear kernel is used to test the predictive performance of the selected genes on the held out subset.

An example of the results of the five-cross-validation stage is shown in the right most table of Figure 13.5. If we look at the first fold iteration we see that SVM classifier based on the five top ranked genes reaches a success rate of 76% on the held out set. The ten top ranked genes (five more genes are added) reach a success rate of 98%.

The number of genes ultimately selected for classification is the one that maximizes the average fivefold cross-validation success rate. This optimal number is denoted N. In our example, the mean success rate (over the five folds), when using the five top ranked genes, is 55.4%. When using the ten top ranked genes we get a success rate of 95%. With the top 100 genes we get 84%. Now, assuming that the highest mean success rate we got is 95%, the optimal number of genes chosen for classification is 10 ($N=10$).

To identify the genes involved in the classification (second stage in Figure 13.5) we re-rank the genes by applying SVM-RFE on the whole working set (and not only on a subset of the data). The N-top genes of the produced ranked gene list comprise the predictive gene set. (The predictive model is constructed by training a SVM classifier on the working set, using the N-top genes chosen in the previous stage and evaluating its performance on the validation set.)

13.3.8
Estimating the Predictive Performance

Since most the samples in our datasets are labeled as lung cancer versus a small number of normal lungs, it is possible to obtain rather good performances simply by classifying all observations by the most frequent category. To counteract that, the classification success rate is measured by the weighted average of true positives and true negatives:

$$\frac{1}{2}\left(\frac{TP}{TP+FP} + \frac{TN}{TN+FN}\right)$$

where TP, FP, TN, and FN are the four possible prediction outcomes: true positives, false positives, true negative, and false negative, respectively.

13.3.9
Constructing a Repeatability-Based Gene List

Based on several predictive gene sets generated by different data samplings we construct the RGL (sampling schemes are often used to increase certainty in the gene ranking). The genes in the RGL are ranked according to their repeatability, that is, their frequency in the different generated predictive gene sets, such that genes that are most frequent are at the top of the list. Whenever a gene is represented by multiple probe sets, we kept for further analysis only one probe set that exhibits its maximal repeatability frequency.

13.3.10
Ranking the Joint Core Genes

The joint core genes are associated with two scores of repeatability frequency originating from the two RGLs obtained from the independent datasets. To rank the joint core genes (which appear in both gene core-sets) we first sort the repeatability scores obtained from the two independent lists, leading to one unified list in which each gene appears twice. The ranking of each gene in the joint core is based on averaging the two positions of the gene in the unified sorted list (see toy example in Section 13.3.2).

13.4
Results

13.4.1
Unstable Ranked Gene Lists in a Tumor Versus Normal Binary Classification Task

It has been previously shown that the instability problem occurs in complex bioinformatics challenges such as finding prognostic gene signatures [20, 21]. Ranked gene lists produced in these studies were unstable and depended strongly on the subgroups of patients on which they were generated. We show that the instability problem is also observed in simpler questions like classification of tumor versus normal tissues. Figure 13.6 demonstrates the instability of the ranked gene lists constructed from repeatedly applying SVM-RFE to the gene expression profiles

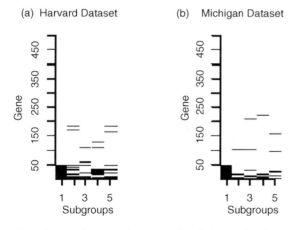

Figure 13.6 Fifty-top ranked genes identified by SVM-RFE in five subgroups of patients drawn at random from the Harvard (a) and Michigan (b) datasets. Each subgroup contains 90% of the samples. Each row represents a gene and each column represents a different subgroup of patients. The genes are ordered by the leftmost column and the top 50 genes are marked by a line.

of different subgroups of patients drawn at random from the Harvard and Michigan datasets separately. Evidently, genes that are ranked high using one subgroup of patients may be ranked low in another (as evident in both datasets).

13.4.2
Constructing a Consistent Repeatability-Based Gene List

Our first challenge is to produce a consistent gene ranking method. Since our ranking procedure uses random samplings of the data [Section 13.3 (Methods)], and hence is not deterministic, it is necessary to determine the number of predictive gene sets, K, sufficient for obtaining a consistent RGL. To this end, we repeat the gene ranking procedure twice, each time using K predictive gene sets, producing two different RGLs.

RGL consistency is evaluated by calculating the Spearman correlation between these two resulting RGLs. A high Spearman correlation obviously testifies to high consistency levels. This consistency test is performed for varying K values, ranging from 50 to 1500 in intervals of 50. The resulting mean Spearman correlation increases with the number K of predictive gene sets used (Figure 13.7). Throughout this work we use $K = 1000$, which evidently yields a consistent ranking. With $K = 1000$ the Harvard dataset exhibits a mean Spearman correlation coefficient of 0.86 with a standard deviation of 0.008 while the Michigan dataset manifest a mean of 0.84 with a standard deviation of 0.01.

Furthermore, the predictive gene sets that construct the RGLs reach high classification success rates. Mean success rates are 90 and 98.6% for the Harvard and Michigan datasets, respectively, testifying to the utility of the RGLs. The mean

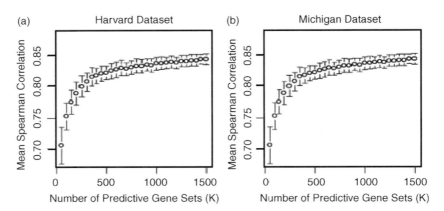

Figure 13.7 Assessing the stability of RGLs (repeatability-based gene lists) in the Harvard (a) and Michigan (b) datasets. The x-axis represents the number of predictive gene sets (K) and the y-axis represents the mean Spearman correlation between two RGLs produced over 100 samplings (Section 13.3). Standard deviations for each number of predictive gene sets are marked.

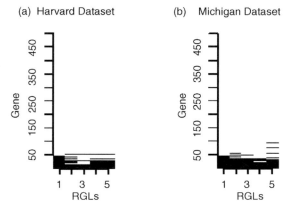

Figure 13.8 Fifty-top ranked genes in five different RGLs produced by five random subgroups of patients drawn from the Harvard (a) and Michigan (b) datasets. Each subgroup contains 90% of the data. Figure layout is similar to Figure 13.6.

number of genes participating in a predictive gene set is 27.8 and 15.8 for the Harvard and Michigan datasets, respectively, with standard deviations of 24.3 and 17.5.

Investigating the two RGLs, we observe that ~90% of the genes in both datasets do not participate in any of the predictive gene sets. Out of 4579 genes included in the two datasets, 547 genes comprise the gene core-set of the Harvard dataset and 411 genes comprise the gene core-set of the Michigan dataset.

13.4.3
Repeatability-Based Gene Lists are Stable

A stable ranked gene list is unsusceptible to random partitioning of the data. Figure 13.8 examines the stability of RGLs produced for the Harvard and Michigan datasets.

In contrast to the large variation in membership of the top 50 genes based on gene rankings by SVM-RFE (Figure 13.6), the top 50 genes in the RGLs are reproducible. The mean overlap between the 50 top ranked genes of the different RGLs is 37 and 40.6 for the Harvard and Michigan datasets, respectively, with standard deviations of 2.86 and 3.23, while the mean overlap between the 50 top ranked genes when using SVM-RFE as a ranking method (Figure 13.6) is 24.1 and 26.8 for the Harvard and Michigan datasets, respectively, with standard deviations of 8.34 and 9.54. These results suggest that indeed RGLs are stable, robust lists (it may be noted, however, that in the improbable case of identical data partitions, our method obviously leads to a less stable ranking than SVM-RFE, as the latter is deterministic).

13.4.4
Comparing Gene Rankings between Datasets

Since the RGL ranking in each dataset separately (Harvard versus Michigan) is rather stable one could expect that genes that are highly discriminative in one dataset would

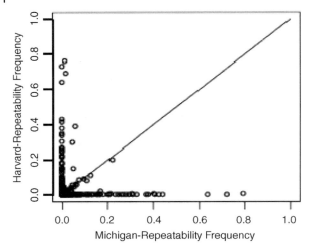

Figure 13.9 Comparison of gene repeatability frequency between the Michigan and Harvard datasets. Each point represents a gene and its repeatability frequency in the Michigan dataset (x-axis) versus its repeatability frequency on the Harvard dataset (y-axis). The diagonal marks the position of genes that have equal repeatability frequencies in both datasets. A gene's repeatability frequency is given as the fraction out of the maximal 1000 repeats possible.

be also highly discriminative in the second dataset. Interestingly, this is not the case: the diagonal in Figure 13.9 marks the position of genes whose repeatability frequency is equivalent in both datasets. Evidently, only a few points are located around the diagonal whereas most points exhibit significant dissimilarity in their repeatability frequencies over the two datasets. Six out of the ten top ranked genes in the Harvard core-set do not appear in Michigan core-set, suggesting that these genes are "dataset specific" and may not be truly reflective of the underlying disease process. The top ranked genes in the Michigan core-set are quite highly ranked in the Harvard core-set (eight out of the ten top ranked genes in Michigan core-set appear in Harvard core-set). These genes are reproducible across the studies, testifying to their reliability.

The dissimilarity between datasets is also demonstrated by the low Spearman correlation of 0.173 between the RGLs of the Harvard and Michigan datasets.

13.4.5
Joint Core Magnitude

Since our goal is to examine whether relevant genes can be more effectively discovered by jointly analyzing two independent datasets, we focus on the joint core genes (obtained as described in Section 13.3, Methods). The magnitude of the joint core of Michigan and Harvard datasets is 118 genes and is statistically significant (p-value < 0.0025 as none of the permutation runs reached the true joint core magnitude). The magnitude of the joint core remains significant across various repeatability frequency thresholds used to determine the genes in the core-sets.

13.4.6
The Joint Core is Transferable

A question remains: Is the joint core more informative than the two independent core-sets? A pertaining test would investigate the transferability of these cores; that is, do they carry predictive information as for a new unseen dataset, preferably even from a different technology? To this end we test the classification performance of the different cores on the Stanford dataset, an independent cross-platform microarray data of lung cancer. To evaluate the classification performance obtained with genes from the three cores (Harvard and Michigan core-sets and the joint core) on the Stanford dataset, an SVM classifier is utilized in a standard train and test procedure. This procedure is repeated for an increasing number of genes selected from the top of the three ranked cores. This enables us to compare the classification performance of the ranked cores for the same number of genes each time.

The results show that the joint core outperforms the two independent core-sets, obtaining a high level of classification already with a very small number of highly ranked genes (<4). As observed in Figure 13.10, the first gene on the top ranked joint core (RAGE) achieves a high success rate of 98% on its own. The Michigan dataset matches the joint core performance with four genes only where the Harvard dataset

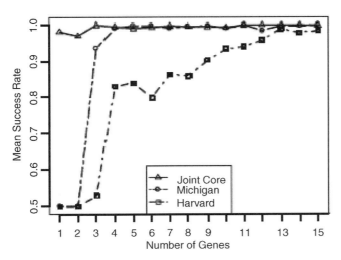

Figure 13.10 Mean success rate of the top ranked genes of joint core (open triangles), Michigan core-set (open circles), and Harvard core-set (open squares) on the Stanford dataset. The top ranked genes include only the genes that appear in the Stanford dataset. The x-axis represents the number of genes utilized by the classifier. For each number of selected genes the procedure is carried out 100 times, on different samplings of the Stanford data into training and test sets. The y-axis represents the mean success rate.

Table 13.2 Ten-top-ranked genes of the joint core, Michigan core-set, and Harvard core-set. Genes that do not appear in the joint-core are marked in bold. Genes that do not appear in the Stanford dataset are marked in italics.

	Joint core	Michigan core-set	Harvard core-set
1	RAGE	TNXB	**SMAD6**
2	TNA	CA4	**GRK5**
3	FABP4	RAGE	**HYAL2**
4	TNXB	FABP4	TEK
5	*COX7A1*	FGR	**CD34**
6	PHLDA2	PHLDA2	***S100A3***
7	FGR	TNA	**FKBP1A**
8	TEK	*COX7A1*	TNA
9	TACSTD1	**CEACAM5**	**TLK1**
10	MAP4	**CASP1**	**EMP2**

requires the top 13 genes to match the joint core performance. As observed in Table 13.2, listing the genes in the different core sets, most genes in the top of the Harvard set are not in the joint core while in the Michigan set this is not the case. Interestingly, a marked increase in the Harvard set's success rate is reached (83%) by adding the fourth gene (TEK), which is the first in the Harvard list to appear in the joint-core.

13.4.7
Biological Significance of the Joint Core Genes

We turn to examine the biological function of the 118 genes composing the joint core, concentrating on their role in cancer. In a prominent review by Hanahan et al. [32], tumorigenesis is presented as a multistep process that manifests several essential alterations in cell physiology; these constitute the "hallmarks of cancer."

In the joint core several representatives of these required alterations are found (their rank in the joint core is indicated in parentheses):

Self-sufficiency in growth signals: In cancer cells many oncogenes activate normal growth signaling pathways that yield uncontrolled proliferation [32]. ErbB3 (rank 72) is a transmembrane receptor tyrosine kinase belonging to the epidermal growth factor (EGF) receptor subfamily. Two members of this family, EGFR (ErbB1) and ErbB2, together with their ligands were shown to constitute a growth stimulatory loop particularly for non-small cell lung cancer (NSCLC) [33]. More recently, it has been shown that ErbB3 forms a heterodimer together with ErbB2 which functions as an oncogenic unit to drive tumor cell proliferation [34].

Insensitivity to antigrowth signals: Antiproliferative signals, such as TGFβ, operate to maintain cellular quiescence and tissue homeostasis within normal cells. Cancer cells must acquire insensitivity to those signals to prosper [32]. Reduced expression of TGFβ receptor type III (TGFBR3, rank 36) is known to be associated with resistance to TGFβ and may play a role in tumorigenesis [35].

Evading apoptosis: Mounting evidence indicates that acquiring resistance towards programmed cell-death (termed apoptosis) is a hallmark of most cancer types [32]. The identified joint core consists of several genes related to apoptosis, as indicated by their Gene Ontology class and KEGG pathway [31]: PHLDA2 (rank 6), SPP1 (rank 21), ZBTB16 (rank 32), DNASE1L3 (rank 38), CSF2RB (rank 60), PML (rank 80), IGFBP3 (rank 81), and TNFRSF25 (rank 82).

Sustained angiogenesis: As the tumor grows rapidly the cancerous cells draw away from the capillary blood vessels that supply oxygen and vital nutrients. Therefore, to invade the surrounding tissue, the tumor must develop angiogenic ability [32]. Several genes in the joint core are related to angiogenesis: TEK (TIE-2, rank 8), MDK (rank 15), EDNRB (rank 23), PECAM1 (CD31, rank 24) ANG1 (rank 35), and CDH5 (rank 65) [36–39]. Interestingly, there may be a clinical potential in targeting these genes' pathways by producing anti-angiogenic agents. For example, it has been shown that blocking the TIE-2/ANG1 pathway inhibits, to a certain extent, tumor angiogenesis [39].

Tissue invasion and metastasis: The final step in the tumor progression is the invasion from the primary tumor mass to adjacent tissues, resulting in its spread and survival in other organs in the body [32]. RAGE, the top ranked gene in the joint core list, was shown to be involved in motility and invasive behavior of cells. Furthermore, inhibition of RAGE-amphoterin signaling suppressed tumor growth and metastases in mice [40]. S100A4 (rank 94) is thought to mediate motility and invasiveness of cancer cells. It is a marker for poor patient prognosis in several cancers [41]. Three other members of the S100 family were found to be in the joint core genes: S100A3 (rank 18), S100G (rank 30), and S100A8 (rank 52). This fact may suggest an association between this family and lung cancer. Other genes in the joint core that are related to tissue invasion and metastases include CAV1 (rank 13), SPP1 (rank 21), and SPINT2 (rank 58) [42–44].

13.5 Discussion

A key component of gene-expression analysis is the identification of genes that play a pivotal role in the biological processes underlying the microarray experiment. With the increasing availability of microarray datasets there is a growing need for integrative computational methods that evaluate multiple independent microarray datasets. Meta-analysis methods are applied to reduce study-specific biases, aiming to yield results that offer improved reliability and validity. We propose a predictor-based meta-analysis approach that generates a robust predictive gene set. The method and results presented here have been reported earlier in journal form [45].

The method has its roots in ensemble learning methods frequently used in prediction and classification, where the underlying base learning algorithm is run multiple times, and a vote is taken on the resulting hypotheses. As confirmed experimentally in numerous cases, ensemble methods can efficiently reduce both the bias and the variance of learning algorithms and improve their overall accuracy [46].

Using this method the genes are first ranked on different datasets, independently, according to their classification power, and then they are combined into a consolidated gene set, the joint core genes. In doing so, we address two main challenges: (i) The instability problem: When dividing a given dataset into training and test sets, different divisions produce different ranked gene lists that subsequently give rise to different predictive gene sets. We show that this phenomenon is not restricted to complex computational challenges such as finding a prognostic gene signatures [20, 21], but is also observed in less challenging questions like binary classification of tumor versus normal tissues. Assuming that genes that are more essential for classification will appear more consistently in different predictive gene sets, we construct a ranked gene list termed RGL. The RGL demonstrates high stability, with an average overlap of approximately 39 genes between the top 50 genes of two RGLs, generated from independent data divisions. (ii) Transferability: How well do features learned in the context of one dataset perform on a second, unseen, dataset? Our results show successful transferability of the joint core genes to the unseen Stanford dataset, in which the top three genes of the ranked joint core yield a classifier with an accuracy of 99.8%.

Applying the suggested gene ranking method to two prominent lung cancer datasets, the Michigan and Harvard datasets, results in a low Spearman correlation ($r = 0.173$) between the two RGLs, although each list by itself is stable. Moreover, genes exhibiting high classification power on one of the datasets (and thus were ranked at the top of the RGL) were ranked at the bottom of the corresponding RGL of the second dataset. Observing that the two independent RGLs produced by our meta-analysis method are stable but exhibit a significant dissimilarity leads us to attribute this dissimilarity to factors like biological differences among samples of different studies, differences in platform generation, and differences in protocols, rather than to inner instability.

The joint core constructed by the meta-analysis approach focuses on genes that appear in the core-sets of both datasets, and hence are likely to be central to the phenomenon studied. The first gene in the ranked joint core, RAGE, exhibits a very high classification performance by itself. RAGE was shown to be strongly downregulated in NSCLC patients compared to their paired normal lung tissues, not only on the transcriptional level (as revealed by this study) but also on a protein level [47]. These results may suggest RAGE as a potential marker for diagnosis of lung cancer.

Studying the transferability to the Stanford dataset confirms that genes that are highly ranked only in one dataset but are not part of the joint core are biased to their dataset and thus exhibit low transferability. The joint core indeed shows improved transferability, demonstrating high classification even with a very small number of genes from the top of the ranked joint core. Although the joint core has better classification capability than the two separate cores, the joint core does not show a significant similarity to the Stanford core set. This may be due to the variation in platforms from which the datasets were produced.

The analysis method demonstrated in this study increases the reliability of identifying powerful predictive genes sets. The putative list of predictive genes identified may hold promise as therapeutic targets and diagnostic markers. Applying the method to other datasets and expanding the method beyond two datasets may enhance our biological understanding of previous microarray studies, with no extra experimental work.

Acknowledgments

We thank Isaac Meilijson, Gideon Dror, Yoav Benjamini, Danny Yekutieli, and Yoram Oron for their valuable comments and suggestions. A. Kaufman was supported by the Yeshaya Horowitz Association through the Center of Complexity Science. E. Ruppin's research is generously supported by the Tauber Fund, the Yeshaya Horowitz Association through the Center of Complexity Science, the Israeli Science Fund (ISF), and the Israeli Ministry of Science and Technology (MOST).

References

1. Allison, D.B., Cui, X., Page, G.P., and Sabripour, M. (2006) Microarray data analysis: from disarray to consolidation and consensus. *Nat. Rev. Genet.*, 7, 55–65.
2. Duggan, D.J., Bittner, M., Chen, Y., Meltzer, P., and Trent, J.M. (1999) Expression profiling using cDNA microarrays. *Nat. Genet.*, 21, 10–14
3. Quackenbush, J. (2006) Microarray analysis and tumor classification. *New Engl. J. Med.*, 354, 2463–2472.
4. Lipshutz, R.J., Fodor, S.P.A., Gingeras, T.R., and Lockhart, D.J. (1999) High density synthetic oligonucleotide arrays. *Nat. Genet.* 21, 20–24.
5. Soinov, L.A. (2003) Supervised classification for gene network reconstruction. *Biochem. Soc. Trans.*, 31, 1497–1502.
6. Brown, M.P.S., Grundy, W.N., Lin, D., Cristianini, N., Sugnet, C.W., Furey, T.S., Ares, M. Jr., and Haussler, D. (2000) Knowledge-based analysis of microarray gene expression data by using support vector machines. *Proc. Natl. Acad. Sci. USA*, 97, 262–267.
7. Mukherjee, S., Tamayo, P., Slonim, D., Verri, A., Golub, T., Mesirov, J.P., and Poggio, T. (1999) Support vector machine classification of microarray data, AI Memo1677, Massachusetts Institute of Technology.
8. Cristianini, N. and Shawe-Taylor, J. (2000) *An Introduction to Support Vector Machines and Other Kernel-Based Learning Methods*, Cambridge University Press.
9. Guyon, I., Weston, J., Barnhill, S., and Vapnik, V. (2002) Gene selection for cancer classification using support vector machines. *Machine Learn.*, 46, 389–422.
10. Golub, T.R., Slonim, D.K., Tamayo, P., Huard, C., Gaasenbeek, M., Mesirov, J.P., Coller, H., Loh, M.L., Downing, J.R., Caligiuri, M.A., Bloomfield, C.D., and Lander, E.S. (1999) Molecular classification of cancer: class discovery and class prediction by gene expression monitoring. *Science*, 286, 531–537.
11. Dopazo, J., Zanders, E., Dragoni, I., Amphlett, G., and Falciani, F. (2001) Methods and approaches in the analysis of gene expression data. *J. Immunol. Methods*, 250, 93–112.
12. Nguyen, D.V. and Rocke, D.M. (2002) Tumor classification by partial least squares using microarray gene expression data. *Bioinformatics*, 18, 39–50.
13. van't Veer, L.J., Dai, H., van de Vijver, M.J., He, Y.D., Hart, A.A.M., Mao, M., Peterse, H.L., van der Kooy, K., Marton, M.J., Witteveen, A.T., Schreiber, G.J., Kerkhoven, R.M., Roberts, C., Linsley, P.S., Bernards, R., and Friend, S.H. (2002) Gene expression profiling predicts clinical

outcome of breast cancer. *Nature*, **415**, 530–536.

14 Shipp, M.A., Ross, K.N., Tamayo, P., Weng, A.P., Kutok, J.L., Aguiar, R.C.T., Gaasenbeek, M., Angelo, M., Reich, M., Pinkus, G.S., Ray, T.S., Koval, M.A., Last, K.W., Norton, A., Lister, T.A., Mesirov, J., Neuberg, D.S., Lander, E.S., Aster, J.C., and Golub, T.R. (2002) Diffuse large B-cell lymphoma outcome prediction by gene-expression profiling and supervised machine learning. *Nat. Med.*, **8**, 68–74.

15 Ein-Dor, L., Zuk, O., and Domany, E. (2006) Thousands of samples are needed to generate a robust gene list for predicting outcome in cancer. *Proc. Natl. Acad. Sci. USA*, **103**, 5923–5928.

16 Lossos, I.S., Czerwinski, D.K., Alizadeh, A.A., Wechser, M.A., Tibshirani, R., Botstein, D., and Levy, R. (2004) Prediction of survival in diffuse large-B-cell lymphoma based on the expression of six genes. *New Engl. J. Med.*, **350**, 1828–1837.

17 Wang, Y., Klijn, J.G.M., Zhang, Y., Sieuwerts, A.M., Look, M.P., Yang, F., Talantov, D., Timmermans, M., Meijer-van Gelder, M.E., and Yu, J. (2005) Gene-expression profiles to predict distant metastasis of lymph-node-negative primary breast cancer. *The Lancet*, **365**, 671–679.

18 Kuo, W.P., Jenssen, T.-K., Butte, A.J., Ohno-Machado, L., and Kohane, I.S. (2002) Analysis of matched mRNA measurements from two different microarray technologies. *Bioinformatics*, **18**, 405–412.

19 Warnat, P., Eils, R., and Brors, B. (2005) Cross-platform analysis of cancer microarray data improves gene expression based classification of phenotypes. *BMC Bioinformatics*, **6**, 265.

20 Ein-Dor, L., Kela, I., Getz, G., Givol, D., and Domany, E. (2005) Outcome signature genes in breast cancer: is there a unique set? *Bioinformatics*, **21**, 171–178.

21 Michiels, S., Koscielny, S., and Hill, C. (2005) Prediction of cancer outcome with microarrays: a multiple random validation strategy. *The Lancet*, **365**, 488–492.

22 Somorjai, R.L., Dolenko, B., and Baumgartner, R. (2003) Class prediction and discovery using gene microarray and proteomics mass spectroscopy data: curses, caveats, cautions. *Bioinformatics*, **19**, 1484–1491.

23 Jiang, H., Deng, Y., Chen, H.-S., Tao, L., Sha, Q., Chen, J., Tsai, C.-J., and Zhang, S. (2004) Joint analysis of two microarray gene-expression datasets to select lung adenocarcinoma marker genes. *BMC Bioinformatics*, **5**, 81.

24 Choi, J.K., Yu, U., Kim, S., and Yoo, O.J. (2003) Combining multiple microarray studies and modeling interstudy variation. *Bioinformatics*, **19**, i84–i90

25 Rhodes, D.R., Barrette, T.R., Rubin, M.A., Ghosh, D., and Chinnaiyan, A.M. (2002) Meta-analysis of microarrays: interstudy validation of gene expression profiles reveals pathway dysregulation in prostate cancer. *Cancer Res.*, **62**, 4427–4433.

26 Rhodes, D.R. and Chinnaiyan, A.M. (2005) Integrative analysis of the cancer transcriptome. *Nat. Genet.* **37** (Suppl.), S31–S37.

27 Beer, D.G., Kardia, S.L.R., Huang, C.-C., Giordano, T.J., Levin, A.M., Misek, D.E., Lin, L., Chen, G., Gharib, T.G., Thomas, D.G., Lizyness, M.L., Kuick, R., Hayasaka, S., Taylor, J.M.G., Iannettoni, M.D., Orringer, M.B., and Hanash, S. (2002) Gene-expression profiles predict survival of patients with lung adenocarcinoma. *Nat. Med.*, **8**, 816–824.

28 Bhattacharjee, A., Richards, W.G., Staunton, J., Li, C., Monti, S., Vasa, P., Ladd, C., Beheshti, J., Bueno, R., Gillette, M., Loda, M., Weber, G., Mark, E.J., Lander, E.S., Wong, W., Johnson, B.E., Golub, T.R., Sugarbaker, D.J., and Meyerson, M. (2001) Classification of human lung carcinomas by mRNA expression profiling reveals distinct adenocarcinoma subclasses. *Proc. Natl. Acad. Sci. USA*, **98**, 13790–13795.

29 Garber, M.E., Troyanskaya, O.G., Schluens, K., Petersen, S., Thaesler, Z., Pacyna-Gengelbach, M., van de Rijn, M., Rosen, G.D , Perou, C.M., Whyte, R.I., Altman, R.B., Brown, P.O., Botstein, D., and Petersen, I. (2001) Diversity of gene expression in adenocarcinoma of the lung. *Proc. Natl. Acad. Sci. USA*, **98**, 13784–13789.

30 Dudoit, S., Fridlyand, J., and Speed, T.P. (2000) Comparison of discrimination

methods for the classification of tumors using gene expression data. *J. Am. Stat. Assoc.*, **97**, 77–87.

31 Dennis, G., Sherman, B., Hosack, D., Yang, J., Gao, W., Lane, H.C., and Lempicki, R. (2003) DAVID: Database for annotation, visualization, and integrated discovery. *Genome Biol.*, **4**, P3.

32 Hanahan, D. and Weinberg, R.A. (2000) The hallmarks of cancer. *Cell*, **100**, 57–70.

33 Fong, K.M., Sekido, Y., Gazdar, A.F., and Minna, J.D. (2003) Lung cancer* 9: Molecular biology of lung cancer: clinical implications. *Thorax*, **58**, 892–900.

34 Holbro, T., Beerli, R.R., Maurer, F., Koziczak, M., Barbas, C.F. III, and Hynes, N.E. (2003) The ErbB2/ErbB3 heterodimer functions as an oncogenic unit: ErbB2 requires ErbB3 to drive breast tumor cell proliferation. *Proc. Natl. Acad. Sci. USA*, **100**, 8933–8938.

35 Copland, J.A., Luxon, B.A., Ajani, L., Maity, T., Campagnaro, E., Guo, H., LeGrand, S.N., Tamboli, P., and Wood, C.G. (2003) Genomic profiling identifies alterations in TGFbeta signaling through loss of TGFbeta receptor expression in human renal cell carcinogenesis and progression. *Oncogene*, **22**, 8053–8062.

36 Ahmed, S.I., Thompson, J., Coulson, J.M., and Woll, P.J. (2000) Studies on the expression of endothelin, its receptor subtypes, and converting enzymes in lung cancer and in human bronchial epithelium. *Am. J. Respir. Cell Mol. Biol.*, **22**, 422–431.

37 Choudhuri, R., Zhang, H.T., Donnini, S., Ziche, M., and Bicknell, R. (1997) An angiogenic role for the neurokines midkine and pleiotrophin in tumorigenesis. *Cancer Res.*, **57**, 1814–1819.

38 Liao, F., Li, Y., O'Connor, W., Zanetta, L., Bassi, R., Santiago, A., Overholser, J., Hooper, A., Mignatti, P., Dejana, E., Hicklin, D.J., and Bohlen, P. (2000) Monoclonal antibody to vascular endothelial-cadherin is a potent inhibitor of angiogenesis, tumor growth, and metastasis. *Cancer Res.*, **60**, 6805–6810.

39 Takahama, M., Tsutsumi, M., Tsujiuchi, T., Nezu, K., Kushibe, K., Taniguchi, S., Kotake, Y., and Konishi, Y. (1999) Enhanced expression of Tie2, its ligand angiopoietin-1, vascular endothelial growth factor, and CD31 in human non-small cell lung carcinomas. *Clin. Cancer Res.*, **5**, 2506–2510.

40 Taguchi, A., Blood, D.C., del Toro, G., Canet, A., Lee, D.C., Qu, W., Tanji, N., Lu, Y., Lalla, E., Fu, C., Hofmann, M.A., Kislinger, T., Ingram, M., Lu, A., Tanaka, H., Hori, O., Ogawa, S., Stern, D.M., and Schmidt, A.M. (2000) Blockade of RAGE-amphoterin signalling suppresses tumour growth and metastases. *Nature*, **405**, 354–360.

41 Li, Z.-H. and Bresnick, A.R. (2006) The S100A4 metastasis factor regulates cellular motility via a direct interaction with myosin-IIA. *Cancer Res.*, **66**, 5173–5180.

42 Ho, C.-C., Huang, P.-H., Huang, H.-Y., Chen, Y.-H., Yang, P.-C., and Hsu, S.-M. (2002) Up-regulated caveolin-1 accentuates the metastasis capability of lung adenocarcinoma by inducing filopodia formation. *Am. J. Pathol.*, **161**, 1647–1656.

43 Rangaswami, H., Bulbule, A., and Kundu, G.C. (2006) Osteopontin: role in cell signaling and cancer progression. *Trends Cell Biol.*, **16**, 79–87.

44 Suzuki, M., Kobayashi, H., Tanaka, Y., Hirashima, Y., Kanayama, N., Takei, Y., Saga, Y., Suzuki, M., Itoh, H., and Terao, T. (2003) Bikunin target genes in ovarian cancer cells identified by microarray analysis. *J. Biol. Chem.*, **278**, 14640–14646.

45 Fishel, I., Kaufman, A., and Ruppin, E. (2007) Meta analysis of gene expression data: a predictor based approach. *Bioinformatics*, **23**, 1599–1606.

46 Dietterich, T. (2002) Ensemble learning, in *The Handbook of Brain Theory and Neural Networks*, MIT Press, Cambridge, MA, pp. 405–408.

47 Schraml, P., Bendik, I., and Ludwig, C.U. (1997) Differential messenger RNA and protein expression of the receptor for advanced glycosylated end products in normal lung and non-small cell lung carcinoma. *Cancer Res.*, **57**, 3669–3671.

14
Kernel Classification Methods for Cancer Microarray Data
Tsuyoshi Kato and Wataru Fujibuchi

14.1
Introduction

Cancer is one of the most malignant diseases affecting almost all tissues of all people of all ages and arising from a group of cells that grow uncontrollably from the normal state. More precisely, a group of cells that show only abnormal but controlled or limited growth is called benign tumor, while cancer refers to malignant tumor cells that show unlimited growth, usually invading other tissues directly or by spreading to distant locations in the body via lymph or blood. The spread of cancer cells is called metastasis and the cells are called metastatic cells, which are considered to be the worst malignancy, leading to high mortality rates. Thus, predicting the state of cancer, that is, whether it is metastatic or not, from specimens is one of the most important studies in cancer diagnosis.

Since the invention of gene expression microarrays in the mid-1990s, classification analyses based on gene expression data from distinct biological groups have become a fundamental approach in various cancer/tumor studies, such as tumor diagnosis [16, 34], anticancer drug response analysis [32, 44], and prognosis analysis [25, 50]. Among various classification methods, kernel-based methods [13] have played important roles in such disease analyses, especially when classifying data with support vector machines (SVMs) [51] by weighting feature or marker genes that are correlated with the characteristics of the groups. In most of those studies, only standard kernels, such as linear, polynomial, and RBF (radial basis function), which take vector data as input and basically convert them into inner-products between vectors, have been popularly used and are generally successful.

Most importantly, however, in microarray analysis designed for cancer study, one of the main issues that limit accurate and practical predictions is the lack of repeat experiments, often due to financial problems or rarity of specimens, such as minor diseases, as well as too much variability of cell types. Some gene expression databases contain disease microarray data (e.g., GEO [2], ArrayExpress [7], and Oncomine [36]) and the use of public or old data together with one's current data could solve this problem; many studies combining several microarray datasets have been

Medical Biostatistics for Complex Diseases. Edited by Frank Emmert-Streib and Matthias Dehmer
Copyright © 2010 WILEY-VCH Verlag GmbH & Co. KGaA, Weinheim
ISBN: 978-3-527-32585-6

performed [29, 35, 53]. Nevertheless, due to the insufficient amount of gene overlaps and consistencies between different datasets, kernels that use vector data as the primary input are often unsuccessful in classifying data from various datasets if naïvely integrated [53].

Instead of the above *vectorial data kernel* family, there is another family called *structured data kernel* family that has been studied in many other fields, including bioinformatics and machine learning [23, 26, 48, 49]. Among them, the synthetic distance-based kernels, or what we call *metrization kernels*, can take any distance data between sample vectors (or samples in short) as primary input without recognizing the original vectorial data from which the distance is calculated while holding positive semidefiniteness of kernel matrices, and is thus applicable to the Euclidean or other distance measures among sample vectors once converted into a distance relationship. Moreover, the metrization kernels have, unlike the RBF kernel, the special property of excluding arbitrary gene values in vectorial data when calculating the distances among samples. Hence, by ignoring only spurious gene values in distinct samples without deleting those genes entirely from a dataset, the metrization kernel can effectively utilize gene expression information in heterogeneous data containing mosaic-like missing or noisy values.

In this chapter, we first describe the general mechanisms of machine learning by kernel methods and SVMs, comparing the properties of standard and metrization kernels as well as referring to two noise handling methods in microarray data. Then, we demonstrate a few machine classification examples using kernel-SVM methods for cancer microarray data, together with different noise-reduction methods, to learn practical issues in handling disease datasets that are noisy and promiscuous. The proofs of Theorems 14.1 and 14.2 are given in Appendix 14.A

14.1.1
Notation

Vectors are denoted by boldface italic lower-case letters and matrices by boldface italic upper-case letters. The transposition of matrix A is denoted by A^T, and the inverse of A is denoted by A^{-1}. The $n \times n$ identity matrix is denoted by I_n. We use E_{ij} to denote a matrix in which (i,j) element is one and all the other elements are zero. The n-dimensional column vector all of whose elements are one is denoted by I_n. We use $\mathbb{R}$ to denote a set of real numbers, $\mathbb{R}^n$ to denote a set of n-dimensional real column vectors, and $\mathbb{R}^{m \times n}$ to denote a set of $m \times n$ real matrices. The set of real non-negative numbers is denoted by $\mathbb{R}_+$, and the set of n-dimensional real non-negative vectors is denoted by $\mathbb{R}_+^n$. We use $\mathbb{S}^n$ to denote a set of symmetric $n \times n$ matrices, $\mathbb{S}_+^n$ to denote a set of symmetric *positive semidefinite* $n \times n$ matrices, and $\mathbb{S}_{++}^n$ to denote a set of symmetric *strictly positive definite* $n \times n$ matrices. We will define positive semidefiniteness and strictly positive definiteness later. $\mathbb{N}$ is a set of natural numbers. $\mathbb{N}_n$ is a subset of $\mathbb{N}$, and is defined by $\mathbb{N}_n \equiv \{i \in \mathbb{N} | i \leq n\}$. Symbols $\leq$ and $\geq$ are used to denote not only the standard inequalities between scalars but also the component-wise inequalities between vectors. Finally, $\langle \cdot, \cdot \rangle$ is the operator of inner-product among vectors.

14.2
Support Vector Machines and Kernels

This section reviews the support vector machine (SVM; e.g., [14]). Nowadays we can find lots of tutorials and introductions about SVM elsewhere [8, 9, 13, 17, 41, 52]. Most of the tutorials describe SVM as a *large margin classifier;* SVM finds a *hyperplane* with the largest margin between two *classes* to determine the classification boundary. Here we attempt to introduce SVM with a different explanation that is based on the literature [3, 12].

14.2.1
Support Vector Machines

SVM is basically a framework that automatically learns a linear classifier to distinguish a positive class from a negative class. For learning, we need a dataset. The dataset used for learning is called a training dataset. Each sample in the dataset has a binary label, $+1$ or -1. In the later section we discuss a case where SVM learns the classifier that discriminates the data of human kidney of normal tissues from those of renal clear carcinoma tissues. In this case, we assign the positive label $+1$ to the normal tissues, and the negative label -1 to the carcinoma tissues. Each sample is represented by a fixed-length vector x often called an input vector. In the case of classification of microarray data, an input vector typically consists of gene expression values. For example, if we use the expression data of d genes, the length of the input vector is d, that is, $x \in \mathbb{R}^d$.

The SVM classifier is a score function of input data. After training the SVM classifier, we compute the score of the data with unknown labels. Unlabeled samples are classified by examining whether the score is greater than a threshold. The threshold is often set to zero. The boundary that distinguishes the positive class from the negative one is a hyperplane. This is because the score function of SVM is a linear function expressed as:

$$f(x; w, b) = \langle w, x \rangle + b,$$

where $w \in \mathbb{R}^d$ and $b \in \mathbb{R}$ are the model parameters of SVM. The score contains a confidence level; a larger value will be a confident prediction of being in a positive class.

Let us consider how to determine the parameters of the classification hyperplane, (w, b). To learn the normal vector automatically, we usually gather training samples first:

$$(x_1, y_1), \ldots, (x_\ell, y_\ell) \in \mathbb{R}^d \times \{\pm 1\}.$$

We then compute some statistics from the samples to determine w. If we have computed the means of the two classes, $m_+ \in \mathbb{R}^d$ and $m_- \in \mathbb{R}^d$, one of the simplest approaches to classification is to classify a new sample x to the class whose mean is closer. The classification boundary of this approach is the hyperplane that is orthogonal to the line segment between m_+ and m_- and bisects the line segment

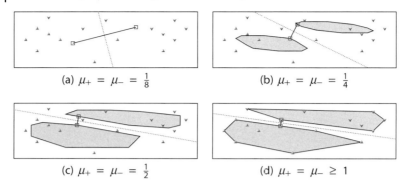

Figure 14.1 Geometrical interpretation of SVM. Positive and negative samples in $\mathbb{R}^2$ are plotted by upward- and downward-pointing triangles, respectively. (a) Shown is the classification boundary designed in a simple way; the boundary bisects the line segment between the means of two classes. (d) The closest points of the two convex hulls are depicted by squares. The convex hulls are obtained by setting $\mu_+ = \mu_- = 1$. Varying the values yields different convex sets and leads to different classification boundaries, as shown in (b)–(d). When $\mu_+ = \mu_-$, all the boundaries can also be produced by SVM with a suitable choice of C.

(Figure 14.1a). The normal vector is obtained from the difference between two points, m_+ and m_-:

$$w = m_+ - m_-$$

and the offset is computed by:

$$b = \frac{1}{2}(\|m_+\|^2 + \|m_-\|^2).$$

Note that the mean of the positive class is close to the new sample if and only if the score is positive. Although the approach is very simple and intuitive, it does not give consideration to how the samples are distributed. We now generalize the simple approach in order to consider the distribution. Let us consider two vector sets, $\mathcal{V}_+$ and $\mathcal{V}_-$, that include the mean of the corresponding class, respectively (i.e., $m_+ \in \mathcal{V}_+$ and $m_- \in \mathcal{V}_-$). We first find the geometrically closest points between the two sets, $v_+ \in \mathcal{V}_+$ and $v_- \in \mathcal{V}_-$, and then construct the hyperplane by:

$$w = v_+ - v_-, \qquad b = \frac{1}{2}(\|v_+\|^2 + \|v_-\|^2).$$

The hyperplane bisects the shortest line connecting the two sets. The simple approach we have introduced first is a special case of the second one in which $\mathcal{V}_+ = \{m_+\}$ and $\mathcal{V}_- = \{m_-\}$. The two closest points can be expressed as the solution of the following minimization problem:

$$\min \ \|v_+ - v_-\|^2 \quad \text{wrt} \quad v_+ \in \mathcal{V}_+ \ \text{and} \ v_- \in \mathcal{V}_-. \tag{14.1}$$

Let us denote the index sets of the positive training set and the negative training set by:

$$\mathcal{I}_+ \equiv \{i \in \mathbb{N}_\ell | y_i = +1\}, \qquad \mathcal{I}_- \equiv \{i \in \mathbb{N}_\ell | y_i = -1\}.$$

Note that $\mathcal{I}_+ \cup \mathcal{I}_- = \mathbb{N}_\ell$. We now focus on the sets expressed as:

$$\mathcal{V}_+ \equiv \left\{ v_+ \in \mathbb{R}^d \,|\, 0 \leq \exists \alpha_i \leq \mu_+, v_+ = \sum_{i \in \mathcal{I}_+} \alpha_i x_i, \sum_{i \in \mathcal{I}_+} \alpha_i = 1 \right\},$$

$$\mathcal{V}_- \equiv \left\{ v_- \in \mathbb{R}^d \,|\, 0 \leq \exists \alpha_i \leq \mu_-, v_- = \sum_{i \in \mathcal{I}_-} \alpha_i x_i, \sum_{i \in \mathcal{I}_-} \alpha_i = 1 \right\},$$

where $\mu_+ \in \mathbb{R}$ and $\mu_- \in \mathbb{R}$ are the predetermined parameters.

Figure 14.1 shows the examples of convex sets, $\mathcal{V}_+$ and $\mathcal{V}_-$, with different values of μ_+ and μ_-. As shown in the figure, we can obtain a variety of classification boundaries by varying the values of μ_+ and μ_-. If we put $\mu_+ = 1/|\mathcal{I}_+|$ and $\mu_- = 1/|\mathcal{I}_-|$, the sets are reduced to $\mathcal{V}_+ = \{m_+\}$ and $\mathcal{V}_- = \{m_-\}$ (Figure 14.1a). If we put $\mu_+ \geq 1$ and $\mu_- \geq 1$, then $\mathcal{V}_+$ and $\mathcal{V}_-$ are the convex hull of the positive training set and the negative training set, respectively (Figure 14.1d). The boundary is the same as that of hard margin SVM [41].

Since every point is represented by using $\boldsymbol{\alpha} \in \mathbb{R}^\ell$ as $v_+ = \sum_{i \in \mathcal{I}_+} \alpha_i x_i$ and $v_- = \sum_{i \in \mathcal{I}_-} \alpha_i x_i$, we wish to find α that represents the closest points. The square Euclidean distance between the two points can be expressed as:

$$\|v_+ - v_-\|^2 = \left\| \sum_{i \in \mathcal{I}_+} \alpha_i x_i - \sum_{i \in \mathcal{I}_-} \alpha_i x_i \right\|^2 = \sum_{i=1}^\ell \sum_{j=1}^\ell \alpha_i \alpha_j y_i y_j \langle x_i, x_j \rangle.$$

To find the closest points, we minimize the distance with respect to α that satisfies:

$$\sum_{i \in \mathcal{I}_+} \alpha_i = \sum_{i \in \mathcal{I}_-} \alpha_i = 1, \quad \text{and}$$

$$\forall i \in \mathcal{I}_+ : 0 \leq \alpha_i \leq \mu_+, \quad \forall i \in \mathcal{I}_- : 0 \leq \alpha_i \leq \mu_-.$$

We can rearrange the first condition to $\sum_{i=1}^\ell \alpha_i = 2$ and $\sum_{i=1}^\ell y_i \alpha_i = 0$. By introducing a predetermined constant ν to rescale the variables by $\nu/2$ and setting $\mu_+ = \mu_- = 2/\nu\ell$, the minimization problem in (14.1) to find the closest points can be rewritten as:

$$\min \sum_{i=1}^\ell \sum_{j=1}^\ell \alpha_i \alpha_j y_i y_j \langle x_i, x_j \rangle \quad \text{wrt } \boldsymbol{\alpha} \in \mathbb{R}^\ell,$$

$$\text{subj to } \sum_{i=1}^\ell \alpha_i = \nu, \quad \sum_{i=1}^\ell y_i \alpha_i = 0, \quad \forall i \in \mathbb{N}_\ell : 0 \leq \alpha_i \leq \frac{1}{\ell}. \tag{14.2}$$

This formulation is well known as the ν-SVM classifier [42], which is a variant of SVM. The algorithm of the original SVM classifier [41] is given by:

$$\min \sum_{i=1}^{\ell}\sum_{j=1}^{\ell} \alpha_i \alpha_j y_i y_j \langle x_i, x_j \rangle - 2\sum_{i=1}^{\ell} \alpha_i \quad \text{wrt} \quad \alpha \in \mathbb{R}^{\ell},$$

$$\text{subj to} \quad \sum_{i=1}^{\ell} y_i \alpha_i = 0, \quad \forall i \in \mathbb{N}_{\ell} : 0 \le \alpha_i \le C. \tag{14.3}$$

The original SVM classifier requires a predetermined parameter C instead of ν. The decision function produced by ν-SVM can be produced by the original SVM classifier with a suitable choice of C [10].

14.2.2
Kernel Matrix

We now express the formulation in Equation (14.3) by using a matrix notation. Suppose we are given $n(>\ell)$ samples and the first ℓ samples are labeled. We train SVM to predict the labels of the remaining $(n-\ell)$ samples. We use an $n \times n$ matrix K to store the values of the inner-product among input vectors:

$$K_{ij} = \langle x_i, x_j \rangle \quad \text{for} \quad i,j = 1, \ldots, n. \tag{14.4}$$

We call $K \in \mathbb{S}^n$ a *kernel matrix* and partition it as:

$$K = \begin{bmatrix} K^{\text{tra}} & K^{\text{tra,tst}} \\ (K^{\text{tra,tst}})^T & K^{\text{tst}} \end{bmatrix} \tag{14.5}$$

where K^{tra} is an $\ell \times \ell$ symmetric matrix, K^{tst} is $(n-\ell) \times (n-\ell)$ and symmetric, and $K^{\text{tra,tst}}$ is $\ell \times (n-\ell)$. The sub-matrix $K^{\text{tra}} \in \mathbb{S}^{\ell}$ corresponds to the kernel matrix of ℓ labeled samples, and is the data inputted to the SVM algorithm. The matrix form of the optimization problem in Equation (14.3) is expressed as:

$$\min \quad \alpha^T D_y K^{\text{tra}} D_y \alpha - 2\alpha^T 1_{\ell} \quad \text{wrt} \quad \alpha \in \mathbb{R}^{\ell},$$
$$\text{subj to} \quad y^T \alpha = 0, \quad 0_{\ell} \le \alpha \le C 1_{\ell} \tag{14.6}$$

where $D_y \in \mathbb{S}^{\ell}$ is a diagonal matrix with the i-th diagonal element y_i. The vector $\alpha = [\alpha_1, \ldots, \alpha_{\ell}]^T$ is the variable to be optimized. Note that input vectors themselves are no longer necessary for SVM learning once the values of the inner-products are computed. In other words, the theory of SVM learning can be applied so long as there exists a set of ℓ vectors that produce the symmetric matrix K. Let us examine an example of the kernel matrix. Can a symmetric matrix:

$$K = \begin{bmatrix} 2 & 2 & 4 \\ 2 & 10 & 12 \\ 4 & 12 & 16 \end{bmatrix}$$

be produced by a set of vectors? The answer is yes. Generally, a symmetric matrix can be produced by different sets of vectors. The set of vectors:

$$x_1 = \begin{bmatrix} -1 \\ -1 \end{bmatrix}, \quad x_2 = \begin{bmatrix} -3 \\ 1 \end{bmatrix}, \quad x_3 = \begin{bmatrix} -4 \\ 0 \end{bmatrix}$$

produces the matrix K, and the set:

$$x_1 = \begin{bmatrix} -1 \\ 1 \end{bmatrix}, \quad x_2 = \begin{bmatrix} 1 \\ 3 \end{bmatrix}, \quad x_3 = \begin{bmatrix} 0 \\ 4 \end{bmatrix}$$

also produces K. One can easily check this using Equation (14.4). Such vectors are called *feature vectors*. On the other hand, there is no set of vectors that produce the following symmetric matrix:

$$K = \begin{bmatrix} 2 & 2 & 4 \\ 2 & 10 & 12 \\ 4 & 12 & 5 \end{bmatrix}.$$

These observations pose the question of how to check whether a symmetric matrix could be applied to SVM learning. This can be done by computing the eigenvalues of the matrix. If all the eigenvalues are non-negative, the matrix can be an input of SVM algorithm. Such a symmetric matrix is said to be *positive semidefinite*, and a formal definition is given as follows:

Definition 14.1 (positive semidefinite, strictly positive definite)
A symmetric matrix $K \in \mathbb{S}^n$ is said to be positive semidefinite if K holds:

$$\forall c \in \mathbb{R}^\ell : c^T K c \geq 0.$$

If $c^T K c > 0$ for all non-zero $c \in \mathbb{R}^\ell$, we say that $K \in \mathbb{S}^n$ is strictly positive definite.

The following two theorems rationalize why we can use the eigenvalues to check whether a symmetric matrix is positive semidefinite and whether there exists a vector set producing the kernel matrix.

Theorem 14.1
A symmetric matrix is positive semidefinite if and only if all the eigenvalues are non-negative.

Theorem 14.2
A symmetric matrix $K \in \mathbb{S}^n$ is positive semidefinite if and only if there exists a set of ℓ vectors that produces K using Equation (14.4).

14.2.3
Polynomial Kernel and RBF Kernel

We have already seen Equation (14.4) which is an algorithm producing a positive semidefinite matrix. Equation (14.4) is called the *linear kernel*. There are many other choices to obtain a positive semidefinite matrix. The widely used polynomial kernel and RBF kernel are defined respectively by:

$$K_{ij}^{\text{poly}} = (c^2 + \langle x_i, x_j \rangle)^p, \quad K_{ij}^{\text{rbf}} = \exp\left(-\frac{D^2(x_i, x_j)}{2\sigma^2}\right) \qquad (14.7)$$

where $p \in \mathbb{N}$ and $\sigma \in \mathbb{R}$ are constants and are called the degree and the width, respectively. The function $D(\cdot, \cdot)$ gives the Euclidean distance:

$$D(x_i, x_j) = \|x_i - x_j\| = \sqrt{\sum_{k=1}^{d} (x_{ik} - x_{jk})^2}, \qquad (14.8)$$

where x_{ik} and x_{jk} are the k-th element of x_i and x_j, respectively. The following two theorems ensure that both kernels always produce a kernel matrix that can be inputted to the SVM algorithm.

Theorem 14.3
Any kernel matrix produced by the polynomial kernel is positive semidefinite.

Theorem 14.4
Any kernel matrix produced by the RBF kernel is positive semidefinite.

Indeed, there exists a mapping function $\phi(\cdot)$ of the input vectors such that the kernel matrix coincides with the inner-products among the feature vectors generated by the mapping function:

$$K_{ij} = \langle \phi(x_i), \phi(x_j) \rangle. \qquad \text{for} \quad \forall i, \forall j \in \mathbb{N}_n.$$

There are several advantages of using the polynomial kernels and the RBF kernels instead of the linear kernel. One advantage of using the polynomial kernels is to incorporate terms of p-th order into a feature vector. Let us examine a simple case of $p = 2$ and $c = 0$. If we define a mapping function:

$$\phi(x) = [x_1 x_1, \ldots, x_d x_1, x_d x_2, \ldots, x_d x_{d-1}, x_1 x_d, \ldots x_d x_d]^T,$$

we have $\langle \phi(x_i), \phi(x_j) \rangle = \langle x_i, x_j \rangle^2$. The derivation is omitted but straightforward.

14.2.4
Pre-process of Kernels

When we analyze data statistically, we often perform pre-processing of the data to remove irrelevant information. We introduce two kinds of pre-processing for analysis with SVM.

14.2.4.1 Normalization
Many studies make the norm of all the feature vectors $\|\phi(x)\|$ unit because norms have little information for classification in many cases. That transformation is called normalization. Any feature vector except zero can be normalized by $\phi(x)/\|\phi(x)\|$. Note that this operation transforms the norm in a unit, although the direction is not changed. This transformation can also be performed only by using the kernel matrix.

The normalized kernel matrix K^{new} is given by:

$$K_{ij}^{new} = \left\langle \frac{\phi(x_i)}{\|\phi(x_i)\|}, \frac{\phi(x_j)}{\|\phi(x_j)\|} \right\rangle = \frac{\langle \phi(x_i), \phi(x_j) \rangle}{\|\phi(x_i)\| \|\phi(x_j)\|} = \frac{K_{ij}}{\sqrt{K_{ii} K_{jj}}}. \quad (14.9)$$

14.2.4.2 SVD Denoising

A particular drawback of the microarray techniques is that running microarray experiments can be technically rather error prone. Microarray devices may contain dust and scratches that may lead to failure of hybridization and image analysis of some spots that represent gene expression levels. Therefore, the microarray data frequently contain noisy values that may seriously disturb subsequent statistical analysis.

For noise reduction, the approach based on principal component analysis (PCA) is often used in many analytical studies, including microarray analysis. PCA is a tool to extract informative subspaces from the dataset. The subspace is called the principal subspace. We project each feature vector to the principal subspace to eliminate the components in the remaining non-informative subspace. Principal subspace is computed by singular value decomposition (SVD), which is a factorization of a matrix given in the following theorem.

Theorem 14.5
Every matrix $X \in \mathbb{R}^{d \times n}$ can be factorized by two orthonormal matrices $U \in \mathbb{R}^{d \times d}$ and $V \in \mathbb{R}^{n \times n}$ and a diagonal matrix $S \in \mathbb{R}^{d \times n}$ such that:

$$X = USV^T, \quad (14.10)$$

where the diagonal matrix forms:

$$S = \begin{bmatrix} \mathrm{diag}\{s_1, \ldots, s_d\}, & \mathbf{0}_{d \times (n-d)} \end{bmatrix},$$

when $d \leq n$; otherwise:

$$S = \begin{bmatrix} \mathrm{diag}\{s_1, \ldots, s_n\} \\ \mathbf{0}_{(d-n) \times n} \end{bmatrix}.$$

The term $\mathrm{diag}\{s_1, \ldots, s_r\}$ denotes an $r \times r$ symmetric diagonal matrix with $s_1 \geq s_2 \geq \cdots \geq s_r \geq 0$.

The factorization in Equation (14.10) is termed singular value decomposition, and s_i are singular values. Each column of U and V is called a left singular vector and a right singular vector, respectively. The k-dimensional principal subspace is spanned by the first k left singular vectors $u_1, \ldots, u_k$. The projection of $x \in \mathbb{R}^d$ onto the principal subspace is given by $(U')^T x$ where $U' \equiv [u_1, \ldots, u_k]$. Substituting the projections into Equation (14.4), we obtain the kernel matrix as:

$$K^{svd} = \sum_{i=1}^{k} s_i^2 v_i v_i^T.$$

The value of s_i^2 is equal to the i-th eigenvalue, and v_i coincides with the i-th eigenvector, as seen in the proof of Theorem 2.2.

However, this approach has a drawback. If the true distribution of data without noise were available, we would be able to obtain the exact principal subspace of the true distribution and, therefore, this approach would work well. Typically, however, we know neither the true distribution nor the true principal subspace in advance. Hence, we have to resort the contaminated data themselves to obtain the principal subspace. In this regard, the principal subspace can still be contaminated, and the resulting projections are not often well-denoised. We will discuss an alternative approach to noise reduction in the next section.

14.3
Metrization Kernels: Kernels for Microarray Data

This section introduces three metrization kernels that are produced from distances among data. The distance designed heuristically for microarray data is often non-metric. Those kernels we review in this section are always valid even if the distance is non-metric. SVM performance depends on the quality of a kernel matrix. Some classes of kernel matrices can be explained as a similarity matrix. One class is normalized kernel matrices because the values are the cosine of the angles among the feature vectors. We can say that the RBF kernel is also regarded as a tool that generates a similarity matrix because of its definition. The kernel is defined by a monotonically increasing function, $\exp(\cdot)$, of the negative Euclidean distance between input vectors. This leads to an additional perspective that the RBF kernel is a transformation from a distance matrix to a valid kernel matrix. This motivates us to devise another distance specialized for gene expression to obtain improved kernel matrices.

14.3.1
Partial Distance (or kNND)

The main issue addressed herein is how to handle noisy and missing values that exist in a large portion of a gene expression profile consisting of heterogeneous data. To effectively eliminate such spurious values without removing the entire gene, we devised the following distance. Assume that we have a gene expression table with d genes and n samples where a sample contains $\nu(\times 100)\%$ of noisy genes on average. In such a case only $(1-\nu)$ of genes in that sample contain no noise. Therefore, for any pair of samples, the ratio of common genes not containing noise is expected to be $(1-\nu)^2$. Based on this observation, we devised the following distance:

$$D_p(x_i, x_j) \equiv \min_{\forall \mathcal{I}, s.t. \mathcal{I} \subseteq \mathbb{N}_d, |\mathcal{I}|=d_p} \sqrt{\sum_{k \in \mathcal{I}} (x_{ik} - x_{jk})^2}, \qquad (14.11)$$

where $d_p < d$ is a predetermined constant. $|\mathcal{I}|$ represents the cardinality of $\mathcal{I}$. The distance can be computed efficiently as follows: First, we compute the one-dimensional

Euclidean distances $d_h = (x_{ih} - x_{jh})^2$ for $\forall h \in \mathbb{N}_d$. Then we select $k = \lfloor (1-\nu)^2 d \rfloor$ of one-dimensional Euclidean distances d_h from the smallest ones. Finally, we take the sum of the selected d_h as the distance between x_i and x_j. We call this distance the partial distance [19], or the k-nearest neighbor distance (kNND) [15]. For instance, if a sample with $d = 100$ genes contains $\nu = 15\%$ of noisy values, $k = \lfloor (1-0.15)^2 \times 100 \rfloor = 72$ of the smallest distance genes out of the 100 genes are only considered in computing the partial distance between samples.

To classify microarray data, we need a kernel matrix. We consider building a kernel matrix from the partial distances. The RBF kernel is a well-known kernel that is computed from distances among samples. In the previous section we chose Euclidean distances as $D(\cdot, \cdot)$ in Equation (14.7). Generally, the RBF kernel produces a positive semidefinite matrix if and only if $-D^2(\cdot, \cdot)$ is conditionally positive semidefinite [4] (the definition is not shown). The negative squared Euclidean distance generates a conditionally positive semidefinite matrix, but $-D_p^2(\cdot, \cdot)$ does not. Hence, we have to employ another approach to metrization from the partial distances to a kernel matrix.

14.3.2
Maximum Entropy Kernel

We here describe an algorithm called the maximum entropy (ME) kernel [15, 49] to construct a kernel matrix from the partial distances. The algorithm was originally devised to represent an undirected graph, such as an enzyme network or a protein–protein interaction network [49].

Unlike the kernels described in the previous section, the ME kernel does not have any predefined functions. Instead, we obtain the ME kernel in matrix form, K, by basically maximizing the von Neumann entropy defined by:

$$H(K) = -\text{tr}(K \log K - K)$$

with respect to a strictly positive definite matrix K subject to the distance constraints:

$$\forall (i,j) \in \mathcal{E} \quad : \quad \|\phi(x_i) - \phi(x_j)\| \leq D_{ij},$$

where $\mathcal{E} \subseteq \mathbb{N}_n \times \mathbb{N}_n$ is a set of pairs, and D_{ij} is the given upper bound of the distance for pair (i,j). Owing to the distance constraints, the kernel matrix is obtained such that a particular pair of feature vectors must not be distant. The distance constraints are constructed from the partial distance defined in Equation (14.11): $D_{ij} = G D_p(x_i, x_j)$ where G is a constant. Since the partial distance is designed for nearby pairs, we remove the distance constraints for distant pairs. To do this, we design $\mathcal{E}$, a set of pairs to form the distance constraints, from the edges of k-nearest neighbor graph[1] [33]. In addition to the distance constraints, we restrict the trace of the kernel matrix to be unit to avoid the unlimited divergence of K.

---

[1] The k-nearest neighbor graph is a graph in which an edge is established if a node of the edge is in k nearest neighbor of the other node.

To obtain the kernel matrix we have to solve the optimization problem. However, it cannot be solved analytically. An efficient numerical algorithm is detailed in Appendix 14 A.

14.3.3
Other Distance-Based Kernels

We present here two other metrization kernels to obtain a kernel matrix from distance matrix D_{ij}. Both approaches are originally devised to convert a non-positive semidefinite similarity matrix $S \in \mathbb{S}^n$ into a kernel matrix. The first approach is to take $S^T S$ as a new kernel matrix. The kernel is sometimes called empirical kernel mapping (EKM) [40]. The second approach is to subtract the smallest negative eigenvalue of the similarity matrix S from its diagonal. We call it the Saigo kernel [39]. We obtain a similarity matrix from distance matrix D_{ij} via $S_{ij} = \exp(-D_{ij}/\sigma^2)$.

14.4
Applications to Cancer Data

In this section we compare the classification performances of the six kernels in various cancer data and discuss the differences between metrization (ME, EKM, and Saigo) kernels and standard vectorial data (linear, RBF, and polynomial) kernels. Again, note that the RBF kernel also uses Euclidean distance as the metric of sample (dis-)similarities but cannot use the partial distance (PD) since it violates the positive semidefiniteness of kernels. Figure 14.2 shows a schematic view of the entire analysis

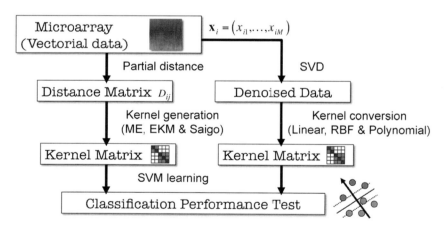

Figure 14.2 Schematic view of the entire process of microarray classification in the metrization (ME, EKM, and Saigo) and vectorial (linear, RBF, and polynomial) kernels. In the metrization kernels, the microarray vectorial data are first converted into a partial distance matrix D_{ij}, generating an optimal kernel matrix that is guaranteed to be positive semidefinite. In the vectorial kernels, the microarray data are first SVD-denoised and directly converted into kernels. Then, the SVM learns the classification boundary from kernel matrices and classifies test samples.

process. We use three examples of cancer datasets: *heterogeneous* human kidney data of normal and renal clear carcinoma tissues, *homogeneous* acute myeloid leukemia (AML) and acute lymphoblastic leukemia (ALL) data with artificial noise, and *heterogeneous* squamous cell carcinoma metastasis in the human head and neck regions.

14.4.1
Leave-One-Out Cross Validation

In the SVM classification analysis, various schemes are available to evaluate accuracies of predictions. In this chapter we simply adopt the standard leave-one-out cross-validation (LOOCV) procedure where each sample is alternatively excluded from the N data and the SVM trained with the remaining $N-1$ samples predicts the excluded one. The exclusion of $1/m \times N$ of data alternatively for use in prediction is generally called "*m*-fold cross-validation test." All accuracies reported in this chapter are calculated with the following formula:

$$\text{Accuracy} = \frac{TP + TN}{TP + FP + TN + FN},$$

where TP, FP, TN, and FN are true positive, false positive, true negative, and false negative frequencies, respectively, in the classification. There are various types of equations to evaluate binary classification performances. For example, there are measurements called "sensitivity" and "specificity" that are frequently used to evaluate the prediction power from more specific aspects:

$$\text{Sensitivity} = \frac{TP}{TP + FN},$$

$$\text{Specificity} = \frac{TN}{TN + FP}.$$

The graph obtained when we plot sensitivity against false positive rate (i.e., 1−Specificity) with various SVM boundary thresholds is called a *receiver operating characteristic* (ROC) curve. The area under an ROC curve is also often used for comparison of prediction performances.

14.4.2
Data Normalization and Classification Analysis

Before testing the performance, all the raw data should be properly normalized by being first log-transformed and then scaled to mean 0 and standard deviation 1 (i.e., Z-normalization) in each sample and then each gene. Practically, many genes have a large number of missing values because heterogeneous data are combined; thus, we might need to estimate those values with the rest of the data beforehand. However, in this chapter, since we do not focus on the missing value estimation issues, we will adopt a simple imputation method that all the missing values are replaced with the mean value, that is, 0. Input genes that show high correlation to class labels, or *feature genes*, are selected by the standard two sample *t*-statistics [38] in each iteration of the LOOCV test. The distance constraint matrices (D_{ij}) are also generated from the same feature genes. If a sample contains missing values, we again adopt a simple imputation method; we replace the one-dimensional Euclidean distance $(x_{ik}-x_{jk})^2$ with the mean value, that is, 2, if x_{ik} or x_{jk} is missing. Once a dataset is ready, the six kernels are tested with SVMs to analyze their classification performance with various numbers of feature genes and various parameters, as in the next section. The maximum accuracy among the tested parameters for each number of feature genes is recorded as the accuracy for each kernel.

14.4.3
Parameter Selection

Since classification accuracies depend on the parameters in the kernel-SVM method, we need to test various parameter values to obtain the best performance possible. In this chapter, for all the six (linear, polynomial, RBF, EKM, Saigo, and ME) kernels tested here, seven SVM parameters, $C = 10^{-3}, 10^{-2}, 10^{-1}, 1, 10, 10^2, 10^3$, are tested. For the polynomial kernel, $D = 1,2,3,4,5,6,7,8,9,10$ are tested. For the RBF, EKM, and Saigo kernels, $\sigma = 10^{-10}, 10^{-9}, 10^{-8}, 10^{-7}, 10^{-6}, 10^{-5}, 10^{-4}, 10^{-3}, 10^{-2}, 10^{-1}, 1$ are tested. In the ME kernel, we use only one parameter G that magnifies the distance constraints D_{ij} to adjust the trade-off between over-learning and generalization of classification models (for details, see Reference [19]). The parameter G has to be chosen carefully. When $G \to 0$, typically $K \to 11^T/N$. When $D_{ij} > 2/N$ for $\forall i, \forall j$, $K \to I/N$. The two are somewhat extreme cases. However, if the value of G is positive but too small, SVM will not be able to find the hyperplane separating the positive class from the negative one clearly. Conversely, if the value of G is too large, the so-called diagonal dominant problem [43] ensues. We test the parameter in the range of $G = 2^{-5}, 2^{-4}, 2^{-3}, 2^{-2}, 2^{-1}, 1, 2, 2^2, 2^3, 2^4, 2^5$. To ensure fairness of comparison, it is also important that the total number of parameter combinations in the ME kernel be equal to those in the RBF, EKM, and Saigo kernels in the study.

14.4.4
Heterogeneous Kidney Carcinoma Data

Data of human renal normal tissues and renal clear carcinoma tissues were collected from the public gene expression database GEO–Gene Expression Omnibus [2]. This dataset consists of ten platforms, two of which are spotted DNA/cDNA arrays and eight are variations of Affymetrix-type oligonucleotide arrays. To uniformly analyze the array data from different platforms, we convert as many probe names as possible into standard UniGene (see Reference [1]) identifiers and combine all the data. The total number of UniGenes in the integrated table is as large as 54 674, all of which contain missing values in some platforms; that is, there are no genes common to all platforms. The total number of normal and carcinoma tissue data is 100 (62 normal and 38 carcinoma) and classification analysis between normal and carcinoma is performed.

Figure 14.3 plots the results of the LOOCV test of 100 samples against various numbers (8–296; increasing 8 genes at each step due to computational limitations) of

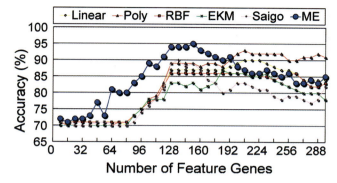

Figure 14.3 Classifications of heterogeneous renal carcinoma data with vectorial and metrization kernels. In most cases, the ME kernel shows much better performance than the linear, polynomial, and RBF kernels and the other two distance-based kernels for various numbers of feature genes. (Modified from Fujibuchi and Kato [15].)

feature genes. The figure shows that the accuracy increases with increasing number of feature genes, plateaus at some region, and decreases, well characterizing typical classification curves. Clearly, the ME kernel performs much better in all cases than the other five kernels for small numbers of feature genes (8–192). In fact, the ME kernel records maximum accuracies of 95.0 (89.5/98.4 sensitivity/specificity)% for 152 feature genes and its accuracies are superior to those of the other five kernels in 64.9% of the tested points (8–296) of feature genes.

14.4.5
Problems in Training Multiple Support Vector Machines for All Sub-data

In the above example of renal carcinoma data, we mix all of the ten sub-data together to train SVMs and predict test samples. As an alternative approach, using vectorial data kernels, it is theoretically possible to train multiple SVMs for all distinct sub-data contained in the composite dataset. However, this approach has practical difficulties in that (i) there are too many heterogeneous sub-data, (ii) some sub-data contain only a few samples, and (iii) some sub-data contain all positive (or negative) samples. The SVMs cannot be trained properly with only a few samples or data with one-sided (positive or negative) labels. In addition, if we do not know the origin (i.e., platform) of the test samples, it would be difficult to determine which SVMs should be used for the classification. Thus, it is very useful to apply the ME kernel to the mixed data because it is much simpler yet quite flexible in this regard.

14.4.6
Effects of Partial Distance Denoising in Homogeneous Leukemia Data

Acute myeloid leukemia (AML) and acute lymphoblastic leukemia (ALL) data for cancer subtype classification have been reported by Golub *et al.* [16] and are often recognized as gold-standard data for microarray classification analysis. There are

72 samples (47 AML and 25 ALL), all of which are quite homogeneous and of good quality, and are thus suitable for artificial noise experiments. To assess the denoising ability of the PD-based ME kernel, we first replace $v_{add} \times 100\%$ of original data in a gene expression profile with artificial white noise. The noise is added according to a normal distribution model by $N(0, (2\sigma_{gene})^2)$; a mean of 0 and a standard deviation of twice that of each gene value distribution in the original dataset. Then, we extract 50 feature genes from the training dataset for each iteration of the LOOCV test by the standard t-test.

As the control experiments use linear and RBF kernels, the standard singular value decomposition (SVD) is applied to reduce noise immediately after artificial noise is introduced. In the SVD denoising, three levels of noise removals by different cumulative proportions, 85, 90, and 95%, of eigenvalues are explored. For the ME kernel, the PD denoising method with the following noise level settings is applied. First, we define the total noise level as the sum of the raw noise and the above artificially added noise as $v_{raw} + v_{add}$, where the raw noise that is assumed to internally exist in the original data is arbitrarily set at $v_{raw} = 0.05$. If 10% artificial noise is added, the total noise level is $v_{raw} + v_{add} = 0.05 + 0.1 = 0.15$ and, according to Equation (14.11), $(1-0.15)^2 \times 100 = 72.3\%$ of the nearest distance genes out of the feature gene set are considered in calculating the PDs between samples.

We repeat the above random noise-adding test ten times and average the highest accuracies among various parameter combinations. Figure 14.4 shows the results. The artificial noise added is within the range of 0–50%. The accuracies decrease gradually with increasing noise levels (10–50%) for the vectorial kernels; for example, the accuracies of the RBF kernel decrease in the order of 96.2, 95.9, 91.0, 82.5, and 79.5%. SVD denoising boosts these accuracies to 98.0, 96.6, 93.2, 91.0, and 86.5%, respectively. Linear and polynomial kernels also show similar accuracies to the RBF kernel when SVD denoising is used.

Interestingly and surprisingly, the three PD-distance-based methods show high accuracies; for example, the PD-ME kernel has an accuracy of 97.8% even at 20%

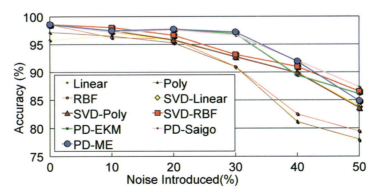

Figure 14.4 AML/ALL classification with artificial noise. The accuracies of standard linear and RBF kernels decrease with increasing noise levels, even with SVD denoising applied, while those of ME and other distance-based kernels with FD denoising are sustained at high levels at 10–30% noise levels. (Modified from Fujibuchi and Kato [15].)

noise level and maintains high accuracies of 97.2 and 92.0% at 30–40% noise levels. The EKM and Saigo kernels using PD-distance also show similar accuracies to the PD-ME kernel. To confirm the superior denoising ability of the PD-based method, results of intensive analysis of the same data with various parameters can be obtained from the author's web site [19].

14.4.7
Heterogeneous Squamous Cell Carcinoma Metastasis Data

We further analyze the total performance of the six kernels with a more practical problem – heterogeneous human squamous cell carcinoma metastasis data. The data consist of four GEO datasets (GSE2280, GSE3524, GSE9349, and GSE2379) from three different platforms (GPL96, GPL201, and GPL91). GSE2280 and GSE3524 are from the same platform (GPL96) but they are from different authors [31, 47]. The four datasets contain 14/8, 9/9, 11/11, and 15/19 metastasis/non-metastasis samples, respectively, and the size of each dataset is too small and not suitable for SVM classification if analyzed separately. However, combining all of the four datasets, we obtain as many as 49 metastasis and 47 non-metastasis samples, making it possible to carry out the SVM classification analysis.

Figure 14.5 shows the results of the LOOCV test for a total of 96 samples against various numbers (1–100; increasing one gene at each step) of feature genes with six different kernels with corresponding denoising methods, namely, SVD-linear, SVD-polynomial, SVD-RBF, PD-EKM, PD-Saigo, and PD-ME. In the PD-ME kernel, five different noise levels, $\nu = 0$ (no noise), $0.05, 0.1, 0.15$, and 0.2 are evaluated. In the SVD denoising, five noise removal levels, 80, 85, 90, 95, and 100 (no noise) % of cumulative proportions, which are equal to the number of parameters of the PD denoising experiment, are tested.

The results indicate that the accuracy of the PD-ME kernel mostly exceeds those of the other kernels. The accuracies increase and plateau at around 20–80 feature genes.

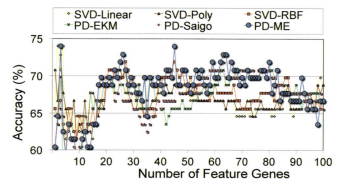

Figure 14.5 Squamous cell carcinoma metastasis classification. Prediction of metastasis by SVMs is performed with gene expression data of squamous cell carcinoma of the human head and neck regions. Classification accuracies of six kernels with corresponding denoising methods are compared.

Note that it is very important to provide robust prediction accuracies in real cancer diagnosis; the regions of 1–20 and 80–100 feature genes give too variant or too low accuracies for use in prediction. The result also indicates that the PD-ME kernel shows relatively stable and high accuracies compared to the other kernels for the proper numbers of feature genes (20–80). The top accuracy rate that the PD-ME kernel performs best among the six kernels in the 20–80 feature gene region is 33 points, which is $33/(80-20+1) = 54.1\%$. An overall maximum accuracy of 74.0 (75.5/72.3 sensitivity/specificity)% is observed for the PD-ME kernel at 45 feature genes, in the 20–80 feature gene region. This accuracy is obtained with the $\nu = 0.15$ denoising parameter.

14.4.8
Advantages of ME Kernel

One of the most remarkable properties of the ME kernel is that the generated kernel matrices always hold positive semidefiniteness, even when the distance matrices for input to the optimization algorithm violate the triangle inequalities at the initial point. This allows us to arbitrarily choose genes from among a set of feature genes to build the distance matrices in a distance-by-distance fashion. Utilizing this property, we introduce the PD denoising method for the distance-based kernels that show better performance than the linear, polynomial, and RBF kernels for leukemia data, even though the data are pre-denoised by SVD. This is quite important in a situation where there are few or heterogeneous samples where SVD may not work properly for denoising because the quality of the eigenvalue decomposition depends on the number of homogeneous samples. Since the PD denoising method only concerns the set of genes between sample pairs, it seems quite robust with regard to the number of samples or the degree of heterogeneity.

Furthermore, the results of kidney carcinoma and squamous cell carcinoma metastasis data in Figures 14.3 and 14.5, respectively, clearly show that the accuracies of the ME kernel exceed those of the other two distance-based kernels, EKM and Saigo. From these observations, the entropy maximization process may work favorably for "heterogeneous" data and allow SVMs to find the discriminant boundaries more easily than the other two distance-based methods, EKM and Saigo.

14.5
Conclusion

Through the analysis presented here, it becomes quite clear that combining similar but distinct data in the microarray analysis may enhance the realistic diagnosis of cancer or other diseases. As shown in our example of metastasis prediction for oral squamous cell carcinoma, each dataset contains only 18–34 samples, which is not suitable for training good SVM predictors. When the datasets are combined, however, the PD-ME kernel demonstrates higher and more robust classification performance than the other kernels, such as linear, polynomial, and RBF kernels regardless of SVD denoising, and even than the other two distance-based kernels, EKM and Saigo.

One weak point of the ME kernel is its scalability. The ME kernel is given by solving a maximization problem. As the solution cannot be given in a closed form, we have to resort to an iterative algorithm to achieve the kernel matrix. The major reason for the heavy computation is the eigendecomposition of an n by n matrix that is required at each iteration. The eigendecomposition takes $O(n^3)$ computation, disabling us from using the ME kernel when the number of samples is huge [18]. Alternatively, we have employed the steepest descent algorithm [5], which is one of the simplest methods for optimization in this textbook. There are some other smart algorithms that may be able to find a better solution. One is the LBFGS (limited-memory BFGS) formula [24], a derivative of the Newton algorithm [30] that needs a Hessian matrix[2] at each iteration. Although the Newton method is very promising because it usually provides a better solution, computation of the Hessian matrix is time-consuming. The LBFGS algorithm [14, 30], which requires and approximates the Hessian matrix at each iteration by using a compact storage, updates the Hessian matrix efficiently. Such techniques may allow us to convert a large-scale dataset into a proper ME kernel matrix. Moreover, if we could devise a new technique to compute the ME kernel for much larger datasets, the ME kernel will benefit from the semi-supervised setting [54] where unlabeled sample data are mixed with labeled ones in learning. The ME kernel is basically designed to use nearest-neighbor graphs [20], pushing unrelated data points away from related cluster of data. As some samples in a class often form clusters in the data space, even unlabeled sample data may help labeled data to establish clusters, which also improves classification accuracies [11].

In the kernel design field, notably, the trade-off between generalization and specialization is always a problem. For example, to obtain better biological results, the creation of specialized kernels to solve specific biological problems may practically be a good solution. However, too specifically designed kernels lose flexibility and thus cannot be applied to many other problems. Therefore, it will be a major task to learn how to create substantial kernels that would be applicable to various problems in various fields, including biomedical analysis.

Although this chapter has shown the use of SVM as an application of the metrization kernels, the SVM is not the only existing algorithm for kernel-based classification; rather, we can use various kernel methods, such as the kernel Fisher discriminant (KFD) [27] and the relevance vector machine (RVM) [46], as well as variants of the SVM. The KFD solves a linear system to obtain values of the model parameters. The coefficient matrix of the linear system is the sum of the kernel matrix and its scaled identity matrix. A naïve approach to solve the linear system is LU decomposition that requires $O(n^3)$ computation. In the case of the ME kernel, a slightly cleverer approach that utilizes the eigendecomposition of the kernel matrix is available. The eigendecomposition can be executed during kernel generation, where the time complexity is only $O(n^2)$. The total complexity is not changed because

---

2) A Hessian matrix is a matrix whose elements are the values of the second derivatives.

generating a kernel matrix requires $O(n^3)$. However, only $O(n^2)$ computation is required in the situation that the same kernel matrix is needed for different discriminant tasks [21, 22].

RVM [46] is formulated by a probabilistic model, allowing us to obtain posterior class probabilities that offer a confidence level of the prediction results. Besides classification, kernel matrices can be used for a wide variety of applications, including clustering [55], regression [46], data visualization [28], and novelty detection [42]. Future work remains in the evaluation of the ME kernel in the above situations to explore its possibilities.

Recently, several new cell types, such as induced pluripotent stem (iPS) cells [45] and cancer stem cells (CSCs) [37], have been either created or found. In these research fields, it becomes increasingly important to characterize the features of cells by computational methods before initiating medical treatments to patients. For example, some iPS cells created from various parts of the human body do not have strong multipotency or proliferation ability and sometimes, even worse, have tumorigenesis characteristics. Thus, cell typing using excellent computational methods, such as the kernel-based discriminant analysis for quality control, is required to realize regenerative medicine using iPS cells. In the future, the number of human cell types, regardless of healthy or diseased, to be discriminated is expected to increase. Kernel or kernel-based methods are expected to make immense contributions to a wide variety of biomedical research areas that require accurate and complex cell typings.

14.A
Appendix

Proof of Theorem 14.1

Any symmetric matrix $K \in \mathbb{S}^n$ has an eigendecomposition:

$$K = \sum_{i=1}^n t_i v_i v_i^T, \qquad (14.\text{A}.1)$$

where $t_i \in \mathbb{R}$ is the i-th eigenvalue and $v_i \in \mathbb{R}^n$ is the corresponding eigenvector: $\langle v_i, v_j \rangle = \delta_{ij}$ where δ_{ij} is the Kronecker delta. For a d-dimensional arbitrary vector $c \in \mathbb{R}^n$:

$$c^T K c = \sum_{i=1}^n t_i c^T v_i v_i^T c = \sum_{i=1}^n t_i \langle c, v_i \rangle^2. \qquad (14.\text{A}.2)$$

Since $\langle c, v_i \rangle^2 \geq 0$ for $\forall i$, the quadratic form $c^T K c$ is non-negative for any c if all the eigenvalue is non-negative. Conversely, suppose at least one of the eigenvalues t_k is negative. If we put $c = v_k$, then:

$$c^T K c = t_k \langle v_k, v_k \rangle^2 + \sum_{i \neq k} t_i \langle v_k, v_i \rangle^2 = t_k < 0 \qquad (14.\text{A}.3)$$

Hence, Theorem 14.1 is established.

Proof of Theorem 14.2

We first prove the necessary condition. From Theorem 14.1, all the eigenvalues of K are non-negative. Letting $t_i \in \mathbb{R}$ be the i-th eigenvalue and $v_i \in \mathbb{R}^n$ be the corresponding eigenvector, K is produced by the set of column vectors in the matrix:

$$X = \left[\sqrt{t_1}v_1, \ldots, \sqrt{t_n}v_n\right]^T.$$

We next show that the sufficient condition is established. Consider the $d \times n$ matrix whose columns are vectors $X = [x_1, \ldots, x_n]$ producing the kernel matrix K. Denote the SVD of X by $X = USV^T$ where $U \in \mathbb{R}^{d \times d}$ and $V \in \mathbb{R}^{n \times n}$ are *orthonormal* and $S \in \mathbb{R}^{d \times n}$ is *diagonal* whose diagonal elements are $\{s_i\}_{i=1}^{\min(d,n)}$. From the definition, $\forall i : s_i \geq 0$. Substituting SVD into X, we obtain the eigendecomposition of the kernel matrix as:

$$K = X^T X = VS^T U^T USV^T = VS^T SV^T = \sum_{i=1}^{\min(d,n)} s_i^2 v_i v_i^T. \tag{14.A.4}$$

Notice that the eigenvalues are s_i^2, which are non-negative. Hence, K is positive semidefinite.

Optimization Algorithm for ME Kernel

We here describe a numerical optimization algorithm to obtain the ME kernel. Let M be the number of pairs in $\mathcal{E}$ and denote $\mathcal{E} = \{(i_k, j_k)\}_{k=1}^M$. Furthermore, for simplicity of notation, we define $U_k \in \mathbb{S}^n$ by:

$$U_k \equiv E_{i_k, i_k} + E_{j_k, j_k} - E_{i_k, j_k} - E_{j_k, i_k} - D_{i_k, j_k} I_n \quad \text{for} \quad k \in \mathbb{N}_M.$$

Then, for any kernel matrix $K \in \mathbb{S}^n$ such that $\text{tr}(K) = 1$, the distance constraints can be rewritten as:

$$\forall k \in \mathbb{N}_M : \quad \|\phi(x_{i_k}) - \phi(x_{j_k})\|^2 - D_{i_k j_k} = \text{tr}(U_k K) \leq 0.$$

There does not always exist a kernel matrix that satisfies all the constraints. To keep the optimization problem feasible, we introduce a slack variable $x \in \mathbb{R}_+^M$ and relax the constraints as $\text{tr}(U_k K) \leq \xi_k$ for $\forall k \in \mathbb{N}_M$. The L1-norm of the slack variable is added to the objective function as a penalty. Then the optimization problem is expressed as:

$$\begin{aligned}
\min \quad & \text{tr}(K \log K) + \lambda \|\xi\|_1 \\
\text{wrt} \quad & K \in \mathbb{S}_{++}^n, \quad \xi \in \mathbb{R}_+^M \\
\text{subj to} \quad & \text{tr}(K) = 1, \quad \forall k \in \mathbb{N}_M : \text{tr}(U_k K) \leq \xi_k,
\end{aligned} \tag{14.A.5}$$

where λ is constant. Since this is a convex problem [6], gradient-based algorithms can easily attain to the optimal solution. An implementation is to solve the dual problem [6] instead of the primal problem given in Equation (14.A.5). The dual problem is described by:

$$\max \; -\log \operatorname{tr}(\exp(-\mathcal{U}\boldsymbol{\alpha})) \quad \text{wrt} \quad \boldsymbol{\alpha} \in \mathbb{R}_+^M \quad \text{subj to} \quad \boldsymbol{\alpha} \leq \lambda \mathbf{1}_M \qquad (14.A.6)$$

where $\boldsymbol{\alpha}$ is a dual variable vector [6] and the operator $\mathcal{U}$ performs $\mathcal{U}\boldsymbol{\alpha} = \sum_{k=1}^{M} \alpha_k U_k$. For optimization, the steepest descent method is used. If we denote the objective function of the problem in Equation (14.A.6) by J, the derivatives are given by:

$$\frac{\partial J}{\partial \alpha_k} = \frac{\operatorname{tr}(U_k \exp(-\mathcal{U}\boldsymbol{\alpha}))}{\operatorname{tr}(\exp(-\mathcal{U}\boldsymbol{\alpha}))} \quad \text{for} \quad \forall k \in \mathbb{N}_M.$$

When the values of some dual variables violate the constraints in (14.A.6) they are forced back into the feasible region. Since the optimization problem is convex, the optimal solution can always be attained from any initial values. Once we obtain the dual optimal solution, we can recover the primal optimal solution as follows:

$$K = \frac{\exp(-\mathcal{U}\boldsymbol{\alpha})}{\operatorname{tr}(\exp(-\mathcal{U}\boldsymbol{\alpha}))}.$$

References

1. NCBI UniGene project at ncbi. http://www.ncbi.nlm.nih.gov/unigene/, 2006.
2. Barrett, T., Suzek, T.O., Troup, D.B., Wilhite, S.E., Ngau, W.C., Ledoux, P., Rudnev, D., Lash, A.E., Fujibuchi, W., and Edgar, R. (2005) NCBI GEO: mining millions of expression profiles-database and tools. *Nucleic Acids Res.*, **33** (Database issue), D562–D566.
3. Bennett, K.P. and Bredensteiner, E.J. (2000) Duality and geometry in SVM classifiers, in *Proceedings of the 17th International Conference on Machine Learning*, Morgan Kaufmann Publishers Inc., pp. 57–64.
4. Berg, C., Christensen, J.P.R., and Ressel, P. (1984) *Harmonic Analysis on Semigroups*, Springer-Verlag, New York.
5. Bertsekas, D.P. (2004) *Nonlinear Programming*, Athena Scientific, Belmont, Mass.
6. Boyd, S. and Vandenberghe, L. (2004) *Convex Optimization*, Cambridge University Press.
7. Brazma, A., Parkinson, H., Sarkans, U., Shojatalab, M., Vilo, J., Abeygunawardena, N., Holloway, E., Kapushesky, M., Kemmeren, P., Lara, G.G., Oezcimen, A., Rocca-Serra, P., and Sansone, S.A. (2003) Arrayexpress-a public repository for microarray gene expression data at the ebi. *Nucleic Acids Res.*, **31** (1), 68–71.
8. Burges, C.J.C. (1998) A tutorial on support vector machines for pattern recognition, in *Data Mining and Knowledge Discovery*, vol. **2**, Kluwer Academic Publishers, pp. 121–167.
9. Campbell, C. (2001) An introduction to kernel methods, in *Radial Basis Function Networks 1: Recent Developments in Theory and Applications*, Physica Verlag Rudolf Liebing KG, Vienna, pp. 155–192.
10. Chang, C.-C. and Lin, C.-J. (2002) Training ν-support vector regression: theory and algorithms. *Neural. Comput.*, **14**, 1959–1977.
11. Chapelle, O., Schölkopf, B., and Zien, A. (2006) *Semi-Supervised Learning*, MIT Press, Cambridge, MA.
12. Crisp, D.J. and Burges, C.J.C. (2000) A geometric interpretation of ν-svm classifiers, in *Advances in Neural Information Processing Systems 12* (eds S.A. Solla, T.K. Leen, and K.-R. Müller), MIT Press.
13. Cristianini, N. and Shawe-Taylor, J. (2000) *An Introduction to Support Vector Machines and Other Kernel-Based Learning Methods*,

Cambridge University Press, Cambridge, UK.
14. Fletcher, R. (1987) *Practical Methods of Optimization*, Wiley-Interscience.
15. Fujibuchi, W. and Kato, T. (2007) Classification of heterogeneous microarray data by maximum entropy kernel. *BMC Bioinformatics*, 8, 267.
16. Golub, T.R., Slonim, D.K., Tamayo, P., Huard, C., Gaasenbeek, M., Mesirov, J.P., Coller, H., Loh, M.L., Downing, J.R., Caligiuri, M.A., Bloomfield, C.D., and Lander, E.S. (1999) Molecular classification of cancer: class discovery and class prediction by gene expression monitoring. *Science*, 286 (5439), 531–537.
17. Hastie, T., Tibshirani, R., and Friedman, J.H. (2003) *The Elements of Statistical Learning*, Springer.
18. Kashima, H., Ide, T., Kato, T., and Sugiyama, M. (2009) Recent advances and trends in large-scale kernel methods. *IEICE T. Inf. Syst.*, 92D, 1338–1353.
19. Kato, T., Fujibuchi, W., and Asai, K. (2006) Kernels for noisy microarray data. CBRC Technical Report, AIST-02-J00001-8. http://www.net-machine.net/~kato/pdf/t-kato-cbrctr2006a.pdf.
20. Kato, T., Kashima, H., and Sugiyama, M. (2008) Robust label propagation on multiple networks. *IEEE T. Neural Network.*, 20, 35–44.
21. Kato, T., Kashima, H., Sugiyama, M., and Asai, K. (2009) Conic programming for multi-task learning. *IEEE T. Knowl. Data Eng.* (in press).
22. Kato, T., Okada, K., Kashima, H., and Sugiyama, M. A transfer learning approach and selective integration of multiple types of assays for biological network inference. *Int. J. Knowledge Discovery Bioinformatics (IJKDB).* (in press).
23. Kondor, R. and Lafferty, J. (2002) Diffusion kernels on graphs and other discrete structures, in *Proceedings 19th International Conference on Machine Learning (ICML) [ICML 2002], San Francisco, CA, USA* (eds C. Sammut and A.G. Hoffmann), Morgan Kaufmann, pp. 315–322.
24. Liu, D.C. and Nocedal, J. (1989) On the limited memory method for large scale optimization. *Math. Program. B*, 45, 503–528.
25. Liu, H., Li, J., and Wong, L. (2005) Use of extreme patient samples for outcome prediction from gene expression data. *Bioinformatics*, 21 (16), 3377–3384.
26. Lodhi, H., Saunders, C., Shawe-Taylor, J., Cristianini, N., and Watkins, C. (2002) Text classification using string kernels. *J. Machine Learn. Res.*, 2, 419–444.
27. Mika, S., Rätch, G., Weston, J., and Schölkopf, B. (1999) Fisher discriminant analysis with kernels, in *Neural Networks for Signal Processing IX* (eds Y-.H. Hu, J. Larsen, E. Wilson, and S. Douglas), IEEE.
28. Mika, S., Schölkopf, B., Smola, A., Müller, K.R., Scholz, M., and Ratsch, G. (1999) Kernel PCA and de-noising in feature spaces, in *Advances in Neural Information Processing Systems 11* (eds M.S. Kearns, S.A. Solla, and D.A. Cohn), MIT Press, pp. 536–542.
29. Nilsson, B., Andersson, A., Johansson, M., and Fioretos, T. (2006) Cross-platform classification in microarray-based leukemia diagnostics. *Haematologica*, 91 (6), 821–882.
30. Nocedal, J. and Wright, S.J. (2006) *Numerical Optimization*, Springer, New York.
31. O'Donnell, R.K., Kupferman, M., Wei, S.J., Singhal, S., Weber, R., O'Malley, B.Jr., Cheng, Y., Putt, M., Feldman, M., Ziober, B., and Muschel, R.J. (2005) Gene expression signature predicts lymphatic metastasis in squamous cell carcinoma of the oral cavity. *Oncogene*, 24 (7), 1244–1251.
32. Okutsu, J., Tsunoda, T., Kaneta, Y., Katagiri, T., Kitahara, O., Zembutsu, H., Yanagawa, R., Miyawaki, S., Kuriyama, K., Kubota, N., Kimura, Y., Kubo, K., Yagasaki, F., Higa, T., Taguchi, H., Tobita, T., Akiyama, H., Takeshita, A., Wang, Y.H., Motoji, T., Ohno, R., and Nakamura, Y. (2002) Prediction of chemosensitivity for patients with acute myeloid leukemia, according to expression levels of 28 genes selected by genome-wide complementary DNA microarray analysis. *Mol. Cancer Ther.*, 1 (12), 1035–1042.
33. Preparata, F.P. and Shamos, M.I. (1985) *Computational Geometry: An Introduction*, Springer.

34 Ramaswamy, S., Tamayo, P., Rifkin, R., Mukherjee, S., Yeang, C.H., Angelo, M., Ladd, C., Reich, M., Latulippe, E., Mesirov, J.P., Poggio, T., Gerald, W., Loda, M., Lander, E.S., and Golub, T.R. (2001) Multiclass cancer diagnosis using tumor gene expression signatures. *Proc. Natl. Acad. Sci. USA*, **98** (26), 15149–15154.

35 Rhodes, D.R., Yu, J., Shanker, K., Deshpande, N., Varambally, R., Ghosh, D., Barrette, T., Pandey, A., and Chinnaiyan, A.M. (2004) Large-scale meta-analysis of cancer microarray data identifies common transcriptional profiles of neoplastic transformation and progression. *Proc. Natl. Acad. Sci. USA*, **101** (25), 9309–9314.

36 Rhodes, D.R., Yu, J., Shanker, K., Deshpande, N., Varambally, R., Ghosh, D., Barrette, T., Pandey, A., and Chinnaiyan, A.M. (2004) Oncomine: a cancer microarray database and integrated data-mining platform. *Neoplasia*, **6** (1), 1–6.

37 Rosen, J.M. and Jordan, C.T. (2009) The increasing complexity of the cancer stem cell paradigm. *Science*, **324** (5935), 1670–1673.

38 Rosner, B. (2000) *Fundamentals of Biostatistics*, 5th edn, Duxbury, Pacific Grove, CA.

39 Saigo, H., Vert, J.-P., Ueda, N., and Akutsu, T. (2004) Protein homology detection using string alignment kernels. *Bioinformatics*, **20** (11), 1682–1689.

40 Schölkopf, B., Weston, J., Eskin, E., Leslie, C., and Noble, W.S. (2002) A kernel approach for learning from almost orthogonal patterns, in *13th European Conference on Machine Learning, Helsinki, Finland* (eds S. Thrun, L. Saul, and B. Schölkopf), Springer, pp. 511–528.

41 Schölkopf, B. and Smola, A.J. (2002) *Learning with Kernels*, MIT Press, Cambridge, MA.

42 Schölkopf, B., Smola, A.J., Williamson, R.C., and Bartlett, P.L. (2000) New support vector algorithms. *Neural. Comput.*, **12**, 1207–1245.

43 Scholköpf, B., Weston, J., Eskin, E., Leslie, C., and Noble, W.S. (2002) A kernel approach for learning from almost orthogonal patterns, in *Proceedings of ECML 2002i, 13th European Conference on Machine Learning, Helsinki, Finland*, Springer, pp. 511–528.

44 Staunton, J.E., Slonim, D.K., Coller, H.A., Tamayo, P., Angelo, M.J., Park, J., Scherf, U., Lee, J.K., Reinhold, W.O., Weinstein, J.N., Mesirov, J.P., Lander, E.S., and Golub, T.R. (2001) Chemosensitivity prediction by transcriptional profiling. *Proc. Natl. Acad. Sci. USA*, **98** (19), 10787–10792.

45 Takahashi, K., Tanabe, K., Ohnuki, M., Narita, M., Ichisaka, T., Tomoda, K., and Yamanaka, S. (2007) Induction of pluripotent stem cells from adult human fibroblasts by defined factors. *Cell*, **131** (5), 861–872.

46 Tipping, M.E. (2001) Sparse Bayesian learning and the relevance vector machine. *J. Machine Learn. Res.*, **1**, 211–244.

47 Torunera, G.A., Ulgera, C., Alkana, M., Galanted, A.T., Rinaggioe, J., Wilkf, R., Tiang, B., Soteropoulosa, P., Hameedh, M.R., Schwalba, M.N., and Dermody, J.J. (2004) Association between gene expression profile and tumor invasion in oral squamous cell carcinoma. *Cancer Genet. Cytogenet.*, **154** (1), 27–35.

48 Tsuda, K., Kin, T., and Asai, K. (2002) Marginalized kernels for biological sequences. *Bioinformatics*, **18** (Suppl. 1), S268–S275.

49 Tsuda, K. and Noble, W.S. (2004) Learning kernels from biological networks by maximizing entropy. *Bioinformatics*, **20** (Suppl. 1), i326–i333.

50 van't Veer, L.J., Dai, H., van de Vijver, M.J., He, Y.D., Hart, A.A.M., Mao, M., Peterse, H.L., van der Kooy, K., Marton, M.J., Witteveen, A.T., Schreiber, G.J., Kerkhoven, R.M., Roberts, C., Linsley, P.S., Bernards, R., and Friend, S.H. (2002) Gene expression profiling predicts clinical outcome of breast cancer. *Nature*, **415** (6871), 530–536.

51 Vapnik, V. (1998) *Statistical Learning Theory*, John Wiley & Sons, Inc., New York.

52 Vert, J.P., Tsuda, K., and Schölkopf, B. (2004) A primer on kernel methods, in *Kernel Methods in Computational Biology*

(eds B. Schölkopf, K. Tsuda, and J.P. Vert), MIT Press, pp. 35–70.
53 Warnat, P., Eils, R., and Brors, B. (2005) Cross-platform analysis of cancer microarray data improves gene expression based classification of phenotypes. *BMC Bioinformatics*, **6** 265.
54 Weston, J., Leslie, C., Zhou, D., Elisseeff, A., and Noble, W.S. (2004) Semi-supervised protein classification using cluster kernels, in *Advances in Neural Information Processing Systems 16* (eds S. Thrun, L. Saul, and B. Schölkopf), MIT Press, Cambridge, MA.
55 Zelnik-Manor, L. and Perona, P. (2005) Self-tuning spectral clustering, in *Advances in Neural Information Processing Systems 17* (eds L.K. Saul, Y. Weiss, and L. Bottou), MIT Press, Cambridge, MA, pp. 1601–1608.

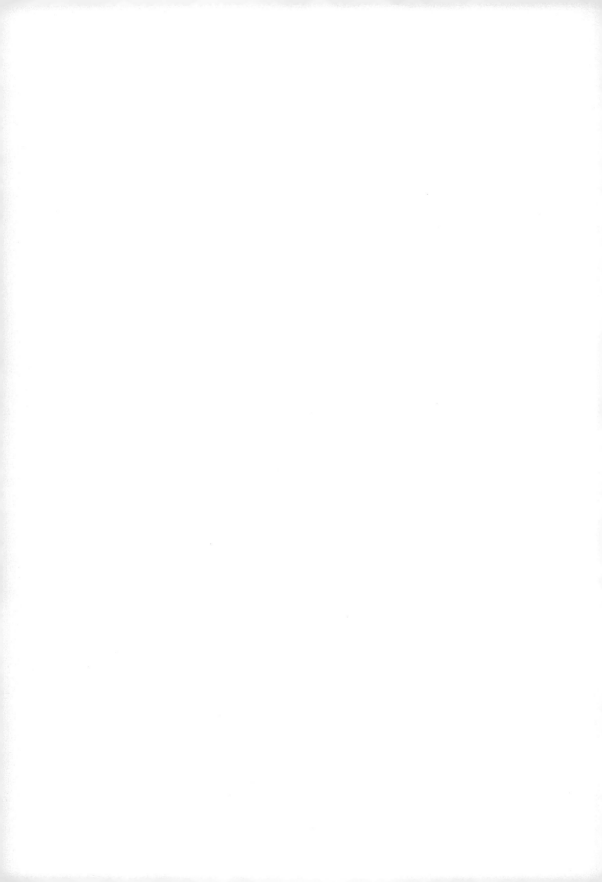

15
Predicting Cancer Survival Using Expression Patterns

Anupama Reddy, Louis-Philippe Kronek, A. Rose Brannon, Michael Seiler, Shridar Ganesan, W. Kimryn Rathmell, and Gyan Bhanot

15.1
Introduction

Cancer causes one in eight deaths worldwide, more deaths than AIDS, tuberculosis, and malaria combined. It is the second leading cause of death in economically developed countries (after heart disease) and the third leading cause of death in developing countries (after heart and diarrheal diseases) (www.cancer.gov). For some cancers (breast, prostate), early detection and vigorous treatment of early stage disease have resulted in effective therapy regimens aimed at preventing recurrence and metastasis. The ultimate goal of cancer research is to make cancer a chronic disease, kept permanently in check by long-term, targeted, individualized adjuvant therapy. For this goal to be realized, the first step is the ability to assign prognostic risk of death, metastasis, or recurrence when the disease is diagnosed or just after surgical intervention.

Focused research over the past 40 years has allowed an identification of the causes of most cancers. It is now well accepted that almost all cancers are caused either by environmental agents (carcinogens, tobacco, radiation, viral infection, etc.) or by genetic/molecular alterations (somatic or germline mutations that alter the function of oncogenes or tumor suppressor genes, loss of function by insertion mutagenesis, chromosomal chaos due to shortened telomeres, regulation error in stem cell differentiation, etc.). The goal of most cancer studies is to identify and understand the genetic and molecular mechanisms that initiate tumorigenesis (allow the tumor to establish itself in the primary tissue) [1] and subsequent changes that allow tumor cells to invade into the surrounding tissue, migrate, and establish in distant organs, and, finally, to sufficiently disrupt intra-organ homeostasis to cause the death of the patient. The hope of all such studies is that there is some identifiable signature in the tumor at biopsy or resection that can be mined to predict the likely course of disease so that an appropriate and effective therapy can be devised that can avoid tumor metastasis.

Medical Biostatistics for Complex Diseases. Edited by Frank Emmert-Streib and Matthias Dehmer
Copyright © 2010 WILEY-VCH Verlag GmbH & Co. KGaA, Weinheim
ISBN: 978-3-527-32585-6

The first step in such an analysis is the ability to place bounds on patient survival using clinical data (IHC, FISH measurements), imaging data, gene expression measurements, SNP analysis, copy number variation, tumor genomic sequence, epigenetic data (methylation, phosphorylation states), miRNA levels, and so on. Such an analysis involves predicting survival time (or time to event) based on recorded variables on studies conducted over a finite interval (typically 10–15 years for the best studies). Most mathematical studies attempt to use the data to determine risk as a continuous function of time from diagnosis, but are often confounded by censored samples. A sample is called censored if it has incomplete "time to event" information. Often, this happens because most studies do not run long enough for the event to be observed in all patients: either the study ends before all patients have an event, or patients opt out of the study after participating for some period, or some of the "event" data turns out not to be reliable. Such a situation is called right censoring and is the most common situation. The converse case is left censoring, when the time of death or the disease progression is known but the time of disease initiation or diagnosis is unknown. This might happen for example if the study recruited patients after metastasis was identified or included patients who died during surgery. In this chapter, we only consider right-censored survival analysis because these constitute the majority of situations in most study designs. A possible (but naïve) approach for handling censored data might be to disregard the censored samples. This would make the analysis much easier and reduce the problem to a classical regression analysis. However, in most studies, a large proportion of samples are censored, so that such a choice often results in an unacceptable loss of predictive power.

In this chapter, using a technique called logical analysis of data (LAD) [2] to find patterns in the data, we develop a new, supervised prognostic algorithm, which we call logical analysis of survival data (LASD), to predict survival time and define a risk score that attempts to account for the effects from censored patients. Other recent techniques include using classification and regression trees for estimating survival functions: for example, relative risk trees [3], neural networks [4], naïve Bayes classifiers [5], splines, and so on. Meta-classifiers, such as bagging, with survival decision trees as base classifiers have also been presented in several papers recently [6–9]. A general flexible framework for survival ensemble techniques is described by Hothorn et al. [10]. Another commonly used method is that of transforming a survival analysis problem into a classification problem involving the prediction of patients at high/low risk of having the event, or good/bad clinical prognosis.

Our algorithm is based on defining high/low risk classes for every time-point t when an event occurs in the dataset, and then building LAD patterns at each time point to distinguish these classes. Each such pattern is associated with a risk score, defined as the area under the survival (Kaplan–Meier) curve for patients covered by that pattern. A patient-specific risk score is defined as the average of the pattern scores satisfied by the patient. Additional mathematical details of our analysis procedure are described in [27].

We illustrate our method on a training dataset of gene expression profiles of clear cell renal cell carcinoma (ccRCC) samples from the University of North Carolina Medical School as well as a validation dataset containing microarray gene expression measurements for 177 ccRCC tumor samples from a previously published study [11]. The outcome that we will try to predict is death due to the cancer. We first identify molecular subtypes of disease in the data [12], with the reasonable expectation that the survival model must depend on the molecular signature of the tumor. Once the subtypes are determined, we build prognostic models within each subtype.

Our method is distinguished from others in the literature not just because of its use of LAD but also because we build the risk model within a molecular subtype. The rationale for a subtype based classification of cancers is slowly gaining acceptance in the clinical community. Although it is common to refer to cancers in the context of the tissues in which they occur, it is well known that clinical outcomes, even within a single tissue, are often heterogeneous. In the case of breast cancer, it is standard practice to determine treatment based on molecular markers for upregulation of the estrogen, progesterone, or the HER2 pathway. Indeed, the levels of these genes are routinely measured by immunohistochemistry tests conducted in the clinic during biopsy or after surgical resection of the tumor [13]. It is also known that most immunohistochemistry measures used in the clinic correlate well with the molecular signature of the tumors [14]. Recent studies have shown that cancers that look identical on pathological or immunohistochemical analysis can be split into molecularly distinct subclasses. Often these classes also have very distinct survival curves and response to therapy [15–25]. Stratifying tumors into subclasses based on similar molecular or genetic profiles is likely to become a routine procedure in the clinic as a method of defining disease classes with significant overlap with clinical outcome. In this chapter we assume that such classes exist and will build our survival model only within these molecular classes of disease.

15.2
Molecular Subtypes of ccRCC

We summarize here the identification of subtypes in ccRCC based on gene expression data collected in a study of 52 ccRCC samples (49 samples and three replicates) collected at the University of North Carolina. The detailed methodology for determining the subtypes from this dataset are presented elsewhere [12].

Principal component analysis (PCA) was performed on the microarray data from these samples after standard normalizing the data per array using the software toolkit ConsensusCluster (http://code.google.com/p/consensus-cluster/). PCA is a feature selection/reduction technique that can be used to identify the features that are most informative. We selected as informative features those with coefficients in the top 25% by absolute value in the highest PCA eigenvalues representing 85% of the variation in the data. In our 52 samples, PCA identified 20 eigenvectors and 281 features useful for further analysis. Unsupervised consensus ensemble clustering was applied using the ConsensusCluster toolkit to identify robust clusters in the data by successively dividing the data into $k = 2, 3, 4\ldots$ clusters. At each value of k, the clusters were made robust by bootstrapping over many randomly chosen subsets of the feature and sample set and averaging over two clustering techniques, K-Means and self-organizing map (SOM). This showed that the samples were composed of two robust disease subtypes, which we call ccA and ccB, distinguished by distinct molecular signatures (Figure 15.1).

Logical analysis of data (LAD) was used to identify patterns to distinguish between the ccA and ccB clusters and identify a small set of genes that can distinguish the two subtypes. Using semi-quantitative RT-PCR we found that five genes – FZD1, FLT1, GIPC2, MAP7, and NPR3, which were overexpressed in ccA – were sufficient to distinguish ccA from ccB with high accuracy (see References [12] for details).

The clusters identified in the UNC data were also identified in the Zhao *et al.* data, which contained survival information [11], using consensus clustering on LAD identified gene sets. As shown in Figure 15.2, there were 84 samples assigned to ccA and 93 assigned to ccB. In Figure 15.3 we plot the Kaplan–Meier (survival) curves for the samples in the ccA and ccB subtypes, demonstrating that the molecular subtype classes have significantly distinct survival curves.

15.3
Logical Analysis of Survival Data

We adapted a method called the Logical Analysis of Survival Data (LASD) described previously [26, 27] to predict patient survival within ccA and ccB subtypes. At each time point t in the data, defined by a recorded event (death), we divided the data into two classes: the *high-risk class* included patients who had an event before time t, and the *low-risk class* included patients who survived beyond t. This reduced the problem to a sequence of two-class classification problems.

For each classification problem (i.e., at each t) we build *patterns* to distinguish the two classes using the principles of logical analysis of data (LAD) [2, 28–30]. Patterns are boxes in multi-dimensional space, that is, combinations of rules on variables. Patterns are also specific to a class, that is, a high-risk pattern covers only high-risk observations and low-risk patterns only low-risk observations. To get meaningful patterns, this constraint is often relaxed to permit a small fraction of errors in the patterns.

The basic algorithm for building a high-risk pattern at event time t is the following: First, define the reference observation to be one that had the event at time t and initialize the high-risk pattern P to cover only the reference observation (by making a grid around that sample in the space where the coordinates are expression values of the features). Next, we extend the coverage of the pattern to include other high-risk samples by iteratively dropping conditions (i.e., extending the cut-point along a randomly chosen coordinate), until coverage cannot be extended further

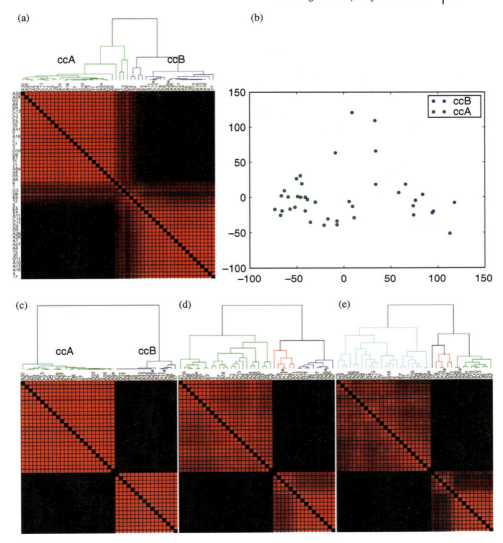

Figure 15.1 Consensus matrices demonstrate the presence of two core clusters within intermediate grade ccRCC. (a) Two core ccRCC clusters are clearly visible; (b) PCA plot showing the data projected onto the first two principal components with the samples from the two clusters drawn in different colors. Clusters obtained from ConsensusCluster for $k = 2$ (c), 3 (d), and 4 (e). Red areas represent sample pairs that cluster together with high frequency in the bootstrap analysis. Parts (c)–(e) show that the two subtypes are stable (retain their sample membership) even when we force the algorithm to try to identify more than two clusters.

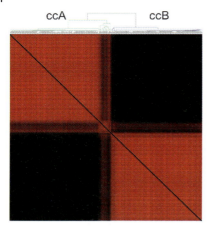

Figure 15.2 Validation of LAD variables in Zhao et al. data [11] show the existence of two ccRCC clusters; consensus matrix of 177 ccRCC tumors determined by 111 variables corresponding to the 120 LAD variables. Two distinct clusters are visible, validating the ability of the LAD variable set to classify ccRCC tumors into ccA (84 samples) or ccB (93 samples) subtypes.

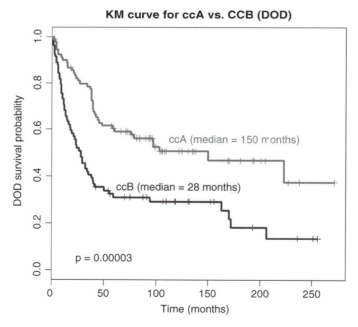

Figure 15.3 Survival curves for tumors in ccA and ccB classes in the Zhao et al. data [11]; 177 ccRCC tumors were individually assigned to ccA or ccB by consensus clustering using LAD genes, and cancer specific survival (DOD) was calculated via Kaplan–Meier curves. The ccB subtype had a significantly decreased survival outcome compared to ccA.

without including low-risk samples. Intuitively, the idea is to build the biggest box (in the space of gene expression data) around the reference observation, such that the box covers the maximum number of high-risk samples and none of the low-risk ones. Low-risk patterns are built in a similar way starting from a randomly chosen sample that has not yet had an event. In practice, requiring that each pattern covers only its target class is sometimes too restrictive. In such cases, we introduce a parameter for fuzziness that represents the maximum fraction of samples of the opposite class that can be covered by the pattern.

Each pattern P is assigned a score $S(P)$, defined as the area under the Kaplan–Meier survival function for samples covered by P. Notably, patterns are not disjoint (or orthogonal) in terms of coverage, and a sample can be covered by multiple patterns. For a sample T covered by patterns $P_1, \ldots, P_k$, the survival score $S(T)$ for sample T is the average of the patterns score $S(P_1), \ldots, S(P_k)$ and the baseline score $S(B)$. The baseline score is simply the area under the survival function for the entire dataset. This is included in the computation because of the possibility that some samples may not be covered by any patterns and must be assigned the baseline score. Thus the survival score is given by:

$$S(T) = \frac{S(B) + \sum_{i=1}^{k} S(p_i)}{k+1} \tag{15.1}$$

This formula can be used for predicting survival score for new (unseen) samples based on pattern coverage, assuming that the new samples come from the same distribution as the training data or can be integrated into the training dataset.

From the pattern building step we obtain a large number of patterns, precisely twice the number of events in the dataset. There is a high degree of redundancy in this large set of patterns, which can lead to overfitting. To account for this, we introduce the notion of a survival model as a subset of patterns that has the same predictive power as the larger set. We select patterns in the survival model by optimizing over the *concordance accuracy* (see [27] for details), which measures the proportion of correctly ranked pairs of samples. Finally, the survival model is used to predict survival scores for the patients in both the training and test sets, and comparisons are made with assignments based on clinical parameters such as stage and grade. A complete description of the LASD algorithm can be found in reference [27].

15.4
Bagging LASD Models

Often, medical datasets are "noisy" because of heterogeneities intrinsic to the disease or population variation. Hence, models built on these datasets tend to have lower accuracies, and may not be robust or applicable to new or unseen data. To overcome these problems, we apply the concepts of bagging for LASD. Bagging, that is, bootstrap aggregating, is a meta-algorithm or ensemble method [31] that improves the stability and robustness of classification models. Bagging improves results mainly when the data is noisy, and the perturbed models have uncorrelated error distributions.

Bagging involves randomly partitioning the training dataset into a "bag" set and an "out-of-bag" set. The regression or classification method is applied on the bag set and predictions are made on the out-of-bag set. This procedure is repeated several times, each time sampling with a uniform probability distribution with replacement. The predictions on out-of-bag set are then aggregated by weighted voting, averaging, and so on to get the final prediction.

For bagging LASD models, we aggregate the results by taking a weighted average of the predicted risk scores, where the weights are the bag accuracies [32]. The output of bagging LASD is an ensemble of LASD models. To predict the risk score for a new observation, we aggregate the results of predictions of all models in the ensemble.

15.5
Results

We illustrate the results of the proposed algorithm on the Zhao et al. [11] dataset. This dataset consists of 177 samples with microarray gene-expression measurements. Missing entries were imputed using the k-nearest neighborhood method ($k = 10$). Distance weighted discriminant (DWD) [33] was used to combine data collected in different batches to remove any systematic bias in the variance. After this, the data was standard normalized for each sample separately. The samples in the two subtypes ccA and ccB were analyzed separately.

Each probe was converted into a binary variable by using the median across samples as a cut-point. Log-rank tests were used for feature selection. To increase the robustness of the selected variables, these tests were run in 1000 bootstrapped experiments, each time randomly selecting 75% of the data. Finally, variables were selected if the p-value was <0.05 for ccA, (<0.025 for ccB) for at least 75% of the tests. There were 41 (79) binary variables selected for the ccA (ccB) subtypes by this method.

After feature selection, we applied LASD as well as Cox regression [34] and random survival forests (RSFs) [9] to the selected variables. Cox regression was performed on the selected variables and validated by bootstrapping 25 times. The parameters in the Cox model were tuned and optimized for c-index. LASD patterns were built for each of the subtypes, pattern coverage was analyzed, and patient-specific scores were computed. We analyzed the accuracy of (i) LASD with model selection, denoted by LASD (model) and (ii) LASD without model selection, denoted by LASD (all patterns). These results were validated based on five five-folding experiments. Bagging was applied to the LASD patterns (without model selection) in 100 bootstrapped experiments. For bagging, no additional validation is required since bagging already involves bootstrapping. The cross-validation estimate for bagging is the out-of-bag accuracy. To compare the performance of bagging LASD, we ran random survival forests (RSFs) also for 100 bootstrapped trees. All the statistical analyses were run using R.2.4.1 [35].

Table 15.1 Cross-validation results (concordance index and 95% confidence interval) of the proposed methods: logical analysis of survival data (LASD) with and without model selection, and bagging LASD. Results from Cox proportional hazards regression and random survival forests (RSFs) are presented for comparison. Analysis was carried out separately on the two ccRCC subtypes, ccA and ccB, and concordance accuracy was computed as the average over cross-validation experiments.

	ccA	ccB
Cox	0.658 ± 0.033	0.516 ± 0.033
LASD (all patterns)	0.758 ± 0.036	0.721 ± 0.023
LASD (model)	0.732 ± 0.037	0.731 ± 0.025
Bagging LASD		
Out-of-bag accuracy	0.759 ± 0.014	0.740 ± 0.013
Final prediction	0.749	0.776
Random survival forests		
Out-of-bag accuracy	$0.757 + 0.006$	0.742 ± 0.004
Final prediction	0.74	0.761

The concordance index (c-index) for LPS, Cox regression, LASD (all patterns), LASD (model), bagging LASD, and RSF is presented in Table 15.1 for ccA and ccB subtypes.

15.5.1
Prediction Results are More Accurate after Stratifying Data into Subtypes

To demonstrate that the prediction results improve if the analysis is done within a molecular class, we also built LASD patterns on the entire dataset of 177 samples (without identifying subtypes) and the results were cross-validated by running five five-folding experiments. Using LASD (all patterns), the concordance accuracy was 0.659, while with LASD (model) it was 0.677. When we used bagging, the concordance accuracy increased to 0.695. This is lower than the accuracies of the models built separately on ccA and ccB (Table 15.1). This shows that we get much more accurate results when we build models on robust subtypes of the disease.

15.5.2
LASD Performs Significantly Better than Cox Regression

Using LASD and building high degree patterns to characterize high and low-risk patients proves to be more accurate than Cox regression. This probably results from a high degree of complexity in the progression and metastasis of tumors. LASD (model) is preferred because it retains accuracy while using fewer patterns to compute survival risk, and eliminating patterns that contribute marginally. Fewer patterns also allow for the possibility of using these methods to create a clinical assay. The LASD (model) also has higher accuracy than Cox regression, which is currently the standard used to judge the usefulness of methods used in predicting clinical survival.

15.5.3
Bagging Improves Robustness of LASD Predictions

Table 15.1 shows that the accuracy of the bagging LASD model is comparable to LASD alone. More importantly, the confidence intervals on the accuracy are significantly reduced, which implies that the results are robust. Bagging LASD also gives results comparable to RSFs, which is known to be a powerful ensemble method, as shown in a recent paper [9]. Note that the out-of-bag accuracies for bagging LASD and RSF cannot be directly compared, since RSF provides out-of-bag accuracy of the k-th bootstrap as an aggregation of results from the first k trees, while bagging LASD provides accuracy of the out-of-bag samples for the k-th tree. This is why the 95% confidence interval for RSF is much lower than that of bagging LASD. We provide the out-of-bag (OOB) accuracy for comparison with the cross-validation accuracy with LASD and Cox regression. The main results here is the final prediction accuracy (aggregate of the out-of-bag predictions for all boot-strapped trees).

15.5.4
LASD Patterns have Distinct Survival Profiles

The model for ccA consisted of nine high-risk and eight low-risk patterns, while the model for ccB had 16 high-risk and six low-risk patterns (Table 15.2). These patterns cover patients who have survival distributions very different compared to the baseline, as indicated by the significant log-rank p-values. Figure 15.4 shows the Kaplan–Meier (KM) plots for LASD patterns in Table 15.2. High risk patterns are colored red, and low risk pattern green. Clearly, from the plot, high-risk patterns cover mostly patients with early events, while low-risk patterns cover mostly patients who had late events. Figure 15.5 shows plots of heat map of the patterns in Table 15.2. The patterns correspond to the rows and samples to the columns. The samples are ordered by their survival time. The horizontal color bar indicates the censoring status for patient (blue indicates event, and grey indicates censoring). The vertical color bar indicates the type of pattern (red indicates high-risk, and blue indicates low-risk). Evidently, from Figure 15.4 the high and low risk patterns in each disease subtype have distinct survival profiles.

15.5.5
Importance Scores for Patterns and an Optimized Risk Score

The bagging procedure generates hundreds of models, which can be used to identify important variables. These are features that occur with high frequency in patterns. Tables 15.3 and 15.4 show the importance score for the top 20 features identified for ccA and ccB, respectively.

Table 15.2 Survival patterns in the LASD model for ccA and ccB subtypes.[a]

Pattern ID	Time	Score	Log-rank p-value	Description
ccA Patterns:				
HR1	4	2.5	3.11×10^{-14}	LOC286 052 ↑ and ATPAF1 ↑ and UCP3 ↑ and N4BP3 ↓
HR2	10	4.96	0.00E + 00	Hs.100 912 ↓ and BPHL ↓ and MR1 ↑ and KCNJ8 ↑ and Hs.102 471 ↑ and Hs.102 471 ↑
HR3	15	5.5	0.00E + 00	ATPAF1 ↑ and CEP57 ↑ and BPHL ↓ and MR1 ↑ and Hs.102 471 ↑ and Hs.102 471 ↑
HR4	14	6.8	7.77×10^{-16}	ATPAF1 ↑ and ATPAF1 ↓ and Hs.100 912 ↓ and BPHL ↓ and LOX ↑
HR5	23	7.33	1.11×10^{-16}	ASNSD1 ↑ and MR1 ↑ and Hs.102 471 ↑ and Hs.102 471 ↑ and Hs.102 471 ↓
HR6	19	7.6	3.45×10^{-14}	ATPAF1 ↑ and Hs.100 912 ↓ and CEP192 ↓ and MR1 ↑ and LOX ↓ and KCNJ8 ↑
HR7	25	9.5	9.47×10^{-14}	ATPAF1 ↓ and MAPT ↑ and ASNSD1 ↑ and LOX ↓ and Hs.102 471 ↑
HR8	38	15.5	4.67×10^{-12}	ATPAF1 ↑ and CEP192 ↓ and BPHL ↓ and KCNJ8 ↑
HR9	48	20.2	4.73×10^{-14}	CEP192 ↓ and MAPT ↑ and LOX ↓
LR1	4	186.55	1.87×10^{-3}	LOC286 052 ↓
LR2	15	186.94	2.98×10^{-3}	Hs.100 912 ↑ and Hs.102 471 ↓
LR3	44	187.37	9.51×10^{-3}	ATPAF1 ↓ and LOX ↓
LR4	10	193.95	1.71×10^{-3}	Hs.102 471 ↑
LR5	38	198.84	9.07×10^{-4}	BPHL ↑ and ASNSD1 ↓
LR6	6	232.85	3.62×10^{-4}	DCUN1D3 ↓ and KBTBD3 ↓
LR7	58	239.8	3.75×10^{-4}	CEP57 ↓ and BPHL ↓
LR8	150	249.02	3.16×10^{-4}	ATPAF1 ↓ and LOX ↑ and Hs.102 276 ↓ and Hs.102 471 ↓
ccB Patterns:				
HR1	2	1.25	0.00E + 00	Hs.102 471 ↑ and Hs.102 572::Hs.602 127 ↓ and Hs.103 183::Hs.596 971 ↓ and ZNF384 ↓ and Hs.103 426 ↓ and C1orf174 ↑
HR2	2	1.4	0.00E + 00	MR1 ↑ and MAN1A1 ↑ and PPARA ↓ and Hs.103 183::Hs.596 971 ↓ and FKBP9 ↑
HR3	4	2	0.00E + 00	Hs.102 471 ↑ and MAN1A1 ↑ and PPARA ↓ and COPE ↑ and C1orf174 ↑
HR4	6	2.5	0.00E + 00	LIG3 ↓ and C1orf166 ↓ and Hs.102 471 ↑ and MAN1A1 ↑ and PPARA ↓ and PPARA ↓
HR5	6	2.71 429	0.00E + 00	LIG3 ↓ and C1orf166 ↓ and BPHL ↓ and MR1 ↑ and LOX ↑ and Hs.102 471 ↑

(*Continued*)

Table 15.2 (Continued)

Pattern ID	Time	Score	Log-rank p-value	Description
HR6	7	2.75	0.00E + 00	C1orf166 ↓ and BPHL ↓ and MR1 ↑ and PPARA ↓ and ZNF384 ↓
HR7	8	3.45 455	0.00E + 00	ASTE1 ↓ and C1orf166 ↓ and BPHL ↓ and PPARA ↓ and ZNF384 ↓
HR8	9	4	5.29×10^{-8}	MR1 ↓ and LOX ↑ and PPARA ↓ and FAM104A ↑ and C1orf174 ↑
HR9	10	4.625	2.05×10^{-10}	MR1 ↓ and Hs.102 471 ↑ and Hs.102 572 ↓ and MAN1A1 ↑
HR10	11	5.07 692	1.11×10^{-16}	C1orf166 ↓ and MAN1A1 ↑ and C1orf174 ↑
HR11	17	6.64 286	3.93×10^{-12}	C1orf166 ↓ and BPHL ↓ and ZNF384 ↓ and FAM104A ↑
HR12	15	7.86 667	3.49×10^{-9}	LIG3 ↓ and Hs.102 607 ↓ and PSMA1 ↑
HR13	24	8.13 636	7.77×10^{-16}	LIG3 ↓ and ASTE1 ↓ and ARL6IP4 ↓
HR14	29	9.85 714	1.45×10^{-5}	BPHL ↓ and Hs.102 471 ↑ and FAM104A ↑
HR15	34	12.1053	3.07×10^{-7}	MCTS1 ↑ and Hs.103 334::Hs.202 872 ↓ and FAM104A ↑
HR16	172	36.0402	4.60×10^{-5}	PSMA1 ↑
LR1	13	150.599	2.00×10^{-5}	C1orf166 ↑ and Hs.103 334::Hs.202 872 ↑
LR2	14	185.628	3.78×10^{-7}	KBTBD3 ↑ and Hs.102 735 ↓ and PPARA ↑
LR3	34	195.028	5.69×10^{-8}	KBTBD3 ↑ and TTC5 ↑ and Hs.102 735 ↓
LR4	50	204.541	8.74×10^{-8}	Hs.100 912 ↓ and Hs.102 471 ↓ and TTC5 ↑
LR5	172	230.958	2.92×10^{-6}	Hs.102 735 ↓ and CUL4B ↓ and Hs.103 822 ↑ and FKBP9 ↓
LR6	206	242.75	6.75×10^{-6}	CUL4B ↓ and Hs.103 183::Hs.596 971 ↑ and Hs.103 822 ↑ and FKBP9 ↓

a) High-risk patterns (HR1–HR9 for ccA and HR1-HR16 for ccB) are those that characterize patients at risk for an event at time t, while low-risk patterns (LR1–LR8 for ccA and LR1-LR6 for ccB) characterize patients who survived beyond time t. "↑" represents up-regulation and "↓" down-regulation based on whether the gene is above or below the median. Note that all patterns have a significant log-rank p-value ($p < 1 \times 10^{-3}$ for ccA and $p < 1 \times 10^{-5}$ for ccB). Time represents the reference time t at which the pattern was built, and the score represents the area under the Kaplan–Meier curve for the patients covered by the pattern.

15.5.6
Risk Scores could be used to Classify Patients into Distinct Risk Groups

Figure 15.6 is a plot of our predicted survival versus the actual survival time. Censored samples are marked " + ". The plot shows that there is a positive correlation between

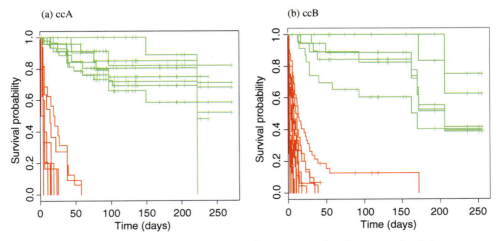

Figure 15.4 Kaplan–Meier survival curves for patterns for (a) ccA samples, (b) ccB samples. Red curves represent high-risk patterns and green represent low-risk patterns. Log-rank test for each of the patterns is highly significant (p-value < 0.001 for ccA and p-value < 0.00001 for ccB).

our risk score and survival time; however, there seems to be considerable scatter. Nonetheless, as Figure 15.7 shows, when we stratify the patients into two risk groups based on the median survival score, the survival distributions of the two risk groups are highly significant (p-value $= 4 \times 10^{-10}$ for ccA, p-value $= 9 \times 10^{-8}$ for ccB).

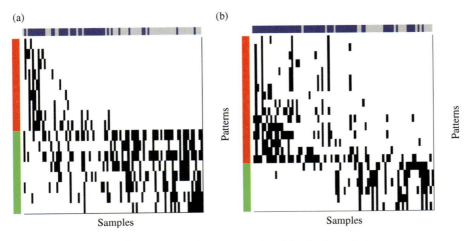

Figure 15.5 Heat maps for the patterns in Table 15.2 for (a) ccA and (b) ccB samples. The patterns (P_i) are along the rows, and samples (S_j) are along the columns (ordered by the survival time). A cell M_{ij} is colored black if pattern P_i covers sample S_j, else it is colored white. The horizontal color bar represents the censoring status for the patients (grey = censored, blue = event), the vertical color bar is red for high-risk patterns and green for low-risk patterns. Samples and patterns are sorted by increasing order of their survival times and survival scores, respectively.

Table 15.3 Top 20 features sorted by their importance score for the ccA subtype, computed as the average of frequency of occurrence of the variable in high, low-risk patterns in the bagging LASD model in the ccA subtype.

UniGene cluster	Gene name	Importance score
Hs.714 295		0.214 051
Hs.648 565	ATF1	0.201 987
Hs.89 497	LMNB1	0.187 964
Hs.531 081	LGALS3	0.176 182
Hs.591 957	DKFZp761E198	0.175 989
Hs.705 395::Hs.703 245		0.167 801
Hs.133 892::Hs.713 685		0.164 325
Hs.483 564	PFDN1	0.163 964
Hs.44 235	C13orf1	0.133 76
Hs.658 510		0.129 822
Hs.194 698	CCNB2	0.123 444
Hs.422 662	VRK1	0.111 522
Hs.557 550	NPM1	0.100 041
Hs.108 106	UHRF1	0.090 153
Hs.657 339	LOC440 295	0.071 901
Hs.648 565	ATF1	0.070 62
Hs.90 756	KLB	0.070 306
Hs.540 469		0.067 632
Hs.654 389	CUX1	0.066 086
Hs.124 696	BDH2	0.063 842

15.5.7
LASD Survival Prediction is Highly Predictive When Compared with Clinical Parameters (Stage, Grade, and Performance)

Stage, grade, and performance are clinical parameters routinely assigned to tumors, and used to assess survival risk and determine treatment. Table 15.5 presents hazard ratios for the LASD score, stage, grade and performance individually (unadjusted), and in a multivariate Cox model (adjusted). Clearly, from Table 15.5, LASD has a very significant hazard ratio not only individually, but also in the adjusted model, showing that it provides additional prognostic value for risk assessment of ccRCC tumors in ccA and ccB subtypes.

15.6
Conclusion and Discussion

We have developed a method, based on Logical Analysis of Survival Data (LASD) [26, 27] to create a score that measures survival risk within molecular classes of cancer and have illustrated its use by employing clear cell renal cell carcinoma (ccRCC) as a

Table 15.4 Top 20 features sorted by their importance score for the ccB subtype, computed as the average of frequency of occurrence of the variable in high, low-risk patterns in the bagging LASD model in the ccB subtype.

UniGene cluster	Gene name	Importance score
Hs.22 047	LOC388 588	0.218
Hs.126 137::Hs.705 753		0.209
Hs.654 668	ARHGAP26	0.157
Hs.81 907	C5orf33	0.139
Hs.518 475	RFC4	0.132
Hs.298 023	AQP5	0.129
Hs.584 801	SFRS2	0.122
Hs.664 750		0.103
Hs.709 753		0.103
Hs.605 712		0.101
Hs.12 967	SYNE1	0.097
Hs.591 852	ADAM9	0.097
Hs.371 823	PRDM2	0.095
Hs.74 052		0.094
Hs.80 305	ARHGAP19	0.094
Hs.7099	PIGG	0.093
Hs.568 613	SLC25A33	0.088
Hs.662 923		0.087
Hs.181 173	GLB1L	0.085
Hs.372 082	TNRC6B	0.080

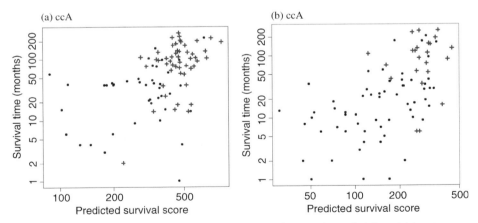

Figure 15.6 Plot of LASD survival score versus actual survival time (in log scales) for ccA (a) and ccB (b). Censored samples are marked with a "+". There is a clear trend in the survival scores, but the individual scores are not very accurate.

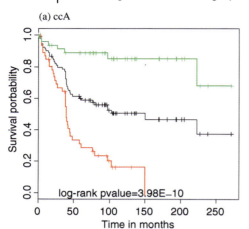
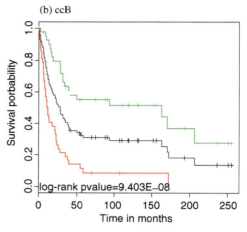

Figure 15.7 Risk stratification of patients into two groups based on the median score. The high risk (red) and low risk (green) groups in both subtypes have very different survival profiles (p-value $= 4 \times 10^{-10}$ and 9×10^{-8} for ccA and ccB, respectively). The middle curve shows survival for all patients in each class.

model system. This tumor type is particularly suited for such an analysis, because most ccRCC patients are assigned into intermediate grade and stage, and it is difficult to assess the outcome. Moreover, renal cell carcinoma (RCC) has undergone a resurgence in interest due to an influx of effective therapies that seem to slow the growth of the disease, which creates the hope that they might be fine tuned or improved to keep the disease at bay in an adjuvant setting.

LASD is an accurate prognostic tool for the estimation of survival functions and event-risk for patients. The main advantage of LASD is that compared to classic

Table 15.5 Hazard ratio (HRa) (p-value) for the LASD score and for the standard clinical measures of stage, grade, and performance; ratios are shown both for each parameter individually (unadjusted) as well as in a multivariate Cox regression model (adjusted).

	Unadjusted HRa (p-value)	Adjusted HRa (p-value)
(A) ccA		
LASD prediction	10.5 (2.3×10^{-7})	10.29 (6×10^{-7})
Stage	0.913 (0.47)	1.00 (0.98)
Grade	1.58 (0.033)	1.84 (0.016)
Performance	1.83 (0.00 032)	1.77 (0.012)
(B) ccB		
LASD prediction	4.1 (6×10^{-7})	3.362 (4×10^{-5})
Stage	0.795 (0.044)	0.938 (0.058)
Grade	1.86 (0.0018)	1.425 (0.093)
Performance	1.5 (0.00 066)	1.252 (0.074)

15.6 Conclusion and Discussion

statistical tools it can detect interactions between variables, that is, patterns, without any prior hypotheses. Survival patterns are meaningful characterizations of groups of observations that are homogenous in terms of survival.

The survival patterns in our analysis are simple rules on the expression levels of genes (or the presence or absence of mutations/deletions/amplifications, levels of proteins, etc.) that are used to stratify patients into risk classes. They are transparent objects that can be easily measured and used in the clinical setting. They also generate potentially useful biological hypotheses for disease progression, which might lead to improved understanding of the disease process if properly interpreted and investigated. For instance, in the case of gene-expression profiles, the expression patterns identified by our method suggest novel interactions of genes (gene-expression signatures), which seem to be linked to survival and probably signal distinct modes of progression within ccA and ccB. To identify the most predictive features and to validate our model, we can use the concepts of bagging. In general, such ensemble methods provide much better performance than simple classifiers.

We can imagine many ways to improve our model. For instance, in our model, a large proportion of the patterns selected are associated with low survival times, because we use concordance accuracy as a measure for selecting patterns into the model. This measure computes the proportion of pairs of samples that are ranked in the correct order by the predicted risk score. Samples that have a very early event contribute to a large proportion of such pairs (since they are compared with all the samples with larger survival). Therefore, our procedure is strongly biased towards accurately identifying samples with potentially early events. While this bias towards early events is clearly important for determining the initial course of therapy, it may be less appropriate for decisions regarding full course of treatment or for the health insurance industry. In these cases, determining risk for later time periods or computing an average risk across all time periods may be more applicable. Indeed, if the patient survives to time t, the clinician would want to estimate the risk for potential events for all time periods after t. Such methods to assess a dynamic risk as a function of t for clinical use are easily devised, using straightforward extensions of the method we illustrate here. For example, one could simply choose patterns more biased towards times greater than t. Similarly, to define an average risk score of interest to the health insurers, one might select patterns uniformly spaced in time. Alternately, it is also possible to use performance measures other than the concordance accuracy within the overall framework we describe here. Overall, our basic analytical method is highly malleable to various different questions, needs, and end users.

In this era of evolving targeted therapies, and their increased use in the adjuvant settings, it becomes more important than ever to be able to precisely assign prognostic risk for death from cancer. For ccRCC, the standard Fuhrman grading system is known to have prognostic value for patients assigned to Grade 1 (low risk) or Grade 4 (high risk). However, intermediate Fuhrman grade ccRCC tumors (Grades 2 and 3) are difficult for pathologists and clinicians to classify into risk categories. Clinical stage also fails to be useful for patients who are in an intermediate disease stage (i.e., who are assigned a clinical Stage of 2 or 3). Our methods provide a score that seems to correlate well with the risk of death from ccRCC and might be useful to urologists and pathologists to improve their ability to assess clinical risk of progression after surgery and assist them in determining the most appropriate therapy for an individual patient.

References

1 Futreal, P.A., Coin, L., Marshall, M., Down, T., Hubbard, T., Wooster, R., Rahman, N., and Stratton, M.R. (2004) A census of human cancer genes. *Nat. Rev. Cancer*, **4** (3), 177–183.

2 Hammer, P.L. and Bonates, T.O. (2006) Logical analysis of data - An overview: From combinatorial optimization to medical applications. *Ann. Oper. Res.*, **148** (1), 203–225.

3 LeBlanc, M. and Crowley, J. (1992) Relative risk trees for censored survival analysis. *Biometrics*, **48** (2), 411–425.

4 Ripley, B.D. and Ripley, R.M. (1998) Neural networks as statistical methods in survival analysis, in *Artificial Neural Networks: Prospects Medicine* (eds R. Dybowsky and V. Gant), Landes Biosciences.

5 Zupan, B., Demsar, J., Kattan, M.W., Beck, J.R., and Bratko, I. (2000) Machine learning for survival analysis: a case study on recurrence of prostate cancer. *Artif. Intell. Med.*, **20**, 59–75.

6 Hothorn, T., Lausen, B., Benner, A., and Radespiel-Troeger, M. (2004) Bagging survival trees. *Stat. Med.*, **23** (1), 77–91.

7 Breiman, L. and Cutler, A. (2002), Available from: www.stat.berkeley.edu/∼breiman/RandomForests/surv_manual.pdf.

8 Ishwaran, H., Blackstone, E., Pothier, C., and Lauer, M. (2004) Relative risk forests for exercise heart rate recovery as a predictor of mortality. *J. Am. Stat. Assoc.*, **99** (467), 591–600.

9 Ishwaran, H., Kogalur, U.B., Blackstone, E.H., and Lauer, M.S. (2008) Random survival forests. *Ann. Appl. Stat.*, **2** (3), 841–860.

10 Hothorn, T., Buhlmann, P., Dudoit, S., Molinaro, A., and van Der Laan, M. (2006) Survival ensembles. *Biostatistics*, **7** (3) 355–373.

11 Zhao, H. et al. (2006) Gene expression profiling predicts survival in conventional renal cell carcinoma. *PLoS Med.*, **3** (1), e13.

12 Brannon, A.R., Reddy, A., Seiler, M., Pruthi, R., Wallen, E., Ljungberg, B., Zhao, H., Brooks, J.D., Ganesan, S., Bhanot, G., and Rathmell, W.K. (2010) Molecular stratification of clear cell renal cell carcinoma using consensus clustering reveals distinct subtypes and survival patterns. Genes and Cancer (in press).

13 Anim, J.T., John, B., Abdulsathar, S.S., Prasad, A., Saji, T., Akhtar, N., Ali, V., and Al-Saleh, M. (2005) Relationship between the expression of various markers and prognostic factors in breast cancer. *Acta Histochem.*, **107**, 87–93.

14 Gruvberger, S., Ringner, M., Chen, Y., Panavally, S., Saal, L.H., Borg, A., Ferno, M., Peterson, C., and Meltzer, P.S. (2001) Estrogen receptor status in breast cancer is associated with remarkably distinct gene expression patterns. *Cancer Res.*, **61**, 5979–5984.

15 van de Vijver, M.J. et al. (2002) A gene-expression signature as a predictor of survival in breast cancer. *New Engl. J. Med.*, **347** (25), 1999–2009.

16 Paik, S. et al. (2004) A multigene assay to predict recurrence of tamoxifen-treated, node-negative breast cancer. *New Engl. J. Med.*, **351** (27), 2817–2826.

17 Percu, C.M. et al. (2000) Molecular portraits of human breast tumours. *Nature*, **406** (6797), 747–752.

18 Sorlie, T. et al. (2001) Gene expression patterns of breast carcinomas distinguish tumor subclasses with clinical implications. *Proc. Natl. Acad. Sci. USA*, **98** (19), 10869–10874.

19 Alexe, G., Dalgin, G.S., Ramaswamy, R., DeLisi, C., and Bhanot, G. (2006) Data perturbation independent diagnosis and validation of breast cancer subtypes using clustering and patterns. *Cancer Informat.*, **2**, 243–274.

20 Sorlie, T. *et al.* (2006) Distinct molecular mechanisms underlying clinically relevant subtypes of breast cancer: gene expression analyses across three different platforms. *BMC Genomics*, **7**, 127.

21 Sotirious, C., Neo, S.Y. *et al.* (2003) Breast cancer classification and prognosis based on gene expression profiles from a population-based study. *Proc. Natl. Acad. Sci. USA*, **100**, 10393–10398.

22 Sotirious, C. *et al.* (2002) Gene expression profiles derived from fine needle aspiration correlate with response to systemic chemotherapy in breast cancer. *Breast Cancer Res.*, **4**, R3.

23 Bertucci, F., Eisinger, F., Houlgatte, R., Viens, P., and Birnbaum, D. (2002) Gene-expression profiling and identification of patients at high risk of breast cancer. *Lancet*, **360**, 173–174.

24 Alexe, G. *et al.* (2007) High expression of lymphocyte-associated genes in node-negative HER2+ breast cancers correlates with lower recurrence rates. *Cancer Res.*, **67** (22), 10669–10676.

25 Dalgin, G.S. *et al.* (2007) Portraits of breast cancer progression. *BMC Bioinformatics*, **8**, 291.

26 Kronek, L.P. and Reddy, A. (2008) Logical analysis of survival data: prognostic survival models by detecting high degree interactions in right-censored data. *Bioinformatics*, **24** (16), i248–i253

27 Reddy, A., Brannon, A.R., Seiler, M., Irgon, J., Ljungberg, B., Zhao, H., Brooks, J.D., Rathmell, W.K., Ganesan, S., and Bhanot, G. (2009) A predictor for survival in intermediate grade clear cell renal cell carcinoma. The 2009 International Conference on Bioinformatics & Computational Biology, Las Vegas.

28 Boros, E. *et al.* (2000) An implementation of logical analysis of data. *IEEE T. Knowl. Data Eng.*, **12** (2), 292–306.

29 Reddy, A. *et al.* (2008) Logical analysis of data (LAD) model for the early diagnosis of acute ischemic stroke. *BMC Med. Inform. Decis. Mak.*, **8**, 30.

30 Boros, E., Hammer, P.L., Ibaraki, T. *et al.* (1997) Logical analysis of numerical data. *Math Program.*, **79**, 163–190.

31 Breiman, L. (2001) Random forests, *Machine Learn.*, **45** (1), 5–32.

32 Alexe, G. and Reddy, A. (2007) Bagging logical analysis of data. Unpublished work.

33 Benito, M., Parker, J., Du, Q., Wu, J., Xiang, D., Perou, C.M., and Marron, J.S. (2004) Adjustment of systematic microarray data biases. *Bioinformatics*, **20**, 105–114.

34 Cox, D.R. (1972) Regression models and life tables (with Discussion). *J. R. Stat. Soc.*, **34** (2), 187–220.

35 Agah, R. *et al.* (2005) Creation of a large-scale genetic data bank for cardiovascular association studies. *Am. Heart J.*, **150** (3), 500–506.

16
Integration of Microarray Datasets
Ki-Yeol Kim and Sun Young Rha

16.1
Introduction

DNA microarrays are useful tools for studying complex systems and are being applied to many areas of biological sciences. However, systematic biases due to handling procedures are often present and are a challenge in these types of experimental studies.

When datasets with limited numbers that were derived from different experimental processes were analyzed individually the results of the analyses were often inconsistent and contained little reliable information. Owing to the limited number of microarray experiments that have been performed, the use of whole datasets is increasing, regardless of the platforms or the experimental procedures used. Therefore, it is necessary to investigate methods that would effectively combine microarray datasets that are derived from different experimental environments in order to minimize systematic bias.

Many studies have analyzed several independently collected microarray datasets. These studies have focused on comparing differentially expressed genes selected from each dataset to find discriminative genes that can classify the different experimental groups [1–7]. These studies have exploited the possibility of identifying more robust datasets through the use of multiple datasets rather than a single dataset. The integration of separate datasets has the same effect as increasing the sample size of a single microarray [8–10], allowing the analysis of multiple microarray datasets in order to overcome the main limitation of single microarray datasets, namely, the small sample size.

In this chapter we introduce several methods for combining microarray datasets derived from different experimental conditions and show the efficiency of combined datasets, using examples.

16.2
Integration Methods

Probe design and experimental conditions are known to influence signal intensities and sensitivities for various high-throughput technologies [11]. Even for similar data

Medical Biostatistics for Complex Diseases. Edited by Frank Emmert-Streib and Matthias Dehmer
Copyright © 2010 WILEY-VCH Verlag GmbH & Co. KGaA, Weinheim
ISBN: 978-3-527-32585-6

types, data from different sources may have varying quality and information depending on the experimental conditions that generated the data. Therefore, in microarray experiments, datasets generated under different conditions cannot be directly compared and integrated [2]. The goal of data integration is to obtain greater precision, higher accuracy, and increased statistical power than any individual dataset would provide. Information from integrated datasets is more likely to be valid and reliable than information from a single dataset [12].

To correct biases caused by differing experimental conditions, normalization can be used. Several methods for adjusting biases between different datasets have been introduced. Singular-value decomposition (SVD) [13, 14] was successfully applied to a microarray and Benito et al. [15] used distance weighted discrimination (DWD) to correct for systematic biases across microarray batches by finding a separating hyperplane between the two batches and adjusting the data by projecting the different batches onto the DWD plane, finding the batch mean, and then subtracting out the DWD plane multiplied by this mean. However, this method could not regulate the dispersion of different datasets. As a mode-based method, ANOVA (analysis of variance) was introduced to select the discriminative genes from several datasets that were derived from different experimental environments [16]. This flexible method can consider any clinical variables as well as genetic information, including several effect factors that represent experimental conditions.

The usage of discretized values of gene expression ratios can reduce biases between datasets because discretization is generally determined by the ranks of gene expressions. Even better, it is also known that the use of discretized values may improve prediction accuracies in classification.

In this section we briefly introduce several methods for integrating microarray datasets, which reduce the biases caused by experimental conditions.

16.2.1
Existing Methods for Adjusting Batch Effects

16.2.1.1 Singular Value Decomposition (SVD) and Distance Weighted Discrimination (DWD)

SVD is a method of removing systematic effects by projecting gene expression ratios onto the directions of large variation. It was successfully applied for batch effect adjustment to a microarray meta-analysis [14]. However, it has been suggested that SVD may be inappropriate to use when the magnitude of the systematic effect variation is similar to the other components of variation [15]. When the magnitude of the systematic effect variation is similar to the other components of variation, the first SVD direction is not appropriate for bias adjustment. In this case, it is natural to choose directions to maximize separation of the bias.

This leads naturally to the development of distance weighted discrimination, which avoids the data piling problem, and data piling can diminish generalizability [17].

Distance weighted discrimination (DWD) [15] is a method to correct for systematic biases across microarray batches by finding a hyperplane between the two different experimental conditions and adjusting the data by projecting the different conditions (or batches) onto the DWD plane, finding the batch mean, and then subtracting the DWD plane multiplied by this mean. There are difficulties associated with both the SVD and DWD methods, and these methods are complicated and usually require many samples (>25) per batch to be implemented [18]. For the SVD adjustment, the eigenvectors in the SVD must be orthogonal, thus the method depends on proper selection of the first several eigenvectors. The DWD method can only be applied to two batches at a time. Benito *et al.* [15] have used a stepwise approach, first adjusting the two most similar batches, then comparing the third batch against the previously adjusted two batches. However, this approach could potentially break down in cases of numerous batches or when batches are not very similar.

16.2.1.2 ANOVA (Analysis of Variance) Model

The ANOVA model was recently introduced to select the discriminative genes from several datasets that were derived from different experimental environments [16]. The ANOVA model, which considers the experimental conditions, can be given by the following equation:

$$y_{ij} = \beta_0 + \beta_T x_{ij}^T + \beta_B x_{ij}^B + \varepsilon_{ij}$$
$$i = 1, 2, 3, \quad j = 1, 2, 3, \ldots, n_i$$

where x_{ij}^T and x_{ij}^B are variables for distinguishing the control and tumor tissues and for the different batches, respectively. In this equation, x_{ij}^B consists of three batches; β_T is the effect of the main interest representing the treatment effect between the control and tumor tissues; β_B represents the batch effect. The goal of this equation is to detect the genes with significant β_T that are differentially expressed between the control and tumor tissues. The error term, ε_{ij}, assumes that the error is normally distributed.

This flexible method can take into account any clinical variables as well as genetic information, including several effect factors that represent experimental conditions. However, using this model, we cannot evaluate how well the datasets are intermixed and we cannot explore the expression patterns of any interesting genes in a combined dataset [19].

16.2.1.3 Empirical Bayesian Method for Adjusting Batch Effect [18]

Suppose the data contains m batches containing n_i samples within batch i for $i = 1, \ldots, m$, for gene $g = 1, \ldots, G$ and for sample j. We assume the model is specified as follows:

$$Y_{ijg} = \alpha_g + X\beta_g + \gamma_{ig} + \delta_{ig}\varepsilon_{ijg}$$

where

Y_{ijg} represents the expression value for gene g, sample j from batch i;
α_g is the overall gene expression;
X is a design matrix for sample conditions;
β_g is the coefficient corresponding to X.

The error term, ε_{ijg}, can be assumed to follow a normal distribution with a mean of zero and variance σ_g^2. The γ_{ig} and δ_{ig} represent the additive and multiplicative batch effects of batch i for gene g, respectively.

The empirical Bayesian method for adjusting batch effect can be executed in the following three steps:

1) **Standardization of data**

   The magnitude of expression values could differ across genes due to mRNA expression level and probe sensitivity. It is implied that α_g, β_g, γ_g, and σ_g^2 differ across genes and that these differences will bias the EB (empirical Bayesian) estimates of the prior distribution of batch effect and reduce the amount of systematic batch information that can be borrowed across genes. To solve this problem we can standardize the data for each gene so that genes have similar means and variances in expression. The standardized data, Z_{ijg}, are calculated by:

   $$Z_{ijg} = \frac{Y_{ijg} - \hat{\alpha}_g - X\hat{\beta}_g}{\hat{\delta}_g}$$

   where $\hat{\alpha}_g$, $\hat{\beta}_g$, and $\hat{\delta}_{ig}$ are estimators of α_g, β_g and δ_{ig}, respectively.

2) **EB batch effect parameter estimates using parametric empirical priors**

   Assume that the standardized data, Z_{ijg}, satisfy the normal distribution, $Z_{ijg} \sim N(\gamma_{ig}\delta_{ig}^2)$, and the parametric forms for prior distributions on the batch effect parameters to be:

   $$\gamma_{ig} \sim N(Y_i, \tau_i^2), \qquad \delta_{ij}^2 \sim \text{inverse gamma}(\lambda_i, \theta_i)$$

   The parameters Y_i, τ_i^2, λ_i, and θ_i are empirically estimated from standardized data using the method of moments. These prior distributions (normal, inverse gamma) can be selected due to their conjugacy with the normal assumption for the standardized data.

   Based on the assumptions of prior distributions, the EB estimates for batch effect parameters, γ_{ig} and δ_{ig}^2, are given by the conditional posterior means:

   $$\gamma_{ig}^* = \frac{n_i \bar{\tau}_i^2 \hat{\gamma}_{ig} + \delta_{ig}^{2*} \bar{\gamma}_i}{n_i \bar{\tau}_i^2 + \delta_{ig}^{2*}}, \qquad \delta_{ig}^{2*} = \frac{\bar{\theta}_i + \frac{1}{2}\sum_J (Z_{ijg} - \gamma_{ig}^*)^2}{\frac{n_j}{2} + \bar{\lambda}_i - 1}$$

3) **Adjust data for batch effect**

   After calculating the adjusted batch effect estimators, γ_{ig}^* and δ_{ig}^{2*}, the EB batch adjusted data γ_{ijg}^* can be calculated as follows:

   $$\gamma_{ijg}^* = \frac{\hat{\sigma}_g}{\delta_{ig}^*}(Z_{ijg} - \hat{\gamma}_{ig}^*) + \hat{\alpha}_g + X\hat{\beta}_g$$

   This method was shown because it allows for the combination of multiple datasets and is robust even with a small sample size [18].

16.2.2
Transformation Method

16.2.2.1 Standardization of Expression Data

To reduce the bias that can occur in each gene expression due to differing conditions, standardization can be applied to each dataset before integration. This method was applied to a microarray dataset in a previous study [20]. The standardized expression ratio Z_{ij} is calculated as follows:

$$Z_{ij} = \frac{(X_{ij}-\bar{X}_i)}{\sqrt{\frac{1}{N_i}\sum_{j=1}^{N_i}(X_{ij}-\bar{X}_i)^2}}$$

where

X_{ij} is the expression level of gene i in experiment j;
$\bar{X}_i$ is the mean expression level of gene i;
the denominator is the standard deviation of expression levels of gene i.
N_i is the number of experiments of gene i.

Figure 16.1 shows the effect of standardization of two datasets derived from different experimental conditions. The dataset shown in Figure 16.1 included two datasets resulting from experiments with different microarray chip batches. M.YCC3 and woSerum experimental groups were experimentally processed in the same batch differing from the remainder groups. When we applied the unsupervised clustering method to the whole dataset, three experimental groups (HUVEC, Matrigel, YCC3) and two experimental groups (woSerum and M.YCC3) were separated and groups in same batch were fastened together. Therefore, we could confirm that some batch effect exists in the dataset (Figure 16.1a). With standardization of data, HUVEC and

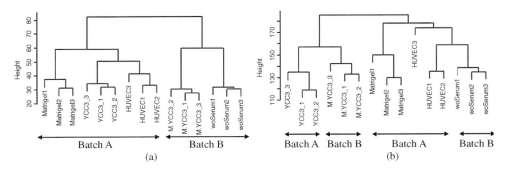

Figure 16.1 Hierarchical clustering analysis of raw data (a) and standardized data (b). HUVEC1–3: HUVEC in conventional culture condition with serum, Martrigel1–3: cultured HUVEC in Matrigel, YCC_1–3: co-cultured HUVEC with YCC-3, woSerum1–3: HUVEC cultured without serum, M.YCC_1–3: cultured HUVEC in Matrigel and co-cultured with YCC-3. The numbers at the end of the experiment labels represent the numbers of replications in the experiment [21].

woSerum experimental groups from different batches were fastened together and other experimental groups were well intermingled (Figure 16.1b), suggesting that the batch effect is negligible through standardization.

16.2.2.2 Transformation of Datasets Using a Reference Dataset

The gene expression intensities of each dataset can be transformed based on the reference dataset by the following three methods, resulting in similar expression patterns in corresponding experimental groups:

1) **A'B**: The gene expression ratios of dataset A are transformed into the form of dataset B, which is considered the reference dataset. The transformed expression ratios of normal and tumor groups in dataset A can be calculated for each gene as follows:

$$AN' = AN(\text{sd}(BN)/\text{sd}(AN)) - [\overline{AN(\text{sd}(BN)/\text{sd}(AN))} - \overline{BN}]$$
$$AT' = AT(\text{sd}(BT)/\text{sd}(AT)) - [\overline{AT(\text{sd}(BT)/\text{sd}(AT))} - \overline{BT}]$$

where AN' and AT' are the transformed expression ratios of normal and tumor groups in dataset A and AN and AT are the normal and tumor groups in dataset A. $\overline{BN}$, $\overline{BT}$ are the mean expression ratios of the tumor and normal groups in dataset B.

The terms $\text{sd}(AN)$, $\text{sd}(AT)$, $\text{sd}(BN)$, $\text{sd}(BT)$ are the standard deviations of the expression ratios of the tumor and normal groups in datasets A and B.

2) **AB'**: The gene expression ratios of dataset B are transformed into the form of dataset A, which is considered the reference dataset. The transformed expression ratios of the normal and tumor groups in dataset B can be calculated for each gene as follows:

$$BN' = BN(\text{sd}(AN)/\text{sd}(BN)) - [\overline{BN(\text{sd}(AN)/\text{sd}(BN))} - \overline{AN}]$$
$$BT' = BT(\text{sd}(AT)/\text{sd}(BT)) - [\overline{BT(\text{sd}(AT)/\text{sd}(BT))} - \overline{AT}]$$

where BN' and BT' are the transformed expression ratios of the normal and tumor groups in dataset B. BN and BT are the normal and tumor groups in dataset B. $\overline{AN}$, $\overline{AT}$ are the mean expression ratios of the tumor and normal groups in dataset A.

3) **A'B'**: The gene expression ratios of datasets A and B are transformed using the pooled standard deviations and mean expression values of the two datasets. The transformed expression ratios of the normal and tumor groups in datasets A and B can be calculated for each gene as follows:

$$AN' = AN(\text{sd}(N))/\text{sd}(AN) - (\overline{AN(\text{sd}(N))/\text{sd}(AN)} - \overline{N})$$
$$AT' = AT(\text{sd}(T))/\text{sd}(AT) - (\overline{AT(\text{sd}(T))/\text{sd}(AT)} - \overline{T})$$

$$BN' = BN(\text{sd}(N))/\text{sd}(BN) - (\overline{BN(\text{sd}(N))/\text{sd}(BN)} - \overline{N})$$
$$BT' = BT(\text{sd}(T))/\text{sd}(BT) - (\overline{BT(\text{sd}(T))/\text{sd}(BT)} - \overline{T})$$

where $\bar{N}, \bar{T}$ are the mean expression ratios of the normal and tumor groups in dataset A and dataset B:

$\mathrm{sd}(N) = \sqrt{\frac{(n_{AN}-1)\mathrm{sd}(AN)^2 + (n_{BN}-1)\mathrm{sd}(BN)^2}{n_{AN}+n_{BN}-2}}$ is the pooled standard deviation of the normal group

$\mathrm{sd}(T) = \sqrt{\frac{(n_{AT}-1)\mathrm{sd}(AT)^2 + (n_{BT}-1)\mathrm{sd}(BT)^2}{n_{AT}+n_{BT}-2}}$ is the pooled standard deviation of the tumor group

$n_{AN}, n_{BN}, n_{AT}, n_{BT}$ are the number of experiments of AN, BN, AT, and BT.

The datasets shown in Figure 16.2 are two microarray datasets from experiments with 154 colorectal tissue samples, consisting of 82 tumor and 72 normal tissues. Dataset A includes 35 normal and 43 tumor tissues; dataset B includes 37 normal and 39 tumor tissues. The only difference between the two microarray datasets is the RNA source, that is, total RNA or amplified RNA (Table 16.4 below). Hierarchical cluster analysis (HCA) clustered the samples into two distinct groups according to the data sources rather than different experimental groups (Figure 16.2a). Figure 16.2b–d shows the results of the transformed datasets by $A'B$, AB', and $A'B'$, respectively. The

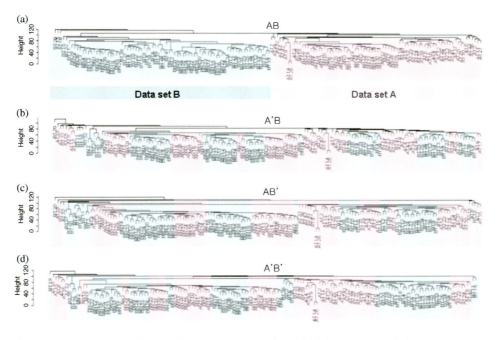

Figure 16.2 Comparison of integration methods using unsupervised hierarchical cluster analysis. All the datasets include two experimental groups, normal and tumor. Euclidean distance and average linkage method were used as a similarity measure and a linkage method for hierarchical cluster analysis, respectively (pink: dataset A; blue: dataset B) [19].

two transformed microarray datasets were well intermixed and the experimental groups (tumor or normal) of the two datasets were more distinctly separated regardless of the transformation methods.

HCA also showed that the two datasets were in fact well intermingled, indicating that the experimental bias had been minimized. Intermingling of different datasets indicates that datasets derived from different experimental conditions are well combined for further analysis.

16.2.3
Discretization Methods

Discretization is the process by which a set of values is grouped together into a range symbol. Usually, the discretization process takes place after sorting data in ascending or descending order with respect to the variables to be discretized.

The use of categorized values of gene expression ratios can reduce the influence of outliers and may improve prediction accuracies in the classification of different experimental classes. The use of discrete values has the advantages of being able to concisely represent and specify, being easier to use, and conducive to improved predictive accuracy [22]. The simplest discretization methods are the "equal interval width" and "equal frequency intervals" methods. Kerber [23] suggested the ChiMerge method. Several entropy-based methods have recently come to the forefront of work on discretization [24]. Fayyad and Irani [24] used a recursive entropy minimization heuristic for discretization and coupled this method with the minimum description length criterion to control the number of intervals produced over continuous space. In addition, a nonparametric scoring method was applied to gene expression data to discretize gene expression ratios [25], which usually transforms expression ratios based on their ranks in each experiment. In this case, some genes are included in the same rank and the score can be calculated differently acccrding to the order of ranks with the same values, which requires more time to score as the number of samples increases.

16.2.3.1 Equal Width and Equal Frequency Discretizations
The equal-width discretization algorithm determines the minimum and maximum of the discretized values and then divides the range into a user-defined number of equal width discrete intervals. If an attribute a is observed to have values bounded by a_{min} and a_{max}, this method computes the interval width with k intervals:

$$\text{width}(k) = (a_{max} - a_{min})/k$$

and constructs thresholds at $a_{min} + I \times \text{width}(k)$ where $i = 1, \ldots, k-1$. Since this method does not utilize decision values in setting partition boundaries, it is likely that classification information will be lost by binning as a result of combining values that are strongly associated with different classes into the same interval. In some cases this could make the effective classification much more difficult. The obvious weakness of this equal-width method is that in cases where the outcome observations are not distributed evenly, a large amount of important information can be lost after the discretization process.

The equal-frequency algorithm determines the minimum and maximum values of the discretized attribute, sorts all of the values in ascending order, and divides the range into a user-defined number of intervals so that every interval contains the same number of sorted values. With the equal-frequency algorithm, many occurrences of a continuous value could cause the occurrences to be assigned into different bins.

16.2.3.2 ChiMerge Method

Chi-squared (χ^2) is a statistical measure that conducts a significance test on the relationship between the values of a feature and the class. In an accurate discretization the relative class frequencies should be fairly consistent within an interval (otherwise the interval should be split to express this difference), but two adjacent intervals should not have a similar relative class frequency (in that case the adjacent intervals should be merged into one) [23]. The χ^2 statistic determines the similarity of adjacent intervals based on some significance level. It tests the hypothesis that two adjacent intervals of a feature are independent of the class. If they are independent they should be merged, otherwise they should remain separate.

The bottom-up method based on chi-squared is ChiMerge [23]. ChiMerge searches for the best merger of adjacent intervals by minimizing the chi-squared criterion applied locally to two adjacent intervals and merges them if they are statistically similar. The stopping rule is based on a user-defined chi-squared threshold to reject the merger if the two adjacent intervals are insufficiently similar.

16.2.3.3 Discretization Based on Recursive Minimal Entropy

A method for discretizing continuous attributes based on a minimal entropy (ME) uses the class information entropy of candidate partitions to select binary boundaries for discretization [24, 26]. If there is a given set of instances S, a feature A, and a partition boundary T, the class information entropy of the partition induced by T, denoted $E(A, T, S)$, is given by:

$$E(A, T; S) = \frac{|S_1|}{|S|} \text{Ent}(S_1) + \frac{|S_2|}{|S|} \text{Ent}(S_2)$$

For a given feature A, the boundary T_{min}, which minimizes the entropy function over all possible partition boundaries, is selected as a binary discretization boundary. This method can be applied recursively to both of the partitions induced by T_{min} until some stopping condition is achieved, thus creating multiple intervals for feature A. There must be $N-1$ evaluations for each attribute with N number of attribute values.

16.2.3.4 Nonparametric Scoring Method for Microarray Data [25]

Microarray data consist of a large number of genes on a relatively small number of samples. Assume that there are n patients in two groups, with n_1 patients in the first group and n_2 in the second group (Figure 16.3).

A scoring method can be processed as follows for identifying informative genes from microarray dataset:

1) Sort the data so that the patients in the first group are on the left and those in the second group are on the right (Figure 16.3) and assign "0" to the patients in the first group and "1" to the patients in the second group.

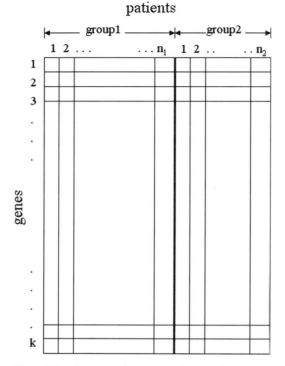

Figure 16.3 Structure of microarray dataset. The dataset is divided into two groups, with n_1 and n_2 patients [25].

2) Sort the expression values from the smallest to the largest, and identify the group index of sorted gene expression. How closely the "0" and "1" are grouped together can be a measure of heterogeneity between two groups.
3) Compute a score statistic that measures the disorder of "0" and "1" for each gene. The gene with small score statistic can be a significant discriminative gene.

For example, suppose we have $n = 6$, $n_1 = 3$, and $n_2 = 3$. Then the score can be calculated as shown in Table 16.1.

The score is 4 in this example and we can write:

$$\text{Score} = \sum_{i \in N_2} \sum_{j \in N_1} h(x_j - x_i)$$

where N_i represents the set of group i and $h(x)$ is the indicator function:

$$h(x) = \begin{cases} 0, & \text{if } x \leq 0, \\ 1, & \text{if } x > 0 \end{cases}$$

The gene with low or high score would be a differently expressed gene in the score method.

Table 16.1 Calculation of the score.

Before sorting:						
Expression values:	0.87	1.21	0.19	0.81	0.52	1.79
Groups:	0	0	0	1	1	1
After sorting:						
Expression values:	0.19	0.52	0.81	0.87	1.21	1.79
Groups:	0	1	1	0	0	1
Score	Data					
	0	1	1	0	0	1
+1	0	1	0	1	0	1
+1	0	0	1	1	0	1
+1	0	0	1	0	1	1
+1	0	0	0	1	1	1

16.2.3.5 Discretization by Rank of Gene Expression in Microarray Dataset: Proposed Method [27]

For transformation of the dataset, gene expression ratios are rearranged in order of expression ratios for each gene and the ranks are matched with the corresponding experimental group. If the experimental groups are homogenous the ranks within the same experimental group will be neighboring. This process can be seen as similar to the first step in the nonparametric Mann–Whitney U test. The process of discretization of gene expressions is summarized in the following steps:

1) Rank the gene expression ratios within a gene for each dataset.
2) List in order of the ranks and assign the order of gene expressions to the corresponding experimental groups.
3) For each gene, summarize the result of (2) in the form of a contingency table.
4) Test the relationship between the gene expression patterns and experimental groups for each gene.

When there are three datasets to be combined, the datasets can each be added by entry, as shown in Table 16.2, after the transformation of each dataset by rank.

Table 16.2 Combination of contingency tables for three datasets ($t_{ij} = a_{ij} + b_{ij} + c_{ij}$). P1, P2, and P3 represent three different phenotypes. E1, E2, and E3 represent three groups by rank of gene expressions; a_{ij}, b_{ij}, and c_{ij} are the numbers of experiments belonging to P_j and E_i at the same time in data A, data B, and data C, respectively.

Dataset A				Dataset B				Dataset C				Combined dataset		
	P1	P2	P3		P1	P2	P3		P1	P2	P3		P1	P2	P3
E1	a_{11}	a_{12}	a_{13}	E1	b_{11}	b_{12}	b_{13}	E1	c_{11}	c_{12}	c_{13}	E1	t_{11}	t_{12}	t_{13}
E2	a_{21}	a_{22}	a_{23}	E2	b_{21}	b_{22}	b_{23}	E2	c_{21}	c_{22}	c_{23}	E2	t_{21}	t_{22}	t_{23}
E3	a_{31}	a_{32}	a_{33}	E3	b_{31}	b_{32}	b_{33}	E3	c_{31}	c_{32}	c_{33}	E3	t_{31}	t_{32}	t_{33}

16.3
Statistical Method for Significant Gene Selection and Classification

For significant gene selection, an independent two-sample t-test or ANOVA could be applied when continuous expression values are used and the sample size is sufficient for a parametric statistical test. However, if the sample size is not large enough, a non-parametric method is suggested, for example, the Mann–Whitney U test or Kruskal–Wallis test. However, when the gene expression is discretized, the categorical data analytical method should be used. In this section we describe the chi-squared test for detecting significant gene sets from the discretized dataset and the random forest (RF) method for calculating the prediction accuracies of the selected significant gene set.

16.3.1
Chi-Squared Test for Significant Gene Selection

When gene expression is discretized by the method shown in Section 16.2.3, the integrated dataset for each gene can be summarized in the form of a contingency table (Table 16.3). To identify the significant gene set from the combined dataset, a nonparametric statistical method, the chi-squared test, can be applied to the dataset for testing the relationship between gene expression patterns and experimental groups.

The test statistics are calculated as follows for each gene:

$$\chi^2 = \sum \frac{[n_{ij} - \hat{E}(n_{ij})]^2}{\hat{E}(n_{ij})}, \quad \hat{E}(n_{ij}) = \frac{r_i c_j}{n}$$

When the sample size for each experiment is small, generally less than five, Fisher's exact test is recommended rather than the chi-squared test.

Table 16.3 Summary of discretized data using rank of gene expressions. The significant genes can be selected by an independency test between the phenotypes and gene expressions using this type of summarized dataset; c_i and r_i represent the marginal sums of the i-th column and row, respectively; n represents the total number of experiments.

Experimental group by rank (or ME[a]) of gene expression	Experimental groups by phenotypes			
	P1	P2	P3	Marginal sum
E1	n_{11}	n_{12}	n_{13}	r_1
E2	n_{21}	n_{22}	n_{23}	r_2
E3	n_{31}	n_{32}	n_{33}	r_3
Marginal sum	c_1	c_2	c_3	N

a) ME: minimal entropy method.

16.3.2
Random Forest for Calculating Prediction Accuracy

To calculate the predictive accuracy of the selected significant gene set, the random forest (RF) test [28] can be used. Random forest grows many classification trees. To classify a new object, put the values of a new object (vector) down each of the trees in the forest. Each tree gives a classification result, and we say the tree "votes" for that class, and the forest chooses the classification having the most votes.

Each tree is grown as follows [28]:

1) If the number of cases in the training set is N, sample N cases at random *with replacement*, from the original data. This sample will be the training set for growing the tree.
2) If there are M input variables, a number $m \ll M$ is specified such that at each node, m variables are selected at random out of the M and the best split on these m is used to split the node. The value of m is held constant during the forest growing.
3) Each tree is grown to the largest extent possible. There is no pruning.

In random forests, there is no need for cross-validation or a separate test set to get an unbiased estimate of the test set error. It is estimated internally as follows: Each tree is constructed using a different bootstrap sample from the original data. About one-third of the cases are left out of the bootstrap sample and not used in the construction of the k-th tree.

Then, put each case left out in the construction of the k-th tree down the k-th tree to get a classification. In this way, a test set classification is obtained for each case in about one-third of the trees. At the end of the process, take j to be the class that got most of the votes every time case n was OOB (out of bag). The proportion of times that j is not equal to the true class of n averaged over all cases is the OOB error estimate.

The program for random forest in the R package can be used for calculation of OOB error in classification:

1) Generate n datasets of bootstrap samples $\{B_1, B_2, \ldots, B_n\}$ by allowing repetition.
2) Use a B_k to build a tree classifier T_k, and classify B_ms ($m \neq k$) data (OOB samples).
3) Calculate classification errors of B_ms and obtain the average, which is the overall classification error (OOB error).
4) Calculate the prediction accuracy of the test datasets using the built-in classifier (2).

16.4
Example

In this example, we evaluate the effect of the combined dataset using classification accuracy. We considered the discretized method described in Section 16.2.3.4 as an integration method.

Table 16.4 Summary of datasets used in this chapter; all are colon cancer related datasets derived from different experimental conditions; genes with missing entries were excluded.

Data name	Experimental sources	Number of genes	Number of total samples	Normal group	Tumor group
Training datasets[a]					
Data A	Total RNA	12 319	78	35	43
Data B	Amplified RNA	12 319	76	37	39
Data AB	Combined dataset by the proposed method	12 319	154	72	82
Test datasets[a]					
Tumor 86	Amplified RNA (Batch I)	17 104	86	0	86
Tumor 211	Amplified RNA (Batch II)	17 104	211	0	211
Training and test dataset [29]					
Affy	Affymetrix HU6800	7464	36	18	18

a) Cancer Metastasis Research Center of Yonsei University, Seoul, Korea.

16.4.1
Dataset

Table 16.4 summarizes the datasets used.

Two cDNA microarray datasets, datasets A and B, determined by experiments with 154 colorectal tissues (82 tumor and 72 normal) were used as training datasets for comparing the prediction accuracies of the ME and proposed methods. These two cDNA microarray datasets were derived from two different RNA sources, total RNA and amplified RNA. Previous studies have concluded that there are differences between the results of these two types of datasets and the sensitivity of detecting differential gene expressions from microarray datasets using amplified RNA is also different compared to those using total RNA [30, 31]. It has also been confirmed, using unsupervised hierarchical cluster analysis [19], that systematic biases exist between these two datasets (Figure 16.2).

Two more cDNA datasets, Tumor 86 and Tumor 211, which included only colorectal tumor tissues, were used in experiments with amplified RNA under different batches as test datasets. These colon cancer datasets determined with cDNA microarrays were from the Cancer Metastasis Research Center at Yonsei University in Seoul, Korea. One additional colon cancer dataset was used; analysis was performed with the Human 6800 Gene Chip Set (Affymetrix). This dataset was obtained from a microarray database at Princeton University [32] and included experiments with adenomas and their paired normal tissue.

To evaluate the performance of the proposed method in different platforms, NCI 60 cell line datasets derived from different platforms were also used. Gene expression datasets for NCI-60 using 9706 cloned cDNA microarrays and 6810 gene Affymetrix HU6800 oligonucleotide arrays were obtained separately from the additional files of a previous study [33]. We used the common 2344 UniGene clusters. Ovarian and colon cancer cell lines were included in the nine tumor cell lines. These two groups included six and seven replications, respectively.

16.4.2
Prediction Accuracies Using the Combined Dataset

16.4.2.1 Data Preprocessing
Gene expression ratios were normalized such that they would have similar distributions across a series of arrays and the normalization process was executed using the "limma" library of the R package [34]. The cDNA data in the NCI 60 cell line datasets included missing entries that were estimated using the SeqKnn (sequential k nearest neighbor) imputation method [35] before analysis.

16.4.2.2 Improvement of Prediction Accuracy Using Combined Datasets by the Proposed Method
The prediction accuracies were compared using two original colon cancer datasets, analyzed with different RNA sources, as training datasets.

While the prediction accuracy of dataset B using dataset A as a training dataset was higher than 95%, the accuracy of dataset A using dataset B as a training dataset was lower than 80% (Figure 16.4a). This indicates that the dataset created using total RNA predicted the dataset using amplified RNA more correctly than the converse. Figure 16.4b shows the prediction accuracies of the two test datasets, Tumor 211 and Tumor 86. The prediction accuracy of the combined dataset was higher than the separated datasets. In addition, dataset B predicted test datasets with higher accuracy than did dataset A. This could be because the two test datasets were also analyzed using amplified RNA. The prediction accuracy was higher in the Batch II-86 tumor dataset than in the Batch I-211 tumor dataset.

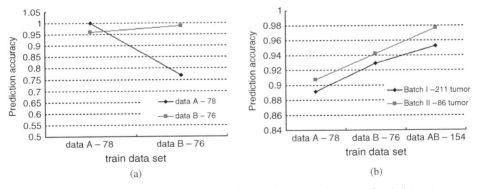

Figure 16.4 Comparison of prediction accuracies. The number next to the name of each dataset represents the sample size. Seven significant genes with high prediction accuracy were used [27].

Table 16.5 Description of six informative genes (one among seven genes is duplicated) selected from the combined dataset after transformation by the proposed method [27].

Gene ID	Gene name	UniGene ID	Symbol	Chromosomal location
AA485 151	Heat shock 105 kDa/110 kDa protein 1	Hs.36 927	HSPH1	13q12.3
AA425 217	Cadherin 3, type 1, p-cadherin (placental)	Hs.354 598	CDH3	16q22.1
AA464 731	s100 Calcium binding protein a11 (calgizzarin)	Hs.417 004	S100A11	1q21
AA504 130	Cytoskeleton associated protein 2	Hs.444 028	CKAP2	13q14
AA455 925	Four and a half lim domains 1	Hs.435 369	FHL1	Xq26
AW050 510	Pyrroline-5-carboxylate reductase 1	Hs.458 332	PYCR1	17q25.3

16.4.2.3 Description of Significant Genes Selected from a Combined Dataset by the Proposed Method

Table 16.5 summarizes the descriptions of six discriminative genes selected from the combined dataset rather than two separated datasets.

AA485 151 was upregulated by over fivefold in colorectal adenocarcinoma [36]. AA425 217 was published as a significant gene in colorectal cancer [37], and 16q22.1, on which AA425 217 is located, is a region that includes CDH1, which encodes a cell–cell adhesion protein and is expressed in gastric cancer and lobular breast cancer. AA464 731 is known to be a downregulated gene in the SW620 metastatic colorectal cancer cell line [38] that is also significantly overexpressed in pancreatic cell lines [39]. AA504 130 is located on 13q12.3, similarly to BRCA2, which is known to be a marker of breast and ovarian cancer. The mutated gene for retinoblastoma is located on chromosome 13q14 [40], on which AA504 130 is also located.

AA455 925 is known to be an E2F-1 regulated gene [41]. Xq26 and Xq25 are two common chromosomal deletion regions [42], and are known to contribute to the malignant progression of gastric epithelial progenitor (GEP) endocrine carcinomas. Colorectal cancer is thought to be more common in men than in women; Xq26 is known to be one of the regions that contain multiple gains-of-function that were significantly more common in males than in females [43]. Since AW050 510 is located at 17q25.3, adjacent to BIRC5 at 17q25 that is known to be a survivin expression colorectal cancer [44, 45], AW050 510 is also expected to have similar characteristics to BIRC5.

16.4.2.4 Improvement of Prediction Accuracies by Combining Datasets Performed using Different Platforms

The prediction accuracies of combined datasets derived from different platforms were investigated. While the prediction accuracies of datasets A and B on affy were low with small numbers of genes, the prediction accuracy increased as the number of genes increased. By combining datasets A and B, the prediction accuracy on affy

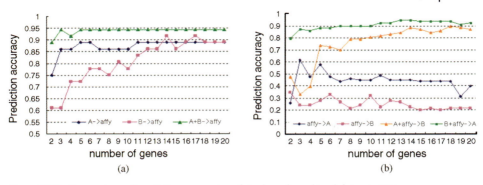

Figure 16.5 Comparison of prediction accuracies of single and combined datasets [27].

improved (Figure 16.5a). When Affymetrix data was used as a training dataset, its prediction accuracies on datasets A and B were lower than 60%. However, after combining with dataset A or dataset B, prediction accuracy improved to greater than 90% (Figure 16.5b).

16.4.3
Conclusions

The designed 25-mer oligochips from Affymetrix provide an absolute value of expression in an RNA sample while cDNA microarrays perform a two-color competitive hybridization that gives the relative transcript expression in two samples. In addition, as long oligonucleotide platforms (typically 60 to 80-mers) also use hybridization, the relative measurements on this platform resulted in higher precision than did absolute measurements [46]. Therefore, experimental biases can occur as a result of the differences in the usage of absolute measurements and ratios.

Additionally, some previous studies have indicated that datasets from different microarray platforms should not be combined directly [33, 47–49]. However, even when the datasets were generated from the same platform, the lab effect, especially when compounded with the RNA sample effect, plays a bigger role than the platform effect on data agreement [50]. Inter-study biases also exist among several microarray datasets tested with different RNA sources, even when they are from the same laboratory and platform. Previous studies have shown that there are some differences in results from datasets tested using different RNA sources. The sensitivity to detecting differential gene expression from a microarray dataset using amplified RNA is also different compared to that using total RNA [30, 31].

One way to attempt to combine these different types of datasets is to use abstraction of expression values such as ranks or discretized values. This method reduces the variability in expression values from different microarray datasets. While there may be a slight loss of information by discretization, the method is robust against outliers, fast, and simple to understand.

In colon cancer datasets derived from cDNA microarrays, a dataset created with total RNA more accurately predicted a dataset created using amplified RNA than the converse (Figure 16.4a). However, the dataset, which was tested using amplified RNA, showed better performance in the prediction of two test datasets than did a dataset from total RNA (Figure 16.4b). It can be interpolated that using the same source can improve prediction power. In addition, the combined dataset predicted two test datasets more accurately than did the separated datasets. The top six discriminative genes selected from a combined dataset, which were not detected from two separated datasets, have been shown in previous studies to be genes associated with colon cancer. Therefore, we believe that the use of a combined dataset is more reliable for the detection of biologically significant genes than the use of separated datasets, due to the increase in sample size.

In the colon cancer dataset derived from oligonucleotide arrays, the prediction accuracies were improved by combination with cDNA datasets. Although two datasets derived from different experimental conditions have different scales in gene expressions, this variation can be compensated for by discretizing gene expression. Therefore, along with the ranking of gene expressions, no other transformation method was required to match these two types of datasets.

16.5
Summary

In this chapter we have introduced several methods for combining microarray datasets derived from different experimental conditions and showed the efficiency of the use of combined datasets after discretization by rank. The combined dataset by rank of gene expression improved prediction accuracy and this method may be especially useful in determining discriminative genes from datasets that have different scales of gene expression ratios.

Numerous gene expression datasets have been accumulated in public databases. It is possible to obtain reliable information using such databases if one can combine datasets derived from different experimental conditions; in such cases it is not even necessary to carry out the microarray experiments, thereby saving time and money. In addition, more reliable information can be obtained, since the sample size would be sufficient for analysis.

References

1 Breitling, R., Sharif, O., Hartman, M.L., and Krisans, S.K. (2002) Loss of compartmentalization causes misregulation of lysine biosynthesis in peroxisome-deficient yeast cells. *Eukaryot. Cell*, **1**, 978–986.

2 Choi, J.K., Yu, U., Kim, S., and Yoo, O.J. (2003) Combining multiple microarray studies and modeling interstudy variation. *Bioinformatics*, **19** (Suppl. 1), i84–i90.

3 Detours, V., Dumont, J.E., Bersini, H., and Maenhaut, C. (2003) Integration and cross-validation of high-throughput gene expression data: comparing heterogeneous data sets. *FEBS Lett.*, **546**, 98–102.

4 Lee, P.D., Sladek, R., Greenwood, C.M., and Hudson, T.J. (2002) Control genes and variability: absence of ubiquitous reference transcripts in diverse mammalian expression studies. *Genome Res.*, **12**, 292–297.

5 Ramaswamy, S., Ross, K.N., Lander, E.S., and Golub, T.R. (2003) A molecular signature of metastasis in primary solid tumors. *Nat. Genet.*, **33**, 49–54.

6 Rhodes, D.R., Barrette, T.R., Rubin, M.A., Ghosh, D., and Chinnaiyan, A.M. (2002) Meta-analysis of microarrays: interstudy validation of gene expression profiles reveals pathway dysregulation in prostate cancer. *Cancer Res.*, **62**, 4427–4433.

7 Xin, W., Rhodes, D.R., Ingold, C., Chinnaiyan, A.M., and Rubin, M.A. (2003) Dysregulation of the annexin family protein family is associated with prostate cancer progression. *Am. J. Pathol.*, **162**, 255–261.

8 Choi, J.K., Choi, J.Y., Kim, D.G., Choi, D.W., Kim, B.Y., Lee, K.H., Yeom, Y.I., Yoo, H.S., Yoo, O.J., and Kim, S. (2004) Integrative analysis of multiple gene expression profiles applied to liver cancer study. *FEBS Lett.*, **565**, 93–100.

9 Jiang, H., Deng, Y., Chen, H.S., Tao, L., Sha, Q., Chen, J., Tsai, C.J., and Zhang, S. (2004) Joint analysis of two microarray gene-expression data sets to select lung adenocarcinoma marker genes. *BMC Bioinformatics*, **5**, 81.

10 Hu, P., Greenwood, C.M., and Beyene, J. (2005) Integrative analysis of multiple gene expression profiles with quality-adjusted effect size models. *BMC Bioinformatics*, **6**, 128.

11 Listgarten, J. and Emili, A. (2005) Statistical and computational methods for comparative proteomic profiling using liquid chromatography-tandem mass spectrometry. *Mol. Cell. Proteomics*, **4**, 419–434.

12 Jansen, R., Lan, N., Qian, J., and Gerstein, M. (2002) Integration of genomic datasets to predict protein complexes in yeast. *J. Struct. Funct. Genomics*, **2**, 71–81.

13 Alter, O., Brown, P.O., and Botstein, D. (2000) Singular value decomposition for genome-wide expression data processing and modeling. *Proc. Natl. Acad. Sci. USA*, **97**, 10101–10106.

14 Nielsen, T.O., West, R.B., Linn, S.C., Alter, O., Knowling, M.A., O'Connell, J.X., Zhu, S., Fero, M., Sherlock, G., Pollack, J.R., Brown, P.O., Botstein, D., and van de Rijn, M. (2002) Molecular characterisation of soft tissue tumours: a gene expression study. *Lancet*, **359**, 1301–1307.

15 Benito, M., Parker, J., Du, Q., Wu, J., Xiang, D., Perou, C.M., and Marron, J.S. (2004) Adjustment of systematic microarray data bases. *Bioinformatics*, **20**, 105–114.

16 Park, T., Yi, S.G., Shin, Y.K., and Lee, S. (2006) Combining multiple microarrays in the presence of controlling variables. *Bioinformatics*, **22**, 1682–1689.

17 Marron, J.S., Todd, M., and Ahn, J. (2007) Distance weighted discrimination. *J. Am. Stat. Assoc.*, **102**, 1267–1271.

18 Johnson, W.E., Li, C., and Rabinovic, A. (2007) Adjusting batch effects in microarray expression data using empirical Bayes methods. *Biostatistics*, **8**, 118–127.

19 Kim, K.Y., Ki, D.H., Jeong, H.J., Jeung, H.C., Chung, H.C., and Rha, S.Y. (2007) Novel and simple transformation algorithm for combining microarray data sets. *BMC Bioinformatics*, **8**, 218.

20 Lee, J.S., Chu, I.S., Mikaelyan, A., Calvisi, D.F., Heo, J., Reddy, J.K., and Thorgeirsson, S.S. (2004) Application of comparative functional genomics to identify best-fit mouse models to study human cancer. *Nat. Genet.*, **36**, 1306–1311.

21 Kim, K.Y., Chung, C.H., Jeung, H.C., Shin, J.H., Kim, T.S., and Rha, S.Y. (2006) Significant gene selection using integrated microarray data set with batch effect. *Genomics Informat.*, **4**, 110–117.

22 Liu, H., Hussain, H., Tan, C.L., and Dash, M. (2002) Discretization: an enabling technique. *Data Min. Knowl. Disc.*, **6** (4), 393–423.

23 Kerber, R. (1992) Chimerge: Discretization of numeric attributes, in *Proceedings of the Tenth National Conference on Artificial Intelligence*, MIT Press, pp. 123–128.

24 Fayyad, U. and Irani, K. (1993) Multi-interval discretization of continuous-valued attributes for classification learning, in *Proceedings of the 13th International Joint Conference on Artificial Intelligence*, Morgan Kaufamann, pp. 1022–1027.

25 Park, P., Pagano, M., and Bonetti, M. (2001) A nonparametric scoring algorithm for identifying informative genes from microarray data. Pacific Symposium on Biocomputing, pp. 52–63.

26 Catlett, J. (1991) On changing continuous attributes into ordered discrete attributes, in *Proceedings of the European Working Session on Learning*, Springer-Verlag, Berlin, Germany, pp. 164–178.

27 Kim, K.Y., Ki, D.H., Jeung, H.C., Chung, H.C., and Rha, S.Y. (2008) Improving the prediction accuracy in classification using the combined data sets by ranks of gene expressions. *BMC Bioinformatics*, **9**, 283.

28 Breiman, L. (2001) Random forest, Statistics Department, University of California, Berkeley, pp. 1–33.

29 Notterman, D.A., Alon, U., Sierk, A.J., and Levine, A.J. (2001) Transcriptional gene expression profiles of colorectal adenoma, adenocarcinoma, and normal tissue examined by oligonucleotide arrays. *Cancer Res.*, **61**, 3124–3130.

30 Feldman, A.L., Costouros, N.G., Wang, E., Qian, M., Marincola, F.M., Alexander, H.R., and Libutti, S.K. (2002) Advantages of mRNA amplification for microarray analysis. *Biotechniques*, **33**, 906–912, 914.

31 Schneider, J., Buness, A., Huber, W., Volz, J., Kioschis, P., Hafner, M., Poustka, A., and Sultmann, H. (2004) Systematic analysis of T7 RNA polymerase based *in vitro* linear RNA amplification for use in microarray experiments. *BMC Genomics*, **5**, 29.

32 Princetown University Microarray-DataBase, Microarray DataBase of Princeton University, www://puma.princeton.edu. Access date: Sep. 20. 2006.

33 Lee, J.K., Bussey, K.J., Gwadry, F.G., Reinhold, W., Riddick, G., Pelletier, S.L., Nishizuka, S., Szakacs, G., Annereau, J.P., Shankavaram, U., Lababidi, S., Smith, L.H., Gottesman, M.M., and Weinstein, J.N. (2003) Comparing cDNA and oligonucleotide array data: concordance of gene expression across platforms for the NCI-60 cancer cells. *Genome Biol.*, **4**, R82.

34 R:A language and environment for statistical computing, http://www.R-project.org. Access date: Feb. 20. 2006.

35 Kim, K.Y., Kim, B.J., and Yi, G.S. (2004) Reuse of imputed data in microarray analysis increases imputation efficiency. *BMC Bioinformatics*, **5**, 160.

36 Choi, K., Park, D.Y., Kim, J.Y., Lee, J.S., and Sol, M.Y. (2003) Overexpression of insulin-like growth factor binding protein 3 in colorectal carcinoma identified by cDNA microarray and immunohistochemical analysis. *Korean J. Pathol.*, **37** (3), 166–173.

37 Han, H., Bearss, D.J., Browne, L.W., Calaluce, R., Nagle, R.B., and Von Hoff, D.D. (2002) Identification of differentially expressed genes in pancreatic cancer cells using cDNA microarray. *Cancer Res.*, **62**, 2890–2896.

38 Kim, B.S., Kim, I., Lee, S., Kim, S., Rha, S.Y., and Chung, H.C. (2005) Statistical methods of translating microarray data into clinically relevant diagnostic information in colorectal cancer. *Bioinformatics*, **21**, 517–528.

39 Futschik, M., Jeffs, A., Pattison, S., Kasabov, N., Sullivan, M., Merrie, A., and Reeve, A. (2002) Gene expression profiling of metastatic and nonmetastatic colorectal cancer cell lines. *Genome Lett.*, **1** (1) 26–34.

40 Friend, S.H., Bernards, R., Rogelj, S., Weinberg, R.A., Rapaport, J.M., Albert, D.M., and Dryja, T.P. (1986) A human DNA segment with properties of the gene that predisposes to retinoblastoma and osteosarcoma. *Nature*, **323**, 643–646.

41 Nowak, K., Kerl, K., Fehr, D., Kramps, C., Gessner, C., Killmer, K., Samans, B., Berwanger, B., Christiansen, H., and Lutz, W. (2006) BMI1 is a target gene of E2F-1 and is strongly expressed in primary neuroblastomas. *Nucleic Acids Res.*, **34**, 1745–1754.

42 Azzoni, C., Bottarelli, L., Pizzi, S., D'Adda, T., Rindi, G., and Bordi, C. (2006) Xq25 and Xq26 identify the common minimal deletion region in malignant

gastroenteropancreatic endocrine carcinomas. *Virchows Arch.*, **448**, 119–126.

43 Unotoro, J., Kamiyama, H., Ishido, Y., Yaginuma, Y., Kasamaki, S., Sakamoto, K., Oota, A., Ishibashi, Y., and Kamano, T. (2006) Analysis of the relationship between sex and chromosomal aberrations in colorectal cancer by comparative genomic hybridization. *J. Int. Med. Res.*, **34**, 397–405.

44 Rohayem, J., Diestelkoetter, P., Weigle, B., Oehmichen, A., Schmitz, M., Mehlhorn, J., Conrad, K., and Rieber, E.P. (2000) Antibody response to the tumor-associated inhibitor of apoptosis protein survivin in cancer patients. *Cancer Res.*, **60**, 1815–1817.

45 Sarela, A.I., Macadam, R.C., Farmery, S.M., Markham, A.F., and Guillou, P.J. (2000) Expression of the antiapoptosis gene, survivin, predicts death from recurrent colorectal carcinoma. *Gut*, **46**, 645–650.

46 Moreau, Y., Aerts, S., De Moor, B., De Strooper, B., and Dabrowski, M. (2003) Comparison and meta-analysis of microarray data: from the bench to the computer desk. *Trends Genet.*, **19**, 570–577.

47 Jarvinen, A.K., Hautaniemi, S., Edgren, H., Auvinen, P., Saarela, J., Kallioniemi, O.P., and Monni, O. (2004) Are data from different gene expression microarray platforms comparable? *Genomics*, **83**, 1164–1168.

48 Kuo, W.P., Jenssen, T.K., Butte, A.J., Ohno-Machado, L., and Kohane, I.S. (2002) Analysis of matched mRNA measurements from two different microarray technologies. *Bioinformatics*, **18**, 405–412.

49 Zhu, B., Ping, G., Shinohara, Y., Zhang, Y., and Baba, Y. (2005) Comparison of gene expression measurements from cDNA and 60-mer oligonucleotide microarrays. *Genomics*, **85**, 657–665.

50 Wang, H., He, X., Band, M., Wilson, C., and Liu, L. (2005) A study of inter-lab and inter-platform agreement of DNA microarray data. *BMC Genomics*, **6**, 71.

17
Model Averaging for Biological Networks with Prior Information

Sach Mukherjee, Terence P. Speed, and Steven M. Hill

17.1
Introduction

In recent years there has been much interest within molecular biology in understanding how multiple genes and proteins act in concert to carry out biological functions (e.g., [1–3]) and how these functions are perturbed in disease states (e.g., [4, 5]). Indeed, it is largely this movement from thinking about one gene or protein at a time to thinking about multiple genes and proteins acting in concert that has characterized so-called "systems" approaches to biology (see e.g., [3, 6]). Networks of molecular components – for example, gene regulatory or protein signaling networks – have been the focus of intense study in both experimental and computational molecular biology [5, 7–15]. This has motivated a need for statistical methods capable of modeling such networks, and doing so under the challenging conditions of small sample size and high variability that are typical of many molecular assays.

At the same time, advances in computationally-intensive statistical methods have allowed statisticians working in biomedical research to perform inference using increasingly realistic, complex data models (e.g., [16]). A specific trend has been an interest in studying systems characterized by multiple interacting components. This has led to much interest in multivariate methods in general, and in graphical models in particular.

Graphical models [17–21] are a class of stochastic models that provide graph-based representations of probabilistic relationships between random variables. A graphical model consists of a graph G (a collection of vertices and linking edges), describing such probabilistic relationships, and parameters Θ that fully specify conditional distributions implied by the graph. The graph G can be regarded as capturing patterns of influence between variables under study (i.e., structural features of the model), whilst the parameters Θ describe the detailed nature of those influences. In molecular biology, we are usually interested in saying something about which molecules or combinations of molecules influence one another. Then, a natural idea is to represent molecular components as random variables and take advantage of the framework provided by graphical models to capture the interplay between them (e.g., [9–12, 14, 15, 22]). This modeling step then allows specific questions concerning features of the underlying biological network to be translated into statistical terms as questions concerning features of the (conditional independence) graph G.

To make inferences regarding features of the network, a method is needed to assess different graphs in light of data. To this end, a "scoring function" over the space of possible graphs is required; here, we take a Bayesian approach and use the posterior distribution over graphs given data $P(G|X)$ as our scoring function. One approach is then to attempt to maximize the scoring function over graphs; this is known as model selection. Alternatively, we can make inferences by averaging over *many* graphs; this is known as model averaging and, for reasons discussed below, is the approach employed here.

Inference on graphical model structure [23–27] is widely recognized to be a daunting task. This is partly because the number of possible graphs grows very rapidly with the number of variables, leading to a vast space of possible models for even a relatively small number of variables. Yet, equally, in many settings, an understanding of the relevant domain may suggest that not *every* possible graph is equally plausible, and that certain features should be regarded as a priori more likely than others; that is, there may be information, not directly contained in the data under study, that can be brought to bear on the questions of interest. Where available, such information, even when uncertain, is surely a valuable resource, making the question of how to exploit it in network inference an important one. This chapter addresses precisely this question, of making inferences regarding biological networks in the presence of prior knowledge concerning network features. We focus on directed graphical models called Bayesian networks, and use Markov chain Monte Carlo (MCMC) for inference. We seek to take account of detailed information concerning network features such as individual edges, edges between classes of vertices, and sparsity. In many settings, such beliefs follow naturally from a consideration of the underlying science or semantics of the variables under study. We present priors for beliefs of this kind and show examples of how these ideas can be used in practical settings.

The remainder of this chapter is organized as follows. Our work builds on a rich body of research in statistics and machine learning; we begin by reviewing key ideas in Bayesian networks and model selection and averaging. We then turn our attention to network priors. We present several examples of the use of our methods, including analyses of challenging synthetic data and of a proteomic dataset pertaining to a biological network of importance in breast cancer. We close with a discussion of the key points covered in the chapter and some ideas for future research.

17.2 Background

17.2.1 Bayesian Networks

Bayesian networks [18, 20, 28] are a type of multivariate statistical model in which a directed acyclic graph (DAG) describing conditional independence statements regarding a group of random variables is exploited to provide a compact description of their joint distribution. "Acyclic" means it is not possible to find a path along directed edges that starts and ends at the same vertex. A Bayesian network consists of two elements: (i) a DAG $G = (V(G), E(G))$, whose vertices V represent random variables $X_1 \ldots X_p$ of interest, and whose edge-set E contains edges describing conditional independences between those variables, and (ii) parameters Θ that specify the conditional distributions implied by the graph. In particular, the graph G implies that each variable is conditionally independent of its non-descendants given its immediate parents. Importantly, this means that the joint distribution $P(X_1 \ldots X_p | G)$ can be factorized into a product of local terms:

$$P(X_1 \ldots X_p | G) = \prod_{i=1}^{p} P(X_i | \mathbf{Pa}_G(X_i)) \tag{17.1}$$

where $\mathbf{Pa}_G(X_i)$ is the set of parents of X_i in graph G.

For example, Figure 17.1 depicts a graph G for a Bayesian network with four variables: X_1, X_2, X_3, and X_4; X_1 and X_2 are root nodes and have no parents, thus $\mathbf{Pa}_G(X_1) = \mathbf{Pa}_G(X_2) = \oslash$, where $\oslash$ denotes the empty set; X_3 has two parents, X_1 and X_2, giving $\mathbf{Pa}_G(X_3) = \{X_1, X_2\}$, whilst X_4 has one parent, X_3, giving $\mathbf{Pa}_G(X_4) = X_3$. From (17.1) we get the overall joint distribution over all four variables as:

$$P(X_1, X_2, X_3, X_4 | G) = P(X_1)P(X_2)P(X_3 | X_1, X_2)P(X_4 | X_3) \tag{17.2}$$

So far, we have only considered the relationships between the variables, but have not specified the conditional distributions on the right-hand side of (17.1). These can, in principle, be freely chosen; common choices include Gaussian for a

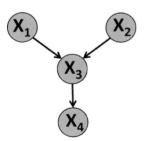

Figure 17.1 An example of a DAG (directed acyclic graph) for a Bayesian network.

continuous variable [29], or multinomial for a discrete variable [23]. The choice of distribution and associated parameters determines precisely how the variables depend on each other. Going back to our example, if each variable in the graph in Figure 17.1 is binary (can only take value 0 or 1) then the conditionals in (17.2) are Bernoulli distributions with parameters that depend on the configuration of the parents. Then, parameters $\theta_{ij} \in [0,1]$ for $i,j = 0,1$ fully specify a Bernoulli distribution for the conditional $P(X_3|X_1, X_2)$ by $P(X_3 = 1|X_1 = i, X_2 = j) = \theta_{ij}$. In the remainder of this chapter we focus on multinomial local conditionals, but note that the framework presented here generalizes, in principle, to any suitable conditional distributions.

17.2.2
Model Scoring

Our goal is to make inferences regarding the graph G that describes relationships between variables. But how can putative descriptions of relationships between variables be assessed? In Bayesian inference, uncertainty regarding an object of interest is described by a probability distribution (the "posterior distribution") over the object, conditioned on the data available. Here the object of interest is the graph G: we therefore seek to characterize the discrete probability distribution $P(G|X)$, where X represents all of the available data. From Bayes' rule:

$$P(G|X) = \frac{P(X|G)P(G)}{P(X)} \tag{17.3}$$

The term $P(X|G)$ is called the marginal likelihood. Let us assume that the form of the local conditional distributions is known, and let Θ represent the full set of model parameters. Then, from the sum rule of probability, we can write the marginal likelihood as an integral over all possible values of the parameters Θ:

$$P(X|G) = \int P(X, \Theta|G) d\Theta \tag{17.4}$$

This process of "integrating out" is known as marginalization in Bayesian inference, hence the name "marginal" likelihood. From the product rule of probability we get (17.4) in the following form:

$$P(X|G) = \int P(X|G, \Theta) p(\Theta|G) d\Theta \tag{17.5}$$

Here, the first term is an explicit likelihood, that is, the joint probability of all the data, under a (now) fully specified model. The term $p(\Theta|G)$ is a prior distribution for the parameters Θ. We will use Dirichlet priors that are conjugate for the multinomial conditionals used here. This has the advantage of yielding a closed-form marginal likelihood (for details see Appendix 17.A):

$$p(X|G) = \prod_{i=1}^{p} \prod_{j=1}^{q_i} \frac{\Gamma(N'_{ij})}{\Gamma(N'_{ij} + N_{ij})} \cdot \prod_{k=1}^{r_i} \frac{\Gamma(N'_{ijk} + N_{ijk})}{\Gamma(N'_{ijk})} \tag{17.6}$$

where, N_{ijk} is the number of observations in which variable X_i takes the value k, given that $\mathbf{Pa}_G(X_i)$ has configuration j; q_i is the number of possible configurations of parents $\mathbf{Pa}_G(X_i)$; and r_i is the number of possible values of X_i. N'_{ijk} are the parameters of the Dirichlet prior distribution, that is, the hyperparameters of the model. Finally, $N_{ij} = \sum_{k=1}^{r_i} N_{ijk}$ and $N'_{ij} = \sum_{k=1}^{r_i} N'_{ijk}$.

The term $P(G)$ in (17.3) is a prior distribution over graphs; we refer to this as a network prior. Appropriate specification of the network prior offers a principled way in which to integrate background information into network inference. We discuss the network prior in detail in Section 17.3.

We note also that graphs G can also be scored using penalized likelihood methods such as the Bayesian information criterion or BIC [30]; see Reference [31] for further details.

17.2.3
Model Selection and Model Averaging

The model score described above provides a way to assess the model represented by a graph G. Such scores can be used to either select a graph or to weight multiple graphs in a process of averaging; these approaches are referred to as model selection and model averaging, respectively. By way of introduction to the inference methods that follow, we now present a brief introduction to these concepts.

In model selection, one is interested in selecting the "best" model M^* from a set of candidate models $\mathcal{M}$. Using the Bayesian posterior score discussed above, a natural idea is to select the model that maximizes posterior probability, that is, $M^* = \text{argmax}_{M \in \mathcal{M}} P(M|X)$, where, as before, X represents the data. We illustrate this idea using a simple linear regression example. Suppose there are two covariates X_1 and X_2 that may influence a response variable Y, but we are uncertain as to which (if any) we should include in our model. Suppose also we have reason to believe that one of the following two models is the most appropriate:

$$M_1 : Y_i = \beta_0 + \varepsilon_i$$
$$M_2 : Y_i = \beta_0 + \beta_1 X_{i1} + \beta_2 X_{i2} + \varepsilon_i$$

where ε_i are i.i.d. (independent and identically distributed) Gaussian with zero mean and variance σ^2. Then, model M_1 is the scenario where Y does not depend on either covariate, whereas model M_2 has Y depending on both X_1 and X_2. Model selection can then be used to determine which of the two models is better, taking into account fit to data as well as number of parameters. Using a Bayesian posterior, this is the model M_j for which $P(M_j|X)$ is larger.

In the linear regression example above, different models are different choices of covariates that influence Y. These two models can be drawn as DAGs G_1 and G_2 as shown in Figure 17.2a. Each model is then a simple Bayesian network containing three variables, X_1, X_2, and Y. G_1 gives the factorization $P(X_1, X_2, Y) = P(X_1)P(X_2)P(Y)$ in which all variables are independent of each other, as in M_1 above. G_2 gives $P(X_1, X_2, Y) = P(Y|X_2, X_1)P(X_2)P(X_1)$. This can be regarded as a

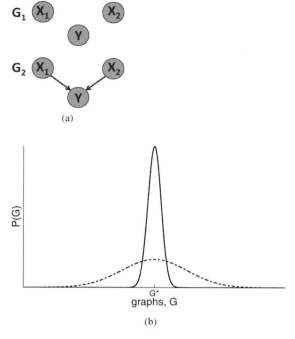

Figure 17.2 (a) Two possible models for three variables, represented as graphs; (b) two posterior distributions $P(G|X)$. The solid line shows a distribution is peaked around the best graph G^* whereas the dashed line shows a distribution that is very diffuse. For ease of illustration, the graph space is represented as continuous.

regression model where Y is the response variable with covariates X_1 and X_2, as in M_2. Then, the posterior probabilities $P(G_j|X)$ (determined using appropriate conjugate parameter priors and a model prior) can be used to choose between models. Consequently, this scenario of variable selection for regression can be viewed as a special case of network inference in which the covariates X are root nodes and the response Y is the only leaf. The graphical approaches that are the subject of this chapter can be thought of as generalizing these ideas to arbitrary DAGs, in which all variables are treated on the same footing.

Model selection can be thought of as trying to find a "winner" from a set of models under consideration. However, in many settings, and especially at small sample sizes, there may be no clear winner, with many models having similar scores. To put this in the context of biological network inference: given a very large number of observations the posterior $P(G|X)$ will become sharply peaked around the "correct"[1] graph (the graph representing the underlying biological network), but, in practice, under conditions of small-to-moderate sample sizes and high variability, the

---

1) Or more correctly, around graphs belonging to the same equivalence class as the "correct" graph G^*.

posterior is likely to be highly diffuse. This is illustrated in Figure 17.2b: the solid and dashed curves represent the "peaked" and "diffuse" regimes respectively. In the diffuse case, the probability $P(G^*|X)$ of the single most probable graph G^* may be small in absolute terms, such that even if we find G^* we cannot be very confident that it is a good representation of the underlying system. Indeed, G^* may not even be the correct graph. An important implication concerns our confidence in network features, such as the presence or absence of specific edges, paths, or subgraphs. Suppose a feature of interest appears in the best graph G^*; the diffuseness of the posterior means that there may be many other graphs with similar scores that do not share that feature. Then, reporting the feature as important would be misleading.

One way to address this issue is by model averaging (e.g., [31–33]). In this approach, we score features of interest by averaging over models, weighting each model by its posterior probability. In such an approach, if a feature appears in many relatively high-scoring models, then the score of this consensus feature is high; in contrast, a feature that appears in the best model G^* but not in most of the other high scoring models gets a low score.

To put these issues in the context of the two illustrative models depicted in Figure 17.2a, suppose we are interested in the presence (or absence) of an edge from X_1 to Y; G_2 contains this edge whereas G_1 does not. If G_2 is the highest-scoring graph, then one might conclude that the edge exists, but if $P(G_2|X) = 0.51$ and $P(G_1|X) = 0.49$ then G_1 is almost as probable as G_2. Averaging over the two models would tell us that the probability of the edge is only 0.51, which gives a better idea of the uncertainty associated with the feature.

More generally, the probability of a feature is just the expectation under the posterior (the "posterior expectation," $\mathbb{E}[\phi(G)]_{P(G|X)}$) of an indicator function $\phi(G)$, which evaluates to unity if the feature is present and zero otherwise. If we could characterize the posterior $P(G|X)$ then the probability of the feature is simply $\mathbb{E}[\phi(G)]_{P(G|X)} = \sum_{G \in \mathcal{G}} \phi(G) P(G|X)$.

Unfortunately, the number of possible graphs grows very rapidly with the number of variables p. Indeed, Robinson [34] has shown that the number $|\mathcal{G}_p|$ of possible DAGs with p vertices is given by the following recurrence formula:

$$|\mathcal{G}_p| = \sum_{i=1}^{p} (-1)^{i+1} \binom{p}{i} 2^{i(p-i)} |\mathcal{G}_{(p-i)}|$$

where, $|\mathcal{G}_1| = 1$ and $|\cdot|$ indicates the cardinality of its argument.

This gives $|\mathcal{G}_2| = 3$, $|\mathcal{G}_3| = 25$, $|\mathcal{G}_{10}| \approx 4.2 \times 10^{18}$, $|\mathcal{G}_{14}| \approx 1.4 \times 10^{36}$ and so on. The number of possible graphs is therefore usually much too large to permit the posterior distribution to be described by exhaustive enumeration of all possible graphs. Thus, while the marginal likelihood and prior probability can be combined to evaluate the posterior probability of a graph up to a multiplicative constant, we cannot actually consider every possible graph in the course of inference. This motivates the use of Monte Carlo methods to perform model averaging for practical problems.

17.2.4
Markov Chain Monte Carlo on Graphs

Markov chain Monte Carlo (MCMC) represents a general class of stochastic simulation methods that are widely used in computational statistics. The basic idea of MCMC is to construct a Markov chain whose state space is the domain of the desired random quantity (here the space $\mathcal{G}$ of DAGs), and whose stationary distribution is the posterior of interest (here $P(G|X)$). Then, simulating the Markov chain (for a sufficiently large number of iterations) allows samples to be drawn from the posterior distribution and hence provides a means by which to carry out inference.

In a Metropolis-Hastings sampler [35], draws are made from a proposal distribution Q, which depends on the current state of the Markov chain, and then accepted or rejected in such a way as to guarantee asymptotic convergence to the desired target distribution. Here, following Madigan *et al.* [24] and Giudici and Castelo [26], we develop a MCMC sampler of the Metropolis-Hastings type for the purpose of simulating the posterior distribution $P(G|X)$ over conditional independence graphs.

Let $\eta(G)$ denote a neighborhood around a DAG G, consisting of every DAG that can be obtained by adding, deleting, or reversing a single edge in G. Define proposal distribution Q as follows:

$$Q(G'; G) = \begin{cases} \dfrac{1}{|\eta(G)|} & \text{if } G' \in \eta(G) \\ 0 & \text{otherwise} \end{cases} \quad (17.7)$$

Then, calculate the following acceptance probability α:

$$\alpha = \frac{P(G'|X)Q(G; G')}{P(G|X)Q(G'; G)}$$

Since the proposal distribution is uniform over the relevant neighborhood, the ratio $Q(G; G')/Q(G'; G)$ may be written in terms of neighborhood size, giving:

$$\alpha = \frac{P(G'|X)|\eta(G)|}{P(G|X)|\eta(G')|}$$

Given current graph G, a proposed graph G', drawn from Q, is then accepted with probability $\min(1, \alpha)$, and otherwise rejected. If accepted, G' is added to the sequence of samples drawn, and becomes the current graph. Else, G is added to the sequence of samples, and remains the current graph. As shown in References [24] and [26], the proposal distribution Q gives rise to an irreducible Markov chain, since there is positive probability of reaching any part of the state space $\mathcal{G}$. Standard results (e.g., [36–38]) then guarantee that the Markov chain must converge to the desired posterior $P(G|X)$. The sampler described above is summarized in Algorithm 17.1.

Algorithm 17.1

A Metropolis-Hastings sampler for structural inference.

1) initialize graph $G^{(1)}$, set $t=1$, $G \leftarrow G^{(1)}$
2) propose $G' \sim Q(G'; G)$
3) accept G' with probability $\min(1, \alpha)$, $\alpha = \dfrac{P(G'|X)Q(G; G')}{P(G|X)Q(G'; G)}$
4) update if G' is accepted, $G^{(t+1)} \leftarrow G'$, $G \leftarrow G^{(t+1)}$ else $G^{(t+1)} \leftarrow G$; set $t \leftarrow t+1$
5) while $t < T$, repeat steps 2–4.

During sampling, we only need the posterior distribution to compute the acceptance ratio α. This means that the unnormalized quantities $p(X|G')P(G')$ and $p(X|G)P(G)$ are sufficient for our purposes. We discussed the marginal likelihood $p(X|G)$ above; we turn our attention to the prior $P(G)$ below.

We can now use the samples obtained from the MCMC algorithm to perform model averaging (as described above) in a computationally tractable manner. As shown in Algorithm 17.1, iterating "propose," "accept," and "update" steps gives rise to samples $G^{(1)} \ldots G^{(T)}$. An important property of these samples is that, provided the Markov chain has converged to its stationary distribution, they allow us to average over graphs and compute the posterior expectation $\mathbb{E}[\phi(G)]_{P(G|X)}$ of essentially any function on graphs $\phi(G)$. Specifically:

$$\hat{\mathbb{E}}[\phi(G)] = \frac{1}{T}\sum_{t=1}^{T} \phi(G^{(t)}) \qquad (17.8)$$

is, by standard results, an asymptotically valid estimator of $\mathbb{E}[\phi(G)]_{P(G|X)}$.

The posterior probability of an individual edge e, or $P(e|X)$ is an important special case of (17.8), which we shall make use of below. We may write $P(e|X)$ as a posterior expectation as follows:

$$\begin{aligned}
P(e|X) &= \sum_{G \in \mathcal{G}} P(e|G, X) P(G|X) \\
&= \sum_{G \in \mathcal{G}} I_{E(G)}(e) P(G|X) \\
&= \mathbb{E}[I_{E(G)}(e)]_{P(G|X)}
\end{aligned}$$

where, I_A is the indicator function for set A.

Then, applying (17.8), we may use samples $G^{(1)} \ldots G^{(T)}$ to obtain an asymptotically valid estimate of $\mathbb{E}[I_{E(G)}(e)]_{P(G|X)}$:

$$\hat{\mathbb{E}}\big[I_{E(G)}(e)\big] = \frac{1}{T}\sum_{t=1}^{T} I_{E(G^{(t)})}(e)$$

where, $G^{(t)} = (V(G^{(t)}), E(G^{(t)}))$

In a similar way, one can assess the posterior probability of essentially any graph feature of interest.

17.3
Network Priors

In this section, we discuss the use of prior information concerning network features. We begin with a motivating example that highlights some of the different kinds of prior beliefs encountered in practice and that we might like to take account of during inference. We then introduce network priors in a general way, before looking at examples of such priors for specific kinds of prior information. Finally, we look briefly at the use of a MCMC proposal distribution based on network priors.

17.3.1
A Motivating Example

We begin with a motivating example taken from cancer biology, which is representative of the type of network inference problem with which this chapter is concerned.

Table 17.1 shows 14 proteins that are components of a biological network called the epidermal growth factor receptor (EGFR) system. Here, each protein is a ligand, receptor, or cytosolic protein; for our present purposes, these may be regarded as well-defined classes of variable.

Our general goal is to infer features of the biological network in which these components participate. We model the relevant biochemical connectivity in terms of conditional independence. Then, questions regarding relationships between molecular components can be expressed, in a natural fashion, as questions regarding features of conditional independence graphs. The biochemistry of the system provides us with some prior knowledge regarding graph features, which we would like to take account of during inference.

Some illustrative examples of the kind of knowledge that might be available include:

(S1) Ligands influence cytosolic proteins via ligand–receptor interactions. As a consequence, we do not expect them to directly influence cytosolic proteins. Equally, we do not expect either receptors or cytosolic proteins to directly influence ligands.

Table 17.1 Some components of the epidermal growth factor receptor system.

Protein	Type	Protein	Type
EGF	Ligand	GAP	Cytosolic protein
AMPH	Ligand	SHC	Cytosolic protein
NRG1	Ligand	RAS	Cytosolic protein
NRG2	Ligand	Raf	Cytosolic protein
EGFR	Receptor	MEK	Cytosolic protein
ERBB2	Receptor	ERK	Cytosolic protein
ERBB3	Receptor		
ERBB4	Receptor		

(S2) Certain ligand–receptor binding events occur with particularly high affinity; these include EGF and AMPH with EGFR, NRG1 with ERBB3, and NRG1 and NRG2 with ERBB4. Equally, the receptors EGFR, ERBB3 and ERBB4 are all capable of influencing the state of ERBB2. Also, there is much evidence indicating that Raf can influence MEK, which in turn can influence ERK.

(S3) Since we observe ligand-mediated activity at the level of cytosolic proteins, we expect to see a path from ligands to receptors, and from receptors to cytosolic proteins.

Without going into a great deal of biological detail it is clear that these beliefs correspond to information regarding graph structure: (S1) contains information concerning classes of vertices; (S2) contains information regarding specific edges and (S3) contains information regarding higher-level network features, pertaining to paths between classes of vertices.

17.3.2
General Framework

We now introduce a general form for our network priors. Let $f(G)$ be a real-valued function on graphs that is increasing in the degree to which graph G agrees with prior beliefs (a "concordance function"). Then, for potentially multiple concordance functions $\{f_i(G)\}$, we suggest a log-linear network prior of the following form:

$$P(G) \propto \exp\left(\lambda \sum_i w_i f_i(G)\right) \tag{17.9}$$

where λ is a parameter used to control the strength of the prior. Here, in the spirit of Reference [39], we use weights w_i to control the relative strength of individual concordance functions, with w_1 set to unity to avoid redundancy. We discuss setting strength parameters below. Note that the only way in which the prior enters into MCMC-based inference is via the prior odds $P(G')/P(G)$ in favor of proposal G'; it is therefore sufficient to specify the prior up to proportionality.

17.3.2.1 Specific Edges

Suppose we believe that certain edges are a priori likely to be present or absent in the true data-generating graph. Let E_+ denote a set of edges expected to be present ("positive edge set") and E_- a set of edges expected to be absent ("negative edge set"). We assume that these two sets are disjoint. Then, we suggest the following network prior:

$$P(G) \propto \exp(\lambda(|E(G) \cap E_+| - |E(G) \cap E_-|)) \tag{17.10}$$

Here, the concordance function is a counting function on individual edges, with the prior attaining its maximum value if and only if G contains all the positive edges and no negative edges.

In the motivating example presented above, (S1) contains negative prior information, while (S2) contains positive prior information regarding individual edges. Such information can be captured in quite a natural way using (17.10). We note also that the notion of specifying a particular prior graph $G_0 = (V_0, E_0)$, and penalizing graphs on the basis of the number of edges by which they differ from G_0 [23] is a special case of (17.10), with $E_+ = E_0$ and $E_- = E_0^c$.

17.3.2.2 Classes of Vertices

The network prior given by (17.10) may also be used to capture beliefs regarding edges between classes of vertices. Examples of knowledge pertaining to vertex classes are abundant in molecular biology, where the classes may represent distinct types of molecule thought to influence one another in specific ways. Let $\{C_k\}$ be a set of classes into which vertices $v \in V$ can be categorized, with $C(v)$ denoting the class to which vertex v belongs. Suppose we wish to penalize graphs displaying edges between vertices of class i and j. This can be accomplished by using the prior specified by (17.10) with a negative edge set E_- containing all such edges:

$$E_- = \{e = (v_l, v_m) : C(v_l) = C_i, C(v_m) = C_j\} \tag{17.11}$$

Positive priors on edges between vertex classes can be defined in a similar fashion.

17.3.2.3 Higher-Level Network Features

In some cases, we may wish to capture prior knowledge concerning higher-level network features that cannot be described by reference to sets of individual edges. To take but one example, we may believe that there ought to be at least one edge between certain classes of vertices, as in (S3) above. Let E_C be a set of ordered pairs of classes such that $(C_i, C_j) \in E_C$ means we believe there ought to be at least one edge from class C_i to class C_j. Then, we suggest the prior in (17.9) with concordance function:

$$f(G) = \sum_{(C_i, C_j) \in E_c} I_{\mathbb{Z}^+} \left[\sum_{(v_1, v_2) \in E(G)} \delta((C(v_1), C(v_2)), (C_i, C_j)) \right]$$

where $\mathbb{Z}^+$ is the set of positive integers and δ the Kronecker delta function.

17.3.2.4 Network Sparsity

In many settings parsimonious models are desirable both for reasons of interpretability and ameliorating overfitting. Since Bayesian networks factorize joint distributions into local terms conditioned on parent configurations, model complexity can grow rapidly with the number of parents. Controlling the in-degree of graphs is therefore a useful means of controlling model complexity. The in-degree, $\text{indeg}(v)$, of a vertex $v \in V$ is the number of edges in edge-set E leading into v, that is:

$$\text{indeg}(v) = |\{v_i, v_j\} \in E : v_j = v\}|$$

Let $\Delta(G) = \max_{v \in V(G)} \text{indeg}(v)$ be the maximum in-degree of graph G. Then, the following network prior penalizes graphs having in-degree exceeding λ_{indeg}, but remains agnostic otherwise:

$$P(G) \propto \exp(\lambda \min(0, \lambda_{\text{indeg}} - \Delta(G))) \tag{17.12}$$

An alternative way to promote sparsity is by penalizing the total number of edges in a graph; for example, using a binomial distribution over the total number of edges, with parameters set to ensure an expected number of edges equal to the number of variables p, and an appropriate maximum number of possible edges [27, 40].

17.3.2.5 Degree Distributions

We may have reason to believe that the degree distribution of the underlying network is likely to be scale-free. The degree, $\deg(v)$, of a vertex v is the total number of edges in which vertex v participates. The degree distribution of a graph G is a function:

$$\pi_G(d) = |\{v \in V(G) : \deg(v) = d\}|$$

describing the total number of vertices having degree d. A graph is said to have a scale-free degree distribution if π_G follows a power-law with $\pi_G(d) \propto d^{-\gamma}, \gamma > 0$ such that $\log(\pi_G(d))$ is approximately linear in $\log(d)$. Accordingly, the negative correlation coefficient between $\log(\pi_G(d))$ and $\log(d)$ is a natural choice for a concordance function for the scale-free property, giving the following network prior:

$$P(G) \propto \exp[-\lambda r(\log(\pi_G(d)), \log(d))]$$

where $r(\cdot, \cdot)$ denotes the correlation coefficient of its arguments.

17.3.2.6 Constructing a Prior

We now consider two aspects of constructing a network prior: the qualitative question of what information to include, and the quantitative question of how to decide upon a value for the strength parameter λ.

In a scientific domain, information to include in the prior must be derived from what is understood regarding the system under study. While this process of extracting domain information is necessarily a subjective enterprise, we favor a conservative approach in which only information about which there is a broad consensus is included in the prior. We provide an example from cancer signaling below.

We address the question of prior strength in two steps. We first engage in a process of elicitation aimed at setting the strength parameter λ roughly to within an order of magnitude; this is accomplished in consultation with collaborators and by reference to the well-known Jeffreys' scale [41] which relates odds ratios to intuitive degrees of belief. We then carry out a sensitivity analysis to check that results obtained are robust to changes in λ around the elicited value; we show examples of sensitivity analysis below. We note that an alternative approach would be to take an "empirical Bayes" approach (e.g., [42]) and attempt to set strength parameters by explicit reference to the data.

Finally, in the present context, we set parameters w_i to unity. However, the formulation presented in (17.9) allows for the weighting of multiple sources of prior information; this is an important topic in its own right but one that we do not address further here.

17.3.3
Prior-Based Proposals

The prior $P(G)$ provides information regarding which graphs are a priori more likely. Yet the proposal distribution (17.7) is uniform over neighborhood $\eta(G)$. A natural idea, then, is to exploit prior information in guiding the proposal mechanism; here, we suggest one way of doing so, which we have found empirically to be useful in accelerating convergence. We suggest a proposal distribution of the following form:

$$Q_P(G'; G) \propto \begin{cases} \lambda_Q & \text{if } P(G') > P(G) \\ 1 & \text{if } P(G') = P(G) \\ 1/\lambda_Q & \text{if } P(G') < P(G) \\ 0 & \text{if } G' \notin \eta(G) \end{cases} \quad (17.13)$$

where, $\lambda_Q \geq 1$ is a parameter controlling the degree to which the proposal mechanism prefers a priori likely graphs.

The proposal distribution specified by (17.13) ensures that all graphs in $\eta(G)$ have a non-zero probability of being proposed, thereby preserving irreducibility and convergence to the desired posterior. Now, large values of λ_Q will result in frequent proposals of a priori likely graphs, but on account of the "Hastings factor" $Q(G; G')/Q(G'; G)$ will also lead to low acceptance rates for such graphs. However, consideration of the form of the acceptance ratio yields a simple heuristic for determining λ_Q. Let Δ_f denote the median non-zero value of the absolute difference $|f(G')-f(G)|$ in the values of the concordance function for G' and G (this can be determined during diagnostic sampling runs). Then, setting:

$$\lambda_Q = \max\left(1, \pi \exp\left(\frac{1}{2}\lambda\Delta_f\right)\right), \pi < 1$$

suffices to ensure that (i) a priori likely graphs do not suffer low acceptance ratios and (ii) if the overall prior is too weak to permit a prior-based proposal, the proposal distribution (17.13) reverts to the uniform distribution (17.7). For example, for the counting function (17.10) and neighborhoods constructed by single edge changes, $|f(G')-f(G)|$ is typically unity, giving $\lambda_Q = \max(1, \pi \exp(\lambda/2))$. In the experiments that appear below, we set $\pi = 1/2$.

17.4
Some Results

17.4.1
Simulated Data

The connectivity of biological networks involved in functions such as gene regulation or signal transduction remains very much an open area of research in molecular biology. For this reason, at the present time it is difficult to rely on biological data for the assessment of network inference methods, because we cannot be certain about the correct connectivity of biological networks.

We therefore simulated data from a known network, and used the methods described above to make inferences regarding the network. All computations were carried out in Matlab, using some elements of Reference [43]. This was done for the $p = 14$ variables described previously in Table 17.1, using the data-generating graph shown in Figure 17.3. Details of our data-generating model are as follows:

- All random variables are binary.
- All conditional distributions are Bernoulli, with success parameter q depending upon the configuration of the parents. In particular, root nodes are sampled with $q = 0.5$, while for each child node, $q = 0.8$ if at least one parent takes on the value 1, and $q = 0.2$ otherwise. This gives each child node a relationship to its parents that is similar to a logical OR.
- Sample size was $n = 200$.

17.4.1.1 Priors

The graph shown in Figure 17.3 is based on the epidermal growth factor receptor system alluded to in the motivating example above. We constructed informative network priors corresponding to the beliefs (S1) and (S2) described above. We used (S1) and (S2) to define a negative edge set E_- and positive edge set E_+ respectively; these edge sets were then used to specify a network prior using (17.10); (S3) was not used in these experiments. To investigate the effects of priors containing erroneous information, we also constructed a mis-specified prior that included incorrect information regarding individual edges. Specifically, it included in its negative edge set edges from Raf to MEK and from MEK to ERK, and in its positive edge set an edge from

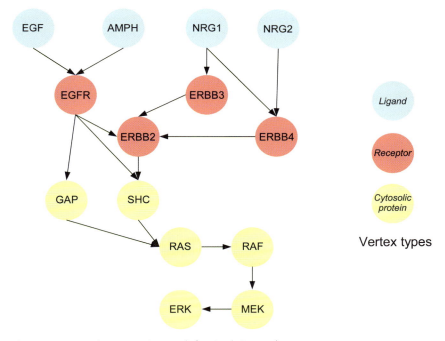

Figure 17.3 True data-generating graph for simulation study.

Ras to ERK. This allowed us to consider a realistic scenario in which the prior is largely reasonable but contains several entirely false beliefs. In all cases, λ was set to unity.

17.4.1.2 MCMC

We based all inferences on a single, long run of $T = 50\,000$ iterations for each prior, with 5000 samples discarded as "burn-in" in each case. For diagnostic purposes, we first performed several short ($T = 10\,000$) runs with different starting points. In each case we found monitored quantities converged within a few thousand iterations, giving us confidence in the results obtained using the subsequent single, longer run.

17.4.1.3 ROC Analysis

Our knowledge of the true data-generating graph allowed us to construct receiver operating characteristic (ROC) curves from calls on individual edges. Let $G^* = (V^*, E^*)$ denote the true data-generating graph. As before, let $P(e|X)$ denote the posterior probability of an edge $e = (v_i, v_j)$. Then, the set of edges called at threshold $\tau \in [0, 1]$ is:

$$E_\tau = \{e : P(e|X) \geq \tau\}$$

The number of true positives called is $|E_\tau \cap E^*|$, while the number of false positives is $|E_\tau \setminus E^*|$. ROC curves were constructed by plotting, for each sampler, the number of true positives against the number of false positives parameterized by threshold τ; these are shown in Figure 17.4. We also show results obtained using absolute log odds ratios $|\psi_{ij}|$ for each pair (i,j) of variables, where $\psi_{ij} = \log(n_{11}n_{00}/n_{10}n_{01})$ and n_{pq} is the number of samples in which $X_i = p$ and $X_j = q$. These are a natural measure of association for binary variables and provide a simple, baseline comparison. Finally, we show results obtained by drawing samples from the prior itself ("prior only").

These ROC curves are obtained by comparison with the true edge-set E^* and in that sense represent "gold-standard" comparative results. The posterior distribution provides substantial gains in sensitivity and specificity over both prior alone and data alone (i.e., the flat prior), suggesting that inference is indeed able to usefully combine data and prior knowledge.

17.4.2
Prior Sensitivity

We investigated sensitivity to the strength parameter λ by performing ROC analyses as described above for a range of values of λ from 0.1 to 10. Figure 17.5 shows the resulting area under the ROC curve (AUC) plotted against λ, for the correctly specified prior. The good results obtained using the informative prior hold up across a wide range of values of λ. Indeed, given the exponential form of the prior, this represents a very wide range of strength regimes.

17.4.3
A Biological Network

Protein signaling networks play a central role in the biology of cancer. There remain many open questions regarding cancer-specific features of signaling networks,

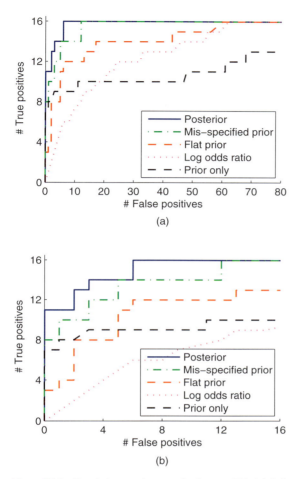

Figure 17.4 Simulation results, sample size $n = 200$: (a) Full receiver operating characteristic (ROC) curves for (i) posterior using informative prior, (ii) posterior using mis-specified prior, (iii) flat prior, (iv) log-odds ratio between pairs of variables, and (v) informative prior alone; (b) a detail of (a).

especially at the level of protein phospho-forms and isoforms. In this section we present some results obtained in an analysis of protein signaling in breast cancer, using the methods introduced above.

17.4.3.1 Data

Proteomic data were obtained for the eleven protein phospho-forms and isoforms shown in Figure 17.6; these included two receptors, PDGF and C-MET (both are receptor tyrosine kinases or RTKs); two phospho-forms of AKT; two isoforms of MKK; two isoforms of ERK; MNK1 and two downstream proteins known to be involved in translational control, ELF4E and EIF2B. The data were obtained from an assay performed by Kinexus Inc. (Vancouver, Canada) on a panel of 18 breast cancer cell lines. Data were discretized, where possible into active and inactive states, or else

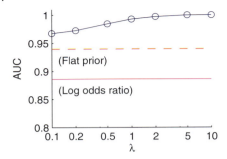

Figure 17.5 Sensitivity analysis for synthetic data. Area under the ROC curve (AUC) is plotted against the strength parameter λ for an informative prior. The AUC captures, as a single number, the correctness of calls on edges across a range of thresholds; higher scores indicate lower error rates. For comparison we show also AUC results for a flat prior and log odds ratios as horizontal lines.

around the median for each protein. This gave rise to binary data for each of the eleven proteins.

17.4.3.2 Priors

Our prior beliefs concerning the network can be summarized as follows. The receptors are expected to have edges going only to ERKs and AKTs. This reflects known biology in which RTKs influence these proteins [44, 45]. The AKTs and ERKs are in turn expected to have edges going only to the downstream proteins ELF4E and

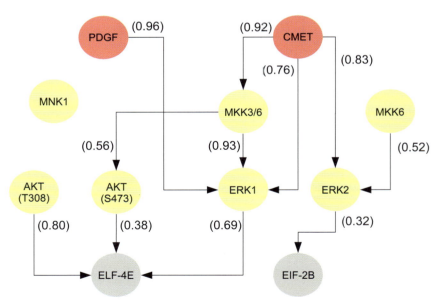

Figure 17.6 Posterior mode for protein data. Edges are annotated with posterior edge probabilities.

EIF2B, and in the case of ERK only, additionally to MNK1; MNK1 is expected to have edges going only to ELF4E and EIF2B [46]. Our prior beliefs concerning MKKs are few: we expect only that they should not have edges going directly to the receptors. We constructed a network prior corresponding to these beliefs using (17.10) and (17.11). In addition, on account of the small sample size, we used sparsity-promoting prior (17.12) with $\lambda_{\text{indeg}} = 3$. Following the prior elicitation strategy discussed above, we set $\lambda = 3$.

17.4.3.3 MCMC
As before, we used short diagnostic runs ($T = 10\,000$) to check for convergence, followed by a single long run of $T = 50\,000$ iterations, with a "burn-in" of 5000 samples. A prior-based proposal (17.13) was used, with λ_Q set (automatically) to $\max(1, \frac{1}{2}\exp(\lambda/2)) = 2.24$. (The resulting acceptance rate was 0.23.)

17.4.3.4 Single Best Graph
Figure 17.6 shows the single most probable graph encountered during sampling. Each edge e is annotated with the corresponding posterior probability $P(e|X)$. Note that some edges in the posterior mode have relatively low probability: this highlights the danger of relying on simple mode-finding rather than posterior simulation and model averaging for inference in problems of this kind.

17.4.3.5 Network Features
Probabilities or posterior odds concerning network features can be computed using (17.8). To take but one example in the present context, a biologically important question concerns the influence of MKK on ERK phosphorylation. We computed the posterior odds in favor of MKK $\to$ ERK connectivity (i.e., at least one edge from MKKs to ERKs) versus no such connectivity (no edge from MKKs to ERKs). The posterior odds in favor of MKK $\to$ ERK connectivity are 42, suggesting that MKK, directly or indirectly, influences ERK activation in the cell-lines under study. Interestingly, the corresponding odds under the flat prior are just under 2. While no prior information was provided concerning MKK $\to$ ERK connectivity specifically, network inferences of this kind are embedded within an overall graph embodying the joint distribution of all variables under study and therefore implicitly take account of specified prior beliefs, even when these concern other parts of the network.

17.4.3.6 Prior Sensitivity
To investigate sensitivity to prior strength we looked at the agreement between results obtained under different values of strength parameter λ. We considered five values of strength parameter λ, as well as a flat prior and samples drawn from the prior only (with $\lambda = 3$). This gave seven different prior settings, each of which led to a set of posterior edge probabilities. Figure 17.7 shows Pearson correlations for these posterior edge probabilities, for all pairs of prior settings: values close to unity indicate posteriors that are effectively very close. Inferences using the informative prior with different values of λ are in very close agreement, yet differ

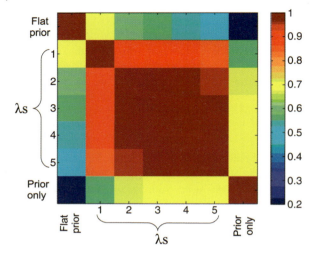

Figure 17.7 Prior sensitivity for protein data. Seven different prior settings (informative prior with strength parameter $\lambda = 1-5$, flat prior, and prior only) each give rise to a set of posterior edge probabilities. The image shows Pearson correlations between these posterior edge probabilities for all pairs of prior settings.

from both the flat prior and from the informative prior alone. This gives us confidence that (i) inference integrates both data and prior information and (ii) results are not too sensitive to the precise value of λ.

17.5
Conclusions and Future Prospects

In this chapter we have discussed model averaging for Bayesian networks, in the context of biological network inference using rich prior information. Our work forms part of a growing trend in the computational biology literature (including References [14, 47, 48]) towards network inference schemes that take account of prior information of various kinds. In our view, informative priors play two related roles. Firstly, they provide a means by which to capture valuable domain knowledge regarding network features. Secondly, they allow us to refine or sharpen questions of interest, in effect playing a role analogous to formulating an initial set of hypotheses, but with much greater flexibility. This flexibility, combined with the well-known robustness of model averaging, means that it is possible to obtain useful results even when priors are mis-specified, essentially by borrowing strength from a large space of models, many of which accord only partially with prior beliefs.

A natural concern regarding informative network priors is whether their use amounts to "putting too much in" during inference. We hold the view that even very strong priors on graphs can play a valuable role in refining or sharpening questions being asked, in a manner analogous to a well thought out set of hypotheses, but with

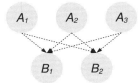

Figure 17.8 Priors for hypothesis formulation. A prior preferring models in which As influence Bs can play a role similar to a hypothesis formulation step in a multiple decision approach.

an added degree of flexibility and generality. Consider, as an example, the five variables illustrated in Figure 17.8. Suppose we knew, from outside knowledge, that the As tend to influence the Bs, and that the main question we were interested in addressing was which combination of As influence each of the Bs. One way of posing this question would be as a multiple decision problem (say, with 2^3 models for each of the Bs). A second approach would be to perform network inference on the variables, with a strong prior in favor of models in which As influence Bs. The network prior would then play a role similar to the hypothesis formulation step in the first approach. Yet the network analysis offers two key advantages. Firstly, it allows for the discovery of unexpected relationships, when such relationships are well-supported by the data. When the variables of immediate interest are embedded in a larger system such relationships could also include outside influences of one kind or another. Secondly, network inference offers a mechanism by which to simultaneously address a range of possible questions concerning relationships between variables: once we have described a posterior distribution over models, we are free to evaluate probabilities or odds concerning essentially any network features of interest.

We saw also that the use of informative priors can lead to very substantive gains at small sample sizes. Much of the literature on MCMC-based structural inference has focused on moderate-to-large sample sizes: for example, Giudici and Castelo [26] analyzed a dataset with $p = 6$ and $n = 1846$. In contrast our experiments focused on the challenging setting in which there is both a greater number of variables and far fewer observations. Although, unsurprisingly, we found that the basic sampling approach does not do well in this setting, we discovered that reasonably well-specified priors do indeed permit effective inference under these conditions, yielding substantive gains even when the features of eventual interest were not described in the prior, or when the priors were partially mis-specified. We note also that the sample size of the protein phosphorylation data analyzed here was orders of magnitude smaller than in a previous application of Bayesian networks to protein signaling [12]; this further motivated a need to make use of existing knowledge regarding the system.

Bayesian formulations can, in general, be viewed as analogous to penalized likelihood, and in that sense they quite naturally promote parsimonious models. An additional penalty on model complexity in the form of a sparsity prior may therefore be unnecessary in many cases. However, when a paucity of data, or a mis-specified model, exacerbates problems of overfitting, explicit sparsity priors can play a useful role.

We note that our network priors do *not* satisfy so-called prior equivalence in that they allow us to express a prior preference for one graph over another even when both graphs imply the same conditional independence statements. Thus, we may express a prior preference for $A \to B$ over $B \to A$, despite the fact that both graphs describe the same likelihood model. This property allows us to express preferences derived from domain knowledge. For example, if we believe that A precedes B in time, or that A is capable of physically influencing B, we may express a preference for $A \to B$ over $B \to A$.

Friedman and Koller [25] proposed an interesting approach to network inference, in which samples are drawn from the space of *orders*, where an order $\prec$ is defined as a total order relation on vertices such that if $X_i \in \mathbf{Pa}_G(X_j)$ then $i \prec j$. The appeal of this approach lies in the fact that the space of orders is much smaller than the space of conditional independence graphs. On the other hand, the use of order space means that network priors must be translated into priors on orders, and inferences on network features must be carried out via order space. This turns out to place restrictions on the kinds of network priors that can be utilized, and moreover makes it difficult to compute the posterior probabilities of arbitrary network features. Furthermore, the authors' own experiments show that sampling in order space offers no advantage at smaller sample sizes. In contrast, we find that remaining in graph space offers real advantages in terms of being able to specify rich priors in a natural and readily interpretable fashion and, just as important, in making inferences regarding essentially arbitrary features of graphs. Also, as we have seen, the use of such priors can lead, in turn, to much improved performance at small sample sizes.

There remains much to be done in extending the methods presented here to higher-dimensional problems. One approach to making such problems tractable would be to place strong priors on some parts of the overall graph. This would, in effect, amount to using background knowledge to focus limited inferential power on the least well-understood, or scientifically most interesting, parts of the graph. Higher dimensions arise, for example, when dynamic models are used for time series data, or when more comprehensive assays are used to probe a greater number of molecular components.

Our current applied efforts are directed towards questions in cancer biology. We have found the ability to specify rich, interpretable priors directly on graphs and make posterior inferences on features of graphs such as edges, groups of edges, and paths to be valuable in casting biologically interesting questions within a statistical framework. We therefore hope that the methods presented here will prove useful in several settings where questions of this kind need to be addressed.

Acknowledgments

The authors acknowledge the support of EPSRC (SM, SH) and the Fulbright Commission (SM) and would like to thank Joe Gray and Paul Spellman of Lawrence Berkeley National Laboratory for a productive, ongoing collaboration and for providing the proteomic dataset used in this chapter.

17.6 Appendix

Here we derive the closed-form marginal likelihood (17.6); a result of using multinomial conditionals $P(X|G, \Theta)$ and conjugate Dirichlet priors $p(\Theta|G)$.

Recall that we have p random variables $X_1, \ldots, X_p$. Let q_i be the number of possible configurations of $\mathbf{Pa}_G(X_i)$ and denote these configurations by j for $j = 1, \ldots, q_i$. When $\mathbf{Pa}_G(X_i)$ has configuration j we write $\mathbf{Pa}_G(X_i) = j$. Let r_i be the number of possible values for X_i. So if X_i is a binary random variable, $r_i = 2$.

Now we define our model parameters. Let Θ_{ijk} be the probability that $X_i = k$ given that $\mathbf{Pa}_G(X_i) = j$, that is:

$$P(x_i = k | \mathbf{Pa}_G(X_i) = j, \Theta_{ijk}) = \Theta_{ijk}$$

More generally:

$$P(X_i | \mathbf{Pa}_G(X_i), \Theta_i) = \prod_{j=1}^{q_i} \prod_{k=1}^{r_i} \Theta_{ijk}^{\delta_{(X_i,k)} \delta_{(\mathbf{Pa}_G(X_i),j)}}$$

where $\Theta_i = \{\Theta_{ijk} : 1 \leq j \leq q_i, 1 \leq k \leq r_i\}$ and:

$$\delta_{(a,b)} = \begin{cases} 1 & \text{if } a = b \\ 0 & \text{otherwise} \end{cases}$$

From the factorization of the joint distribution (17.1) we have:

$$P(X_1, \ldots, X_p | G, \Theta) = \prod_{i=1}^{p} \prod_{j=1}^{q_i} \prod_{k=1}^{r_i} \Theta_{ijk}^{\delta_{(X_i,k)} \delta_{(\mathbf{Pa}_G(X_i),j)}}$$

where $\Theta = \{\Theta_{ijk} : 1 \leq i \leq p, 1 \leq j \leq q_i, 1 \leq k \leq r_i\}$

Now, let X be a $p \times n$ data matrix, where X_{im} is the i-th variable in the m-th sample. We define N_{ijk} to be the number of samples in X that have $X_i = k$ and $\mathbf{Pa}_G(X_i) = j$. Then, assuming that the samples are independent and identically distributed given the graph G and parameters Θ, it follows that:

$$P(X|G, \Theta) = \prod_{m=1}^{n} P(X_{1m}, \ldots, X_{pm} | G, \Theta) = \prod_{i=1}^{p} \prod_{j=1}^{q_i} \prod_{k=1}^{r_i} \Theta_{ijk}^{N_{ijk}}$$

This is the full likelihood for all the data. We also need to define a prior distribution over parameters, $p(\Theta|G)$ [see (17.5)]. A Dirichlet prior is chosen:

$$p(\Theta_{ij1}, \ldots, \Theta_{ijr_i} | G) = \frac{\Gamma(N'_{ij})}{\prod_{k=1}^{r_i} \Gamma(N'_{ijk})} \prod_{k=1}^{r_i} \Theta_{ijk}^{N'_{ijk} - 1}$$

where N'_{ijk} are Dirichlet hyperparameters and $N'_{ij} = \sum_{k=1}^{r_i} N'_{ijk}$. Assuming prior independence of parameters then gives:

$$P(\Theta|G) = \prod_{i=1}^{p} \prod_{j=1}^{q_i} p(\Theta_{ij1}, \ldots, \Theta_{ijr_i} | G) = \prod_{i=1}^{p} \prod_{j=1}^{q_i} \frac{\Gamma(N'_{ij})}{\prod_{k=1}^{r_i} \Gamma(N'_{ijk})} \prod_{k=1}^{r_i} \Theta_{ijk}^{N'_{ijk} - 1}$$

We can now explicitly calculate the marginal likelihood using (17.5):

$$P(X|G) = \prod_{i=1}^{p}\prod_{j=1}^{q_i} \frac{\Gamma(N'_{ij})}{\prod_{k=1}^{r_i}\Gamma(N'_{ijk})} \int \prod_{k=1}^{r_i} \Theta_{ijk}^{N_{ijk}+N'_{ijk}-1} d\Theta_{ijk}$$

The integrand is an unnormalized Dirichlet distribution with parameters $N_{ijk} + N'_{ijk}$.

Hence the integral evaluates to the inverse of the Dirichlet normalizing constant, giving closed-form marginal likelihood (17.6).

References

1 Sharan, R. and Ideker, T. (2006) Modeling cellular machinery through biological network comparison. *Nat. Biotechnol.*, **24** (4), 427–433.

2 Zhu, X., Gerstein, M., and Snyder, M. (2007) Getting connected: analysis and principles of biological networks. *Gene. Dev.*, **21**, 1010–1024.

3 Ideker, T. and Lauffenburger, D. (2003) Building with a scaffold: emerging strategies for high-to low-level cellular modeling. *Trends Biotechnol.*, **21** (6), 255–262.

4 Chuang, H.Y., Lee, E., Liu, Y.T., Lee, D., and Ideker, T. (2007) Network-based classification of breast cancer metastasis. *Mol. Syst. Biol.*, **3** (140), published on-line, doi: 10.1038/msb4100180.

5 Kolch, W. (2000) Meaningful relationships: the regulation of the Ras/Raf/MEK/ERK pathway by protein interactions. *Biochem. J.*, **351** (2), 289–305.

6 Kitano, H. (2002) Systems biology: A brief overview. *Science*, **295** (5560), 1662–1664.

7 Yarden, Y. and Sliwkowski, M.X. (2001) Untangling the ErbB signalling network. *Nat. Rev. Mol. Cell Biol.*, **2** (2), 127–137.

8 Oda, K., Matsuoka, Y., Funahashi, A., and Kitano, H. (2005) A comprehensive pathway map of epidermal growth factor receptor signaling. *Mol. Syst. Biol.*, published on-line, doi: 10.1038/msb4100014.

9 Mukherjee, S. and Speed, T.P. (2008) Network inference using informative priors. *Proc. Natl. Acad. Sci. USA*, **105** (38), 14313–14318.

10 Yu, J., Smith, A., Wang, P.P., Hartemink, A.J., and Jarvis, E.D. (2004) Advances to Bayesian network inference for generating causal networks from observational biological data. *Bioinformatics*, **20** (18), 3594–3603.

11 Friedman, N., Linial, M., Nachman, I., and Pe'er, D. (2000) Using Bayesian networks to analyze expression data. *J. Comput. Biol.*, **7** (3–4) 601–620.

12 Sachs, K., Perez, O., Pe'er, D., Lauffenburger, D.A., and Nolan, G.P. (2005) Causal protein-signaling networks derived from multiparameter single-cell data. *Science*, **308** (5721), 523–529.

13 Segal, E., Shapira, M., Regev, A., Pe'er, D., Botstein, D., Koller, D., and Friedman, N. (2003) Module networks: identifying regulatory modules and their condition-specific regulators from gene expression data. *Nat. Genet.*, **34** (2), 166–176.

14 Tamada, Y., Kim, S.Y., Bannai, H., Imoto, S., Tashiro, K., Kuhara, S., and Miyano, S. (2003) Estimating gene networks from gene expression data by combining Bayesian network model with promoter element detection. *Bioinformatics*, **19** (ii), 227–236.

15 Husmeier, D. (2003) Reverse engineering of genetic networks with Bayesian networks. *Biochem. Soc. Trans.*, **31** (6), 1516–1518.

16 Husmeier, D., Dybowski, R., and Roberts, S. (eds) (2005) *Probabilistic Modeling in Bioinformatics and Medical Informatics*, Springer-Verlag.

17 Darroch, J.N., Lauritzen, S.L., and Speed, T.P. (1980) Markov fields and log-linear inter action models for contingency tables. *Ann. Stat.*, **8** (3), 522–539.

18 Pearl, J. (1988) *Probabilistic Reasoning in Intelligent Systems: Networks of Plausible Inference*, Morgan Kaufmann.

19 Lauritzen, S.L. and Spiegelhalter, D.J. (1988) Local computations with probabilities on graphical structures and their application to expert systems. *J. R. Stat. Soc. B Method.*, **50** (2), 157–224.

20 Lauritzen, S.L. (1996) *Graphical Models*, Oxford University Press.

21 Jordan, M.I. (2004) Graphical models. *Stat. Sci.*, **19**, 140–155.

22 Friedman, N. (2004) Inferring cellular networks using probabilistic graphical models. *Science*, **303** (5659), 799–805.

23 Heckerman, D., Geiger, D., and Chickering, D.M. (1995) Learning Bayesian networks: the combination of knowledge and statistical data. *Machine Learn.*, **20** (3), 197–243.

24 Madigan, D., York, J., and Allard, D. (1995) Bayesian graphical models for discrete data. *Int. Stat. Rev.*, **63** (2), 215–232.

25 Friedman, N. and Koller, D. (2003) Being Bayesian about network structure. A Bayesian approach to structure discovery in Bayesian networks. *Machine Learn.*, **50** (1), 95–125.

26 Giudici, P. and Castelo, R. (2003) Improving Markov chain Monte Carlo model search for data Mining. *Machine Learn.*, **50** (1), 127–158.

27 Jones, B., Carvalho, C., Dobra, A., Hans, C., Carter, C., and West, M. (2005) Experiments in stochastic computation for high-dimensional graphical models. *Stat. Sci.*, **20** (4), 388–400.

28 Kiiveri, H., Speed, T.P., and Carlin, J.B. (1984) Recursive causal models. *J. Aust. Math. Soc. A*, **36** (1), 30–52.

29 Geiger, D. and Heckerman, D. (1994) Learning Gaussian networks, in *Proceedings of the Tenth Conference on Uncertainty in Artificial Intelligence*, (eds R. López de Màntaras and D. Poole) Morgan Kaufmann, pp. 235–243.

30 Schwartz, G. (1978) Estimating the dimension of a model. *Ann. Stat.*, **6**, 461–464.

31 Claeskens, G. and Hjort, N.L. (2008) *Model Selection and Model Averaging*, Cambridge University Press.

32 Hoeting, J.A., Madigan, D., Raftery, A.E., and Volinsky, C.T. (1999) Bayesian model averaging: A tutorial. *Stat. Sci.*, **14** (4), 382–417.

33 Wasserman, L. (2000) Bayesian model selection and model averaging. *J. Math. Psychol.*, **44** (1), 92–107.

34 Robinson, R.W. (1973) Counting labeled acyclic digraphs, in *New Directions in Graph Theory* (ed. F. Harary), Academic Press.

35 Hastings, W.K. (1970) Monte Carlo sampling methods using Markov chains and their applications. *Biometrika*, **57** (1), 97.

36 Tierney, L. (1994) Markov chains for exploring posterior distributions (with discussion). *Ann. Stat.*, **22** (4), 1701–1762.

37 Gilks, W.R., Richardson, S., and Spiegelhalter, D.J. (1996) *Markov Chain Monte Carlo in Practice*, Chapman & Hall/CRC.

38 Robert, C.P. and Casella, G. (2004) *Monte Carlo Statistical Methods*, Springer.

39 Jensen, S.T., Chen, G., and Stoeckert, C.J. Jr. (2007) Bayesian variable selection and data integration for biological regulatory networks. *Ann. Appl. Stat.*, **1** (2), 612–633.

40 Buntine, W. (1991) Theory refinement on Bayesian networks in *Proceedings of the Seventh Conference on Uncertainty in Artificial Intelligence* (eds B. D'Ambrosio and P. Smets), Morgan Kaufmann, pp. 52–60.

41 Jeffreys, H. (1961) *The Theory of Probability*, 3rd edn, Oxford.

42 Carlin, B.P. and Louis, T.A. (2000) *Bayes and Empirical Bayes Methods for Data Analysis*, Chapman & Hall/CRC.

43 Murphy, K. (2001) The Bayes Net toolbox for Matlab. *Comput. Sci. Stat.*, **33**, 331–351.

44 Östman, A., Heldin, C.H., and Rönnstrand, L. (1998) Signal transduction via platelet-derived growth factor receptors. *Biochim. Biophys. Acta*, **1378**, F79–F113.

45 Jeffers, M., Bellacosa, A., Mitsuuchi, Y., Vande Woude, G.F., Xiao, G.H., and Testa, J.R. (2000) Anti-apoptotic signaling by hepatocyte growth factor/Met via the phosphatidylinositol 3-kinase/Akt and

mitogen-activated protein kinase pathways. *Proc. Natl. Acad. Sci. USA*, **98** (1), 247–252.

46 Sonenberg, N. and Gingras, A.C. (1998) The mRNA 5′ cap-binding protein eIF4E and control of cell growth. *Curr. Opin. Cell Biol.*, **10** (2), 268–275.

47 Bernard, A. and Hartemink, A.J. (2005) Informative structure priors: joint learning of dynamic regulatory networks from multiple types of data. Biocomputing 2005: Proceedings of the Pacific Symposium, Hawaii, USA, 4–8 January 2005.

48 Werhli, A.V. and Husmeier, D. (2007) Reconstructing gene regulatory networks with Bayesian networks by combining expression data with multiple sources of prior knowledge. *Stat. Appl. Genetics Mol. Biol.*, **6** (1), 15.

Index

a

achieved significance level (ASL) 192
acute lymphoblastic leukemia (ALL) 66, 91, 97
– age categorization 107
– age vs. phenotype, confounding 106, 107
– aneuploidies 102, 103
– BCR/ABL residuals 99
– chromosome sub-bands, list of 108
– dataset 97
– gene-ltering 97–99
– GSEAlm, diagnostics in 99–102
– hyperdiploidy 107
– NEG residuals 99
– signal-to-noise evaluation 103–106
acute lymphoblastic leukemia dataset 91
– expression matrix 110
– gene expression 99
– map of suspected aneuploidies 104
– positive inter-gene correlations, demonstration of 96
adenocarcinoma tumors 263
ad hoc measurement 102
adjusted batch effect estimators 328
adjusted *p*-values 52
adult stem cells 25
Affymetrix Microarray Suite 118
Akaike information criterion (AIC) 232, 241
Akt genes 11
AKT pathway 83
analysis of covariance (ANCOVA) test 169, 177
– analysis of variance model 177
analysis of variance (ANOVA) model 155, 157, 326, 327
aneuploidy detection outlier method, demonstration 103
angiogenesis 10

annotation analysis 133
anthracycline 39
anti-apoptotic proteins 248
anticancer drug response analysis 279
anticancer treatment 231
APC gene 83
– inactivation 76
apoptin 244
apoptosis 8, 14, 17, 231
– cancer-perturbed PPI network for 239–241
– – cancer drug targets prediction 241, 244, 246
– mechanism at systems level 247
– regulators 244, 245
– – at systems level 248
area under the ROC curve (AUC) 362
Arf mutation 17
ArrayExpress 279
augmentation 59, 60
autoregressive coefficients 211, 213
auxiliary proteins, deregulation 16, 17

b

Bax vectors 245
Bayesian information criterion (BIC) 351
Bayesian networks 187, 188, 348, 349, 358
– dependency network, graph 187
– directed acyclic graph (DAG) 349
– elements 349
– marginalization 350
– model averaging 366
– structure 188
B-cells 8
– BCR/ABL mutation 97
– lymphomas 16
BCL2 apoptosis drug target 244
BCL-2 inhibitors 244
Bcl-2 related proteins 248

BCR signaling 15, 16
– ABL inhibitors 33
– ABL phenotype 97
Bernoulli distribution 350
BIND database 232
BioLattice 149
biological network 185, 347, 352, 362
– appendix 369
– background 349–355
– – Bayesian networks 349
– – Markov chain Monte Carlo on graphs 354
– – model scoring 350
– – model selection/model averaging 351–354
– components 356
– conclusions/future prospects 366–369
– connectivity 360
– data 363
– – sensitivity analysis 364
– experiments and results 192–198
– – breast cancer dataset analysis 196
– – *in utero* excess E2 exposed adult mammary glands analysis 198
– – simulation of 192
– features 356
– general framework 357
– – constructing a prior 359
– – degree distributions 359
– – higher-level network features 358
– – network sparsity 358
– – specific edges 357
– – vertices, classes 358
– inference 352
– introduction 347
– MCMC 365
– method 188–192
– – DDN, local dependency model 188
– – DDN, network/extraction, hot spots identification 192
– – local structure learning 189
– – statistically significant topological changes, detection 191
– model averaging, with prior information 347
– network features 365
– network priors 356–360
– – general framework 357–359
– – motivating example 356
– preliminaries 187
– – graph structure learning/l_1-regularization 188
– – probabilistic graphical models/dependency networks 187
– priors 364
– – proposals 359
– – sensitivity 362, 365
– – results 360–366
– simulated data 360–362
– – data-generating graph 361
– – MCMC 362
– – priors 361
– – ROC analysis 362
– single best graph 365
– topological changes identification 185
– – differential dependency network analysis 185
biological processes 205, 222
BIRC2 gene 220
B-lymphocytes 12
bone marrow niche, importance 30, 31
Bonferroni correction 139
Bonferroni solution 45, 46
breast cancer 36, 307
– biological network 348
– molecular markers 307
– cell line, differential dependency network 197
– dataset analysis 196
– – application of DDN analysis 197
– – experiment background/data 196
Burkitt's lymphoma 13, 17

c

cancer 75, 231, 305
– biology of 232, 356
– data, applications to 290, 291
– – classification analysis 291, 292
– – data normalization 291, 292
– – effects of partial distance denoising 293–295
– – heterogeneous kidney carcinoma data 292, 293
– – leave-one-out cross validation 291
– – parameter selection 292
– death rate 305
– drug targets, prediction of 246
– environmental agents 305
– patient survival prediction 305, 306
– – bagging LASD models 311
– – clear cell renal cell carcinoma (ccRCC), molecular subtypes 307
– – clinical data 306
– – Kaplan–Meier curve 306
– – results 312
– – survival data, logical analysis 308
– – using expression patterns 305
– perturbed PPI networks 232
– research, goal 259, 305

cancer stem cells (CSCs)   25–28, 298
– diagnostic relevance of   38, 39
– hallmark   205
– hypothesis   37, 38
– in solid tumors   35
– phenotype of   34, 35
– therapeutic relevance   39, 40
– tools for the detection of   33, 34
caspase family   247, 248
– caspase-3   244
– – activation   248
– caspase-8   248
– caspase-9   244
– regulators   247, 248
β-catenin   84
– signaling   85
causality concept, definition   207
cDNA microarray   253, 254, 341, 342
– datasets   338
– oligonucleotide probes   89
celastrol   40
cell
– adhesion   7
– illustrator   224
– metabolism   6
cell-cycle   7, 206, 208, 216, 218
central limit theorem (CLT)   92
chi-square distribution   227
chi-squared test   336
chronic fatigue syndrome   186, 198
chronic myeloid leukemia (CML) disease   32, 33
clear cell renal cell carcinoma (ccRCC)   307, 321
– consensus matrices   309
– gene expression profiles   307
– molecular subtypes   307
– patients   319
– risk assessment   318
– risk of death   322
– samples   307
– tumors   321
clustering algorithms   131
c-Myc function   5
– as survival factor in hematopoietic cells   10
– gain of function   10, 11
– loss of function   9, 10
– – implicating Epo signaling   10
Cochrane–Orcutt procedure   215
coefficient matrices   212
coefficient of determination (COD)   190
– definition   190
coexpression analysis   131
colon cancer   37, 64

– data   66
– – p-values for   65
– – selected genes   66
– – set   342
– – t-statistics   65
– gene identification in   64
– – classification of leukemia   64, 66
colon cancer initiating cells (CC-IC)   37
colony forming cells-spleen(CFU-S)   29
colorectal cancer
– model of deregulation in   81
– progression model   76
comparative pathway analysis   186
computationally-intensive statistical methods   347
computational molecular biology   347
concanavalin A,   14
concordance accuracy, see concordance index (c-index)
consensus cluster toolkit   308
consistent repeatability-based gene list   268, 269
conventional dependency network approach   188
covariance matrix, procedure   215
cyclin-dependent kinases (CDKs)   7
– inhibitor-1,   245
cytotoxic drugs   231

d

D4-GDI signaling pathway   142, 149
data
– collection   76
– matrix   369
– normalization   291, 292
– pre-processing   263, 264
– reduction process   90
– standardization   76, 77
DAVID database   264
dCoxS algorithm   135
– Fisher's Z-transformation   136, 137
– interaction score (IS)   136
– lung cancer, pathophysiology   147
– overview   135
– Rényi relative entropy   136
dCoxS analysis   140
death-receptor pathway   248
diabetes, data over-representation analysis   174
diabetes dataset   173, 177
– gene set analysis   177, 178
– – MAP00252_alanine_and_aspartate_metabolism, GCT-plots   179
– – P53_Down, GCT-plots   179

differential coexpression analysis, types   134
differential coexpression of gene sets (dCoxS)   135, 136
– algorithm   135
differential dependency network (DDN) analysis   186, 188, 194, 199
– algorithm   192, 195
– analysis   192, 193, 195–197, 200
– – flowchart   193
– – precision-recall curve   195, 196
– local dependency model   188, 189
differentially coexpressed gene clusters, identification   134
differentially expressed (DE) analysis   110
– chromosome sub-bands, list of   108, 109
– detection   93
– gene-sets   93
differentially expressed genes (DEGs)   103, 113, 131
– bioinformatics analyses   121
– error rates of discriminant analyses   123
– grouping categories of   121, 122
– Hotelling's T^2 test   114, 115, 122
– human liver cancers   120
– – pathophysiological pathways   121
– identification   119–122
– multiple forward search (MFS) algorithm   116, 117
– resampling   117, 118
– two-sample T^2 statistic   115, 116
– Wishart distribution   114, 115
diffuse large B-cell lymphomas (DLBCL)   13, 16
directed acyclic graph (DAG)   223, 349, 351, 354
– recurrence formula   353
Dirichlet distribution, prior distribution   351
Dirichlet normalizing constant   370
discretization methods   332
– ChiMerge method   333
– discretization based on recursive minimal entropy   333
– equal-width discretization algorithm   332
– microarray data, nonparametric scoring method   333
– microarray dataset, proposed method   335
– – dicretization by rank of gene expression   335
disease microarray data   279
disease-related pathways   192
distance-based kernels   290
distance metric   140
distance weighted discrimination (DWD) method   312, 326, 327

DNA
– damage   8, 17, 231
– microarrays   46, 206, 253, 325
– – data analysis, different statistical strategies   132
– protein interaction   232
– sequence   163
Duchenne's muscular dystrophy (DMD)   139
– data analysis   142–145
– dataset   142
– – differential coexpression   144, 145, 148
– – dZIS   146
– – IS   149
– – lung cancer dataset   149
dynamic vector autoregressive (DVAR) model   207, 208, 211, 214, 217
– actual data, application   218
– application   219, 220, 222
– covariance matrix estimation   215
– DVAR(p) model   212
– estimation procedure   214
– hypothesis testing   216
– single realization   218
– wavelet-based   224

e

embryonic stem cells (ESCs)   25
empirical Bayesian method   327, 359
– adjusted data for batch effect   328
– batch effect parameter estimation, using parametric empirical priors   328
– for adjusting batch effect   327
– standardization of data   328
enrichment score (ES)   175
epidermal growth factor receptor (EGFR) system, components   356
equal-width method   332
estrogen receptor
– alpha (ER-alpha) protein   197
– positive (ER+) breast cancer cell   187, 196

f

false discovery exceedance (FDX)   51
– control   62, 63
– procedures controlling   59
false discovery rate (FDR)   62, 63, 91, 167, 196, 219
– error   168
family-wise error rate (FWER) control   62
farnesyltransferase inhibitor   33
FAS (TNFRSF6)-associated death domain (FADD)   248
Fisher's exact test   151, 168, 172, 174
follicular lymphoma   16

g

gastric epithelial progenitor (GEP) endocrine carcinomas 340
– malignant progression 340
Gaussian distribution 210, 217
GCT statistics 172
– applications
– – diabetes dataset 177, 180
– – p53 dataset 180, 181
– one-sided test
– – gene set enrichment analysis (GSEA) test 175
– – OLS global test 174, 175
– two-sided test
– – ANCOVA test 177
– – MANOVA model 175, 176
– – SAM-GS test 176
gene 205
– clusters, biological knowledge-based annotation 133
– differential expression 116
– functional disruption of classes 205
– hills 75
– identification in colon cancer 64
– level microarray inference 97
– mountains 75
– – colorectal cancer 76
– network modeling/analysis 185
– pair-wise differential coexpression 138, 139, 142
– rankings 269, 270
gene class testing (GCT) 167
– analysis 182
– approach 169
– competitive *vs.* self-contained tests 169–171
– tests 177
gene expression 4, 93, 113, 216, 335, 336
– discretization process, steps 335
– discretized data using rank 336
– databases 222, 279
– – exponential growth of 124
– – time series 216
– – time-varying properties 222
– microarrays 186
– – high-dimensional data 186
– ratios 326, 335, 339
– – discretized values 326
– signals 224
gene-gene correlations 95
gene ontology (GO) 131
– analysis 153
– annotations of proteins 246
– database 151, 161, 186

generalized augmentation (GAUGE) 60, 61, 63
generalized least-squares (GLS) estimator 215
gene regulatory networks 185, 205
– DVAR method to actual data application 218
– final considerations 222–224
– regulatory networks/cancer 205–207
– simulations 216–218
– statistical approaches 207–216
– structure 205
– time-varying connectivity estimation 205
gene set analysis (GSA) 110, 152, 167
– challenge 89, 90
– correlation 156
– detection step 109
– differential expression analyses 131–133
– expression 90, 107
– gene-specific *t*-statistics 91
– methods 91–97, 105
– – correlations/permutation tests 95–97
– – motivation 91, 92
– on phenotype 101
– plots of 154
– *p*-values 154
– residuals 101
– SAM statistics 176
– schematic overview of 153
– type of 92
gene set enrichment analysis (GSEA) 93, 133, 168, 175
– one-sided test 171
– two-sided test 171
– statistic 171
– tests, *p*-values 178
gene set models 83, 84, 97, 139
– datasets 139
– differential expression analysis method 133, 134
– GNF_Female_Genes, GCT-plots 180
– measuring coexpression of 136, 137
– measuring differential coexpression 137, 138
– Rényi relative entropy of 137
– residuals 101
– signal detection 89, 92
– studies 139, 140
– wide expression 96
– with *p*-values 181
Gleevec pathway-genes 85
Granger causality 207–209, 220, 223, 224
– definition 224
– direction 210

– interpretation 224
– non-causality 210
– relationships, diagram 218
– time series 208
graphical Gaussian models (GGMs) 223
graphical models 188, 347, 348
– structure 188, 348
GSEAlm package 94
– modeling options 95
gsealmPerm function 94, 95
gut associated lymphoid tissue (GALT) 15

h

Hastings factor 360
HDGF expression 122
HectH9 ubiquitin ligase 6
HeLa cell cycle 218
– gene expression data 219
hematological malignancies 11, 12
hematopoietic stem cells (HSCs) 12, 28
hepatocellular carcinoma (HCC) 119
– p53 mutations 120
– tumors 127
– venous invasion 120
– vs. non-tumor tissues 119, 123
hepatoma-derived growth factor (HDGF) 122
heterogeneous kidney carcinoma data 292, 293
heterogeneous squamous cell carcinoma metastasis data 295, 296
hierarchical cluster analysis (HCA) 329, 331, 332
– gene expression 81
– integration methods, comparison 331
high-scoring models 353
high-throughput gene expression experiments 205
high-throughput genomic technologies 185
– gene expression microarrays 185
Histone modification 6
Homeostasis 8
Hotelling's T^2 statistic 115, 127
– validation of
– – DEGs, identification of 118
– – human genome U95 spike-in dataset 118
Hotelling's T^2 test
– average error rates 123
human 6800 gene chip set 338
human breast cancers
– cluster analysis 124
– dataset 124
human genome U95 spike-in dataset 119
human liver cancers
– dataset 118–120

– DEG, identification of 120–122
– gene expression 118
– human liver tissues, classification 122, 123
– sub-datasets 122
human protein reference database (HPRD) 232
4-hydroxy-2-nonenal (HNE) 39
hyperdiploid samples 100
hypergeometric test 93
hypothesis formulation 367
hypothesis testing 211, 216
hypoxia 6

i

idarubicin 39
individual gene analysis (IGA)
– GSA 152
– ORA approach 172
– p-values of 171
IgH/Myc fusion loci 13
imatinib 33
imatinib mesylate 85
immunohistochemical analysis 307
induce pluripotent stem cells (iPSs) 6
inhibitor of apoptosis (IAP) 244
initial protein-protein interaction (PPI) networks 233
– identification of interactions 236–238
– modification of 238, 239
– prediction of apoptosis drug targets 241, 244
– – flow chart for drug target identification 243
– – gain/loss-of-function proteins 242
instability phenomenon 261
interaction score (IS)
– Fisher's Z-transformed values 138
– gene expression profiles 146
interferon-α (IFN-α) 33
inter-quartile range (IQR) 98
in utero excess E2 exposed adult mammary glands analysis 198
– DDN analysis, application 198
– experiment background/data 198
in vivo repopulation 30
islet beta-cells 10

j

Jeffrey's scale 359
J genes 116
joint core
– biological significance of genes 272, 273
– genes, ranking 267
– magnitude 270, 271

– of genes 261
– transferable 271, 272

k

Kaplan–Meier curves 306, 308
Kaplan–Meier survival function 311
kernel Fisher discriminant (KFD) 297
Kernels 280
– for microarray data 288
– matrices 280
– pre-process of 286
–– normalization 286, 287
–– SVD denoising 287, 288
– SVM methods, for cancer microarray data 280
k-nearest neighborhood method 312
Kolmogorov–Smirnov statistic 175
KRAS activation 76
Kronecker product 210, 225
Kyoto encyclopedia of genes and genomes (KEGG) 120

l

lactate dehydrogenase A (LDH-A) 6
Lasso estimator 190
Lasso method 186
least angle regression (LARS) method 188, 190
least-square method 190
leave-one-out cross validation 291
leave-one-out error 79, 80
leukemia 12
– data 67
– tool for cancer research 28, 29
leukemic stem cell 31
– in bone marrow niche 31, 32
Lid/Rpb2 H3-K4 demethylase 6
likelihood methods 351
– Bayesian information criterion (BIC) 351
linear model 226
local dependency models 186
local structure learning algorithm 200
logarithmic transformation 264
logical analysis of data (LAD) technique 306, 308
– consensus clustering 308
– principles 308
– use 307
– variables, validation 310
logical analysis of survival data (LASD) 306, 308, 313, 318
– accuracy analysis 312
– advantage 320
– algorithm 311

– bagging models 311, 312, 319
–– accuracy 314
–– performance 312
–– robustness improvement of LASD predictions 314
– cross-validation results 313
– Hazard ratio (HRa) 320
– survival patterns 314–316
–– distinct survival profiles 314
–– heat maps 317
–– Kaplan–Meier (KM) plots 314, 317
–– optimized risk score 314, 318
–– prediction, with clinical parameters 318
–– risk scores 316
– survival score $vs.$ actual survival time plot 319
– $vs.$ Cox regression 313
log-linear network 357
long-term self-renewing HSC (LT-HSC) 12
lung cancer
– data analysis 140–142
– dataset 143
–– differential coexpression 144
– microarray datasets 263

m

machine learning 255, 280
Mad-Max/Mnt-Max complexes 5
Mahalanobis distance 123
MALT lymphoma 15
Mann–Whitney test 79
– U test 335, 336
multivariate analysis of variance (MANOVA) model 158, 159
– application of 160
– based scoring method 162, 164
– distributional assumptions 159
– matrix inversion 159
– microarray data 160
– permutation test 160
– tests 175, 182
Mantel statistics 145
MAPK signaling pathways 11
mapping, to gene sets 77, 78
marginal likelihood 350, 369, 370
– advantage 350
Markov chain 354
Markov chain Monte Carlo (MCMC) 348, 354, 362, 365
– based inference 357
– based structural inference 367
– use 356
Markov random field model 186
matrix, estimation procedure 210

maximum entropy kernel   289, 290
mean square error (MSE)   190
MedGene database   127
MEK (MAPK kinase) inhibitors   245
ME kernel
– advantages of   296
– optimization algorithm for   299, 300
– scalability   297
metastasis   205
metrization kernels   280, 288
Metropolis–Hastings sampler   354
– for structural inference   355
– MCMC sampler   354
microarray analysis   90
– data analysis   113, 124, 131, 333
– – MANOVA, applying   159, 160
microarray datasets   325, 338
– contingency tables, combination   335
– example   337–342
– – conclusions   341
– – dataset   338
– – prediction accuracies, using combined dataset   339–341
– gene expression ratios   330
– integration methods   325–335
– – adjusting batch effects, existing methods   326–328
– – discretization methods   332
– – transformation method   329–332
– limitation   325
– prediction accuracies, comparison   341
– score, calculation   335
– scoring method   333
– significant gene selection/classification, statistical method   336
– – calculating prediction accuracy, random forest   337
– – chi-squared test   336
– structure   334
microarray expression measurements   102
microarray gene expression profiling   185
– data analysis, demands/challenges   185
microarray quality control (MAQC)   90
– oligonucleotide's   98
– studies   98
microarray technology   103, 113, 151, 259
– differentially expressed genes (DEGs)   103
– – Hotelling's T^2 test   114
microRNAs (miRNAs)   9
– binding sites   133
minimal entropy (ME)   333
minimum mean squared error (MSE)   208
mitochondrial proteins   231
mitogen-activated protein kinase(MAPK)   245

model statistics, development and validation   82, 83
molecular biology   347, 348
Monte Carlo methods, use   353
Monte Carlo simulation   216
mucosal associated lymphoid tissue (MALT)   15
multiple endpoints, in clinical trials   58
multiple forward search (MFS)   116, 128, 160, 161
– algorithm   114, 116
– structure of   117
multiple gene approach
– correlation, importance of   152–155
– multivariate analyses   154
multiple testing procedure (MTP)   47
– and characteristics   68
– categories of   52, 53
– procedures controlling
– – FDR, 56–58
– – FWER, 55, 56
– to gene discovery   63, 64
– – gene identification in colon cancer, classification of leukemia   64–67
multivariate analysis of variance (MANOVA)   152, 155–159, 169
– analysis of variance (ANOVA)   156, 157
– case studies, application of
– – identifying disease specific genes   160, 161
– – pathways   161, 162
– – protein-protein interaction data, subnetworks identification   162, 163
multivariate statistical analysis   157
MYC function   4
– cell cycle   7
– cellular transformation   12
– down regulation of N cadherin   8
– dysregulation in hematological malignancies   13
– family genes, deregulation   11
– gene in hematological cancers   14
– influencing cell metabolism   6
– locus, amplification   13
– oncogene   3
– overexpression   4, 8, 11
– – in lymphoid malignancies   15, 16
– phosphorylation   14
– proteins   16
– – mutations in   14
– proto-oncogene   13
– recruit transcriptional coregulators   6
– ribosomal genes affected by   7
– RNA pol I, II, and III activation   7
– role in

– – cell cycle regulation   14
– – gene expression   5
– – lymphoid cancers development   15
– – MicroRNA, regulation of
– – regulate transcription.
– to induce glutaminolysis and   6
– tumor biology   11, 12
Myc-Max complexes   5

n

NCI 60 cell line   180
– cDNA data in   339
– datasets   338, 339
NEG group, ages   106
network priors   368
network topology   193, 194
non-Hodgkin's lymphomas (NHLs)   12
nonlinear stochastic interaction model   233–236
nonlinear vector autoregressive (NVAR) model   206
nuclear factor-χB (NF-χB)-mediated survival signals   39
nuclear factor-kappa B (NFϰB)   220
– pathway activation   221
– signaling pathways   221
– subunits   198
nucleosome instability   6
null hypothesis   47, 48, 191, 211, 216

o

O'Brien's OLS statistic   174
oligonucleotide microarray   255
oncogenes   305
– function   305
oncomine   279
ordinary least-squares (OLS) analysis   181
ornithine decarboxylase   6
out-of-bag (OOB) accuracy   314
over-representation analysis (ORA)   168, 171, 172

p

p53-dependent forms of apoptosis   8
p53 mutations   17
partial directed coherence (PDC)   223
– use   223
partial distance   288, 289
pathway mountains   76
Pearson's correlation coefficient   137
Philadelphia chromosome   97
PI3 kinase/AKT   17
Pim1-kinase   6
pluripotent stem (iPS) cells   298
polymerase chain reaction (PCR)   47
polynomial kernel   285, 286
predictive model
– construction   264
– gene sets, construction   264–266
predictive performance, estimation   266
primary human breast tumors
– hierarchical clustering analyses   125, 126
principal component analysis (PCA)   128, 161, 181, 307
prior equivalence   369
pro-apoptotic Bax protein   245
probabilistic graphical models   187
– examples   187
– probabilistic nature   187
probability   350, 353, 369
– joint probability   350
– posterior probabilities   352, 355
– product rule   350
probe set reduction   264
programmed cell death   8
proof theorems   280
proportion of false nulls, estimation   53–55
prostate cancer   36, 37
proteasome inhibitor   39
protein data   364
– posterior mode   364
– prior sensitivity   366
– single best graph   365
protein-protein interaction (PPI)   231
– data   162
– networks   233
protein signaling networks   362
protein synthesis   7
PTC1 pathway   84
PTDINS gene set   83
p-value   47, 49, 64

r

radial basis function (RBF) kernel   285, 286
Rényi relative entropy
– multivariate kernel density   146
random errors   217
random forests (RFs)   337
– classification trees   337
– OOB error, calculation program   337
random survival forests (RSF)   312
– confidence interval   314
ranked genes lists   261
Ras genes   11
Ras proto-oncogene   17
receiver operating characteristic (ROC) curves   362
receptor tyrosine kinases (RTKs)   363, 364

regression process 200
regularized multi-task learning (RMTL) 75, 78, 79
renal cell carcinoma (RCC) 320
– influx of effective therapies 320
repeatability-based gene list 266
– stable 269
resampling-based LBH, 60, 61
resampling based testing 49, 50
rheumatoid factor 15
right-censored survival analysis 306
RNA 338, 339, 342
– sample effect, role 341
robust multi-array analysis (RMA) 118, 139
row-Kronecker product 226
Roy's largest root 158
RT-PCR, semi-quantitative 308

s

Saccharomyces cerevisiae 193
– signaling network 193
Sample's cells 100
Significance analysis for microarrays (SAMs)
– DNA microarray data 58
– GS statistic 168
– GS test 176
– statistic 176
Scott's rule 137
seed protein, mRNA expression 163
self-organizing map (SOM) 308
sequential k nearest neighbor (SeqKnn) imputation method 339
sex differences 105
Shuffling sample 138
significance analysis of microarray for gene set reduction (SAMGSR) 182
simulation experiment 192
– algorithm analysis 195
– DDN analysis, application 193
– experiment data 193
single gene model 83
singular-value decomposition (SVD) method 326, 327
sonic hedgehog (SHH) signaling 84
space program 28
sparse vector autoregressive (SVAR) model 206
stability condition 225
standardized expression ratio 329
statistical hypothesis testing 45
stem cells 25
step-down LR, 60, 61
stochastic models 347
– class 347

stochastic process, *see* weakly stationary process
stratification 77
stress-induced signaling 245
structural equation modeling (SEM) 223
structured data kernel 280
supervised learning 256
support vector machines (SVM) 256–258, 281–284
– and kernels 281
– classifying data with 279
– problems in training 293
– recursive feature elimination 258
survival model 311
– concordance accuracy 311
SynTReN software 193

t

T cell 10
– leukemias 14
– receptor 13
test statistics 49
TETRAD software 207
TGFb BMP signaling pathway 121
thresholding 263
time-varying connectivity function 219, 220
Tip60 complex 6
T-lymphocytes 12
topology-based cancer classification method 186
toy example 261–263
TP53 signaling pathways 221, 222
– inactivation 76
transcription factor 7, 221
transcription regulation 4
transferring receptor (TFRC1) 6
transformation method 329–332
– standardization of expression data 329
– transformation of datasets using reference dataset 330–332
TRRAP coactivator 6
tumorigenesis 84
tumornecrosis factor (TNF) 244
– stress 147
tumors 221, 310
– ccA/ccB classes 310, 312, 313
– metastasis 313
– metastatic properties 221
– progression 313
– survival curves 310
tumor suppressor genes, *see* oncogenes
type I error 46–48, 52
– control under dependence 61, 62
type II errors 48
tyrosine phosphorylation 85

u
unstable ranked gene lists 267, 268

v
vec operator 225
vector autoregressive (VAR) models 206, 208, 209
– generalization 211
– k-dimensional, equations system 209
vectorial data kernel family 280

w
Wald statistics 226, 227
Wald test 211, 215, 216, 226
Watson, t-statistic 134
wavelet coefficients 213
wavelet functions 213
weakly stationary process 225
Western blot analyses 122
Wilks' Λ, *see* Hotelling's T^2
Wilks' Λ test, distribution of 176
Wishart distribution 114, 115
WNT signaling pathway 84

x
X-chromosome genes 104

y
Y-chromosome genes 104
– effect 107
yeast 185
– condition-specific transcriptional networks 185